Handbook of Measurement and Evaluation in Rehabilitation

Handbook of Measurement and Evaluation in Rehabilitation

Edited by

Brian Bolton
Arkansas Rehabilitation Research
and Training Center
University of Arkansas

University Park Press
Baltimore · London · Tokyo

UNIVERSITY PARK PRESS
International Publishers in Science and Medicine
233 East Redwood Street
Baltimore, Maryland 21202

Typeset by The Composing Room of Michigan, Inc.
Manufactured in the United States of America by Universal Lithographers,
Inc., and The Maple Press Co.
Second printing, October 1978

Library of Congress Cataloging in Publication Data

Main entry under title:

Handbook of measurement and evaluation in
rehabilitation.

Bibliography: p.
Includes index.
1. Rehabilitation counseling—Addresses, essays,
lectures. 2. Psychometrics—Addresses, essays,
lectures. I. Bolton, Brian F.
HD7255.5.H35   361'.06   76-6479
ISBN 0-8391-0861-3

Contents

Contributors

Mary K. Bauman is a graduate of the University of Pennsylvania and for more than 10 years served on the staff of the Psychological Clinic of that University. She is a Diplomate of the American Board of Examiners in Professional Psychology, a Fellow of the American Psychological Association, and is licensed as a psychologist in private practice in Pennsylvania. She has been director of two psychological service organizations over a span of nearly 30 years, but her special interest and the center of her many years of research and writing has been psychological and rehabilitation problems of the blind and visually handicapped. Well known as a lecturer, consultant, and author in this field, she is currently Director of the Nevil Interagency Referral Service in Philadelphia.

Nancy E. Betz is Assistant Professor of Psychology at Ohio State University. She received her Ph.D. from the University of Minnesota where she was a research assistant in the Psychometric Methods program. Dr. Betz has coauthored several publications in the area of computerized ability testing. Her research interests are in the area of the psychometric and psychological effects of adaptive (or tailored) measurement of abilities.

Brian Bolton is Associate Professor of Rehabilitation and Adjunct Associate Professor of Psychology at the University of Arkansas. He was formerly Assistant Professor of Psychology at the Illinois Institute of Technology and Research Associate at the Chicago Jewish Vocational Service. He received his Ph.D. from the University of Wisconsin and is a licensed psychologist in Illinois and Arkansas. Mr. Bolton wrote *Introduction to Rehabilitation Research* and is the author of more than 100 publications in rehabilitation, deafness, and psychometrics. He has received six ARCA research awards and is currently Associate Editor of the *Rehabilitation Counseling Bulletin* and serves on the Editorial Board of *Rehabilitation Psychology*.

Ray H. Brown is presently a graduate student in vocational rehabilitation at Texas Tech University where he received his M.A. degree. He has special interests in rehabilitation processes involving therapeutic involvement of the family unit within a community setting. Another area of interest is the development of training programs for paraprofessionals within the rehabilitation setting.

René V. Dawis is currently Professor in the Departments of Psychology and Industrial Relations, Director of the Counseling Psychology Program, and Co-Principal Investigator of the Work Adjustment Project at the University of Minnesota, the institution which awarded him his Ph.D. Professor Dawis is coauthor of *Adjustment to Work* and is author or coauthor of over 60 publications in vocational rehabilitation, vocational psychology, and psychometrics, including the award-winning *Minnesota Studies in Vocational Rehabilitation.*

Robert C. Droege is a Research Psychologist with the Manpower Administration of the U.S. Department of Labor. Mr. Droege, who received his M.A. from the University of North Carolina, is the author or coauthor of 30 articles published in psychological, educational, and personnel journals. Most of these publications are concerned with research on USES tests.

Herbert W. Eber is president of two companies, one of which maintains offices for clinical diagnostic services in Birmingham and Gadsden, Alabama, and in Atlanta, Georgia. The other company provides computer based services to that practice and to other psychologists. He obtained his Ph.D. in clinical psychology from the University of North Carolina and taught at Alabama College until 1960 when he entered private practice, specializing in rehabilitation efforts and in consultation to rehabilitation agencies. Dr. Eber, who is a Fellow of the APA, has authored numerous articles in professional journals, oriented primarily toward vocational rehabilitation and toward systems approaches to diagnosis, and several chapters in recent textbooks dealing with psychological measurements.

William Gellman has been Executive Director of the Chicago Jewish Vocational Service since 1946. He is also Director of the Easter Seal Research Foundation and serves on the advisory boards of many rehabilitation councils, organizations, and institutions. Dr. Gellman, who received his Ph.D. from the University of Chicago, is a Fellow of the American Psychological Association and past president of its Division on Psychological Aspects of Disability and the American Rehabilitation Counseling Association. He received the W. F. Faulkes Award in 1959 from the National Rehabilitation Association for his pioneering work on behalf of handicapped persons.

Carl Hansen completed his doctorate degree at the University of Northern Colorado. From 1965 through 1967 he worked as a rehabilitation counselor in California. Since 1968 he has been with the University of Texas at Austin and is currently Director of the Rehabilitation Counselor Education Program. During the last 16 years he has served in the capacity of president of the National Rehabilitation Counseling Association, secretary for the American Rehabilitation Counseling Association, Coeditor of the *Journal of Applied Rehabilitation Counseling,* served on numerous professional committees, and published broadly within the field of rehabilitation.

Lenore W. Harmon is Professor of Educational Psychology at the University of Wisconsin-Milwaukee. She was formerly Director and Counselor in the Department of Student Counseling at the University of Wisconsin-Milwaukee and Assistant Professor and Counselor in the Student Counseling Bureau at the University of Minnesota. Dr. Harmon received her Ph.D. from the University of Minnesota. She serves on the editorial board of *The Counseling Psychologist* and is editor of *The Journal of Vocational Behavior*. Dr. Harmon has written numerous articles on interest measurement and the career development of women.

Marvin S. Kivitz has been Director of Education, Vocational Training, and Rehabilitation at Elwyn Institute since 1961. He completed his doctorate degree in clinical psychology at the University of Pennsylvania in 1959 and served an internship at the VA Hospital at Coatesville, Pennsylvania. Dr. Kivitz is a consultant at the Lansdowne Association for Retarded Children and has served on several advisory committees to regional and national organizations. He has served as Chairman of the Vocational Rehabilitation Section of the American Association on Mental Deficiency and was a Consulting Editor of the *American Journal of Mental Deficiency*.

G. Frank Lawlis is Associate Professor of Psychiatry at the University of Texas Health Science Center at San Antonio. Dr. Lawlis, who received his Ph.D. from Texas Tech, is coauthor of *Multivariate Techniques for the Behavioral Scientist* and has recently authored a book on the measurement of interpersonal relationships. He has also published more than 50 articles, chapters, and professional papers on counseling process, methodology, vocational aspects of poverty, and personality research. Dr. Lawlis is a diplomate in Counseling Psychology and a clinical member of American Association for Marriage and Family Counseling. Currently, he is conducting research on troubled families and developing effective methods of intervention.

Edna S. Levine is Professor Emeritus of New York University. She was formerly Professor of Educational Psychology and Director of the SRS Project Explorations in the Psychology of Deafness, Director of the Deafness Research and Training Center and Director of the Multidisciplinary Training Program in Deafness, New York University. Dr. Levine received her Ph.D. from New York University and the Litt. D. from Gallaudet College. She is a Fellow of the American Psychological Association and a Diplomate in Clinical Psychology. She initiated the mental health project for the deaf at New York State Psychiatric Institute and the theatre project for the deaf, now National Theatre of the Deaf. Dr. Levine is the author of *Youth in a Soundless World, The Psychology of Deafness, Lisa and Her Soundless World,* and coeditor of *Psychological Practices with the Physically Disabled* and *Rehabilitation Practices with the Physically Disabled* and has authored numerous journal articles.

Ralph K. Meister is Chief Psychologist and directs the in-service training program at the Chicago Jewish Vocational Service. He completed his Ph.D. in psychology at the University of Chicago. The first 15 years of his career were spent in the positions of research assistant, associate, and finally assistant director at a laboratory for child research. The next 10 years he served as director of a child guidance clinic. Dr. Meister is a member of the American Association for the Advancement of Science, the American Psychological Association, Sigma Xi, and Psi Chi.

Gregory A. Miller is Professor of Rehabilitation Counseling at Michigan State University, the institution which granted him his Ph.D. He was formerly Chief Psychologist for the Michigan Department of Corrections and the Michigan Department of Mental Health. Dr. Miller has been a visiting professor at several colleges and universities throughout the country, including the University of Florida and New York University, and has been a consultant on numerous occasions to other universities in regard to their graduate rehabilitation counselor education programs. He is the author or coauthor of several publications in rehabilitation psychology and has served as President of the American Rehabilitation Counseling Association for 1970–1971.

Hendrik D. Mugaas is a Manpower Development Advisor at the Bureau of International Labor Affairs of the U.S. Department of Labor. He has worked in this capacity in several countries overseas. Formerly he was Chief, Branch of Services to the Handicapped in the Headquarters Office of the U.S. Employment Service. He was previously a career employee of the North Dakota State Employment Service, where he was Supervisor of Counseling, Testing, Test Development, and Services to the Handicapped. Mr. Mugaas is a member of the American Rehabilitation Counseling Association.

Randall M. Parker is Associate Director of the Rehabilitation Counselor Education Program at the University of Texas at Austin. He received his Ph.D. in counseling psychology from the University of Missouri-Columbia in 1970. His previous positions were intern and staff counselor at the University of Missouri Testing and Counseling Center and rehabilitation counselor for the Wisconsin Rehabilitation Division. He is presently coeditor of the *Journal of Applied Rehabilitation Counseling.*

Jack M. Plummer is a psychologist in private practice in Hot Springs, Arkansas and an instructor at Garland County Community College. Dr. Plummer, who received his Ph.D. from Texas Tech, was formerly Director of Training, Arkansas Rehabilitation Research and Training Center. Dr. Plummer is the author of various publications in rehabilitation, corrections, and psychometrics.

Kenneth W. Reagles is Associate Professor of Rehabilitation Counseling at Syracuse University. He was formerly Research Director at the University of Wisconsin-Madison Regional Rehabilitation Research Institute. Dr. Reagles has served as President of the Wisconsin Rehabilitation Association, Chairman of the National Research Committee of the American Rehabilitation Counseling Association, and Member of the National Research Committee of the National Rehabilitation Counseling Association. Dr. Reagles, who received his Ph.D. from Wisconisn, has coauthored a book, *Rehabilitation in Israel* (1974), six monographs, and numerous research journal articles and reports. He has frequently presented formal papers at professional meetings. Dr. Reagles' research has centered on rehabilitation counselor roles and functions, and evaluation techniques and effectiveness measures.

Marvin Rosen has been Director of Psychology at Elwyn Institute in Media, Pennsylvania since 1963. At Elwyn he supervises Psychology services at a large school and rehabilitation center for the mentally handicapped. He also directs behavioral research programs and has been responsible for a long-term follow-up investigation of mentally retarded adults discharged from the institution to independent community living. Dr. Rosen completed his doctoral work in clinical psychology at the University of Pennsylvania in 1961, and he served an internship at the VA Hospital at Perry Point, Maryland. Prior to working at Elwyn Dr. Rosen worked as Child Psychologist at the Albert Einstein Medical Center in Philadelphia and taught at the University of Pennsylvania. He is a consultant for special education programs at a local school district and conducts a private practice in clinical psychology. Dr. Rosen is the author of over 30 articles in professional journals dealing with the adjustment of the mentally retarded. He has also authored several chapters in recent textbooks dealing with mental retardation, and has edited a history of mentàl retardation.

Stanford E. Rubin is Senior Research Scientist, Arkansas Rehabilitation Research and Training Center, and Associate Professor of Education, University of Arkansas. He received his Ed.D. in Counseling and Rehabilitation from the University of Illinois. In 1970–1971 he was a staff psychologist at the Office of Psychological Services at Wright State University. Dr. Rubin is coauthor of *Facilitative Management in Rehabilitation Counseling: A Casebook* and author or coauthor of over 40 articles and monographs. He has also been the recipient of two ARCA Research Awards. Dr. Rubin was Project Director of a national program evaluation project in state rehabilitation agencies and serves on the editorial board of the *Journal of Rehabilitation*.

Vijay Sharma is Assistant Professor in the Rehabilitation Counselor Education Program at the University of Wisconsin-Milwaukee. She was formerly Associate Director and Assistant Professor in the Department of Counselor Education and Counseling at San Jose State University and Visiting Professor in the Department of Psychology, Counseling, and Guidance at the University of Northern Colorado. Dr. Sharma, who received her Ph.D. from the University of Oregon, has published several articles on counseling women and on test construction. Her professional presentations have focused on the status of women and the recruitment of ethnic minority rehabilitation workers.

Asher Soloff has been Research Coordinator at the Chicago Jewish Vocational Service since 1960 and has supervised the CJVS Research Utilization Laboratory since 1968. Mr. Soloff, who received his M.A. in sociology from the University of Chicago, has authored or coauthored many publications in rehabilitation including *A Work Therapy Research Center* which received an ARCA Research Award in 1972.

Robert M. Thorndike is Associate Professor in the Department of Psychology and the Center for Cross-Cultural Research at Western Washington State College. He was formerly a Research Associate with the Work Adjustment Project at the University of Minnesota, the institution which granted him his Ph.D. Mr. Thorndike is coauthor of *Cross-Cultural Research Methods* and author of the forthcoming book *Correlational Procedures for Research*. He has published numerous papers on psychometrics and multivariate statistics.

Ann B. Trotter is Coordinator of the Rehabilitation Counselor Education Program and Professor of Educational Psychology at the University of Wisconsin-Milwaukee. Dr. Trotter received her Ph.D. from the University of Wisconsin and is a licensed psychologist in Wisconsin. Dr. Trotter was formerly a rehabilitation counselor at the University of Washington and an instructor at the University of Minnesota. She is active in professional organizations, including the National Rehabilitation Counseling Association and the Council of Rehabilitation Counselor Educators. Dr. Trotter has contributed numerous articles to the professional literature in counseling and rehabilitation, and she coauthored *Rehabilitation Research*.

M. S. Tseng is Research Associate at the West Virginia Rehabilitation Research and Training Center and Professor of Educational Psychology at West Virginia University. Professor Tseng did postdoctoral work in educational research and computer applications from 1964 to 1966 at Indiana University, the institution which granted him his Ed.D. He is the author of three research monographs, 30 research articles published in various professional journals, and 30 research papers presented to various professional association conventions.

Richard T. Walls is Research Associate at the West Virginia Rehabilitation Research and Training Center and Professor of Educational Psychology at West Virginia University. Dr. Walls, who received his Ph.D. from Pennsylvania State University, has received Standard Oil Corporation and West Virginia University awards for teaching excellence and is the author of more than 40 publications in rehabilitation and human learning.

David J. Weiss has been Director of the Psychometric Methods Program at the University of Minnesota since 1970 and is currently Professor of Psychology. He received his Ph.D. in psychology from the University of Minnesota in 1963 where he was a Vocational Rehabilitation Administration Fellow in couseling psychology for 2 years. Dr. Weiss directed the Work Adjustment Project at the University of Minnesota from 1963 through 1970. Dr. Weiss was corecipient of an ARCA Research Award in 1964 and the Special Research Award of the American Personnel and

Guidance Association. He is a Fellow of the American Psychological Association and serves as a Consulting Editor for the *Journal of Counseling Psychology*. Dr. Weiss is author or coauthor of more than 80 publications in psychometrics and vocational psychology, including four book chapters, and is editor of the journal *Applied Psychological Measurement*.

Preface

During the past decade rehabilitation counseling has achieved a professional identity separate from other areas of counseling practice. Concurrent with the emergence of a professional specialization is the delineation of a systematic body of knowledge which is transmitted to succeeding generations of practitioners in formal training programs. The developing body of knowledge which characterizes a new profession consists, to a great extent, of information, techniques, and procedures which are adopted from established professions. Psychological and vocational evaluation techniques which are utilized in rehabilitation illustrate well the process of borrowing (from clinical, counseling, educational, and vocational psychology) and synthesizing to produce a new professional specialty.

The *Handbook of Measurement and Evaluation in Rehabilitation* summarizes the current status of one major area of the discipline of rehabilitation counseling: psychological measurement principles and practices as they are applied in the evaluation of disabled clients. The title of the book accurately reflects an emphasis on the application of psychological testing procedures in rehabilitation counseling. The primary objective of this volume is to prepare rehabilitation counselors to understand the results of psychological evaluations and use the information as a basis for program planning with clients. A second purpose is to provide a handbook for clinical psychologists who conduct psychological evaluations of disabled persons. The third purpose for which the book was designed is to serve as a reference volume for researchers who conduct projects to evaluate the effectiveness of rehabilitation programs.

The *Handbook* can be profitably read by practitioners who have had no previous coursework or experience in psychological measurement or effectively utilized in undergraduate and graduate courses in rehabilitation counseling. However, the counselor or student with no previous exposure to psychological tests may want to obtain a copy of *How to Select, Administer, and Interpret Psychological Tests: A Guide for the Rehabilitation Counselor,* published by the West Virginia Rehabilitation Research and Training Center. Another useful introductory source is the Studies in Continuing Education for Rehabilitation Counselors Project carried out at the University of Iowa. Nine of the 30 learning units developed in conjunction with the Project address topics in psychological testing and evaluation.

In a very real sense, this volume is the product of the many years of clinical and research experience of the authors of the chapters, whose credentials and achievements are summarized in their biographical citations. They are acknowledged authorities in psychometrics, clinical assessment, and counselor education and their contributions to the advancement of rehabilitation counseling are greatly appreciated. Special thanks are due Diane Graham who assisted with preparation of the manuscript and assembled the indexes for the book. Preparation of the *Handbook of Measurement and Evaluation in Rehabilitation* was supported in part by SRS Grant No. RD 16-5681216-07 to the Arkansas Rehabilitation Research and Training Center.

Introduction

The primary objective of the vocational rehabilitation process is the optimal vocational adjustment of disabled clients. The rehabilitation process consists of planning and providing the necessary services that will prepare the client for successful job placement and subsequent vocational adjustment. The implicit assumption underlying the focus on vocational functioning is that adequate vocational adjustment will foster satisfactory adjustment in other life spheres.

PSYCHOLOGICAL EVALUATION
IN REHABILITATION COUNSELING

The basic rehabilitation services are evaluation, counseling, medical treatment, training, and job placement. A comprehensive evaluation, which includes medical, psychological, vocational, and social appraisal, constitutes the foundation for planning the client's rehabilitation program. The medical examination is required of all clients who apply for vocational rehabilitation services. However, assessment of the client's psychological status is usually important and may be essential for adequate rehabilitation program development. McGowan and Porter (1967, pp. 65–67) list several situations in which psychological evaluation services are needed and other situations in which they may not be necessary.

Psychological evaluation services *are needed* when:

1. Mental retardation has to be determined, and testing will include a valid test of intelligence and an assessment of social functioning and educational progress and achievement
2. Psychiatric disorders are suspected, and a determination has to be made whether psychological evaluation, as an alternative to psychiatric evaluation, is appropriate
3. Long-term or expensive training is involved in a rehabilitation
4. Client or counselor needs information or confirmation of the client's abilities, aptitudes, achievements, interests, and personality patterns
5. Data on the client's capacities and abilities are lacking, ambiguous, or contradictory

6. Important talents, capacities, abilities, or disabilities are suspected by the counselor or client
7. A person is known to have or suspected of having certain disabilities that require specialized evaluations of his capacities, abilities, skills, interests, and personality

Psychological evaluation services *may not be needed* when:

1. The person has very recently been successfully employed and intends to return to his work as soon as physical restoration services have been rendered
2. The person has been successfully employed, is now unable to find similar work because of the prejudice of employers toward the handicapped, and it is necessary for the counselor to convince the employer that the client has the abilities required for the position
3. The person has been successfully employed, and only a minor shift is contemplated in the type of work that he will do in the future
4. The person has a long and rich background of information on the jobs he held, the jobs are in related types of work, and the person has changed jobs for reasons beyond his control
5. The person has a long and rich background of education, the caliber of the school in which he matriculated is well established, the caliber of the teachers in important subjects is well established, and the client does not plan to study or work in areas unrelated to his background
6. The person is not cooperative and does not desire to be tested

Vocational and social appraisal, which overlap to a considerable extent with psychological assessment, are equally important. Additional specialists such as the vocational evaluator and social case worker may contribute to the evaluation of the client's vocational potential and psychosocial status.

Client evaluation includes two phases: 1) collection of adequate diagnostic information, and 2) realistic interpretation of the data, i.e., translation of the information into a comprehensive rehabilitation plan. The counselor may be involved to some extent in the conduct of the first phase (e.g., taking case histories, administering standard inventories) but he assumes complete responsibility for working with the client to develop a mutually acceptable rehabilitation plan based on the knowledge derived through client evaluation procedures.

ARE PSYCHOLOGICAL EVALUATIONS USEFUL?

A thorough diagnostic study is an integral aspect of rehabilitation program planning, and psychological evaluation often constitutes a major phase of the diagnostic process. Given the expense of psychological assessment procedures and the questionable validity of many instruments, it is not unreasonable to ask how useful psychological evaluations are to rehabilitation counselors. Sindberg, Roberts, and Pfeifer (1968) conducted a study to find out to what extent counselors actually follow the recommendations made by psychologists and the degree to which psychologists' predictions are subsequently confirmed.

Thirty-five cases were selected from the files of a psychological consulting agency which routinely evaluated candidates for rehabilitation services. The psychological reports were reviewed and every statement that could be considered to be either a specific recommendation or a prediction was extracted. The rehabilitation counselor's case files were also reviewed, and summaries of each client's outcome were prepared. Three independent judges, all experienced psychologists, evaluated the extent to which each recommendation was followed and each prediction was confirmed. A total of 67 specific recommendations and 79 predictions were rated on four point scales.

Two thirds of the psychologists' recommendations were rated as having been followed to some extent, with over one half rated as followed to a large extent or definitely followed. Thus, in a large proportion of the cases, the counselors planned and acted along the lines recommended in the psychological reports. For the reports to be truly useful, however, they must be predictive of subsequent client behavior. One half of the predictions were tested, and of these three fourths were rated as confirmed to a large extent or strongly confirmed. These results further suggest the value of psychological reports in rehabilitation planning.

In addition it was found that predictions based on a battery of tests were more useful than predictions based on single tests. The study generally supports the usefulness of psychological evaluations to rehabilitation counselors in planning services for their clients.

USING TEST RESULTS IN COUNSELING

There is no substitute for practice in learning how to utilize psychological test results in counseling with rehabilitation clients. Nevertheless, some preliminary suggestions and guidelines can facilitate the learning process. McGowan and Porter (1967) offer the following general suggestions for interpreting test results to clients (p. 120):

1. Develop short, clear, concise methods of *describing* to the client the purpose of the test he has taken and the meanings of the results—do this before you go into the interpretation of his actual test scores—then, you can concentrate on his *reactions* to the test scores rather than run the risk of being trapped into a technical discussion of the purpose of the test, its construction, etc., during the interpretation period.
2. Make test data meaningful in terms of the *client's behavior*—make the transfer from the test score to the client's behavior. Ask yourself the following questions: "What does the score mean in terms of client behavior?" and, "How can I express the scores to him in such a way that he can relate them to past, present, and anticipated behavior?"
3. Do not become *overidentified* with the client's test scores. The test

scores are his, not yours. Present test material in such a way that he can question it, discuss it, reject it, or accept it without having to reject or accept you by doing so.

4. Know how you *perform yourself* on objective tests and try to work out, as best you can, a reasonable acceptance of your own test scores. Generally this will mean you are able to work with test scores and to interpret them objectively to clients. If you think test scores are either very good or no good, you will be communicating this in many ways to the clients that you are working with. Avoid projecting too many of your own subjective feelings into the objective tests that you are using.

McGowan and Porter (1967) provide 19 specific suggestions for test interpretation (p. 121):

1. Have confidence in the client's problem-solving ability—even if he has shown little

2. Remind girls of both career and homemaking plans—not just one or the other

3. Make alternate plans sound respectable—not like impending failure

4. Open new educational and vocational doors—do not just close them to the client

5. Relate test data to other experiences—do not discuss them as abstractions

6. Reflect a client's rejection of low test scores—do not write off low performance

7. Get clients involved in test interpretation—do not just recite the results

8. Explain the purpose of the test in functional terms—not in psychological jargon

9. Distinguish carefully between interest and aptitude—do not use the terms loosely

10. Use test results in context with all other data—not as goals in themselves

11. Use test results for client planning—not for the counselor's diagnosis

12. Refresh the client's memory on each test before discussing it—do not discuss it cold

13. Let tests add to the client's picture of himself—not be a mysterious magic formula

14. Explain test results simply—do not use elaborate statistical devices

15. Express low test performance or unpleasant information honestly—but with perspective

16. Remember expressed and demonstrated interests—not just interest inventory results

17. Have the client summarize often—do not deprive him of the chance to review and organize

18. Have the client summarize the whole interview—do not do it for him

19. End on a positive note—even if some of the interview has been unpleasant

The single most comprehensive source in this area is the book by Goldman (1971), which includes detailed treatments of the topics of test selection, administration, interpretation, and reporting. The longest chapter (eleven) of his book presents several illustrative cases that are both interesting and instructive. Finally, the counselor should be familiar with the 1974 revision of *Standards for Educational and Psychological Tests,* which includes, for the first time, a lengthy section entitled "Standards for the Use of Tests."

REFERENCES

American Psychological Association. 1974. Standards for Educational and Psychological Tests. APA, Washington, D. C.

Goldman, L. 1971. Using Tests in Counseling (Second Edition). Appleton-Century-Crofts, New York.

McGowan, J. F., and T. L. Porter. 1967. An Introduction to the Vocational Rehabilitation Process (Revised). Department of HEW, Washington, D. C.

Sindberg, R. M., A. F. Roberts, and E. J. Pfeifer. 1968. The usefulness of psychological evaluations to vocational rehabilitation counselors. Rehabilitation Literature 29:290–294.

I
FUNDAMENTALS
OF MEASUREMENT

1 | Scores and Norms

BRIAN BOLTON, G. FRANK LAWLIS, and RAY H. BROWN

Most psychological tests and inventories generate numerical scores that indicate the extent to which a person possesses a defined trait or characteristic, such as intelligence, spatial ability, clerical aptitude, mechanical interest, introversion, dominance, etc. However, test scores by themselves are almost meaningless. Norms and other interpretative devices are employed to translate scores into meaningful information that can be used to improve decision-making processes in counseling. This chapter will introduce the concept of a test score and discuss the use of normative data in interpreting test scores.

Several topics pertaining to the development and interpretation of test scores are discussed in subsequent chapters and, therefore, will only be mentioned briefly here: 1) The error-based interpretation of test scores is discussed in Chapter 2; 2) predictive or functional interpretative devices (cutting scores, expectancy tables, etc.) are discussed in Chapters 5 and 11; and 3) the issue of general versus special norms is discussed in Chapters 5, 0, and 14. Several other topics are not considered in this and other chapters because of their technical nature, e.g., normalization of score distributions, calibration and equating of test scores, development of norms, and others. The interested reader is referred to Angoff (1971) for a detailed presentation of these and related topics.

PSYCHOLOGICAL MEASUREMENT DEFINED

Psychological measurement may be defined as the process of assigning numbers to persons in such a way as to represent quantities of attributes.

3

Thus, measurement and quantification are often used synonomously in the psychometric literature. When assessed by scientific standards, psychological tests are relatively unsophisticated measuring instruments. Of course, some psychological measuring instruments are more sophisticated than others and generate numerical scores of a higher quality, i.e., scores with more desirable statistical properties.

LEVELS OF MEASUREMENT

Four levels of psychological measurement can be distinguished: nominal, ordinal, interval, and ratio. Each of these types of measurement is described and illustrated below.

Nominal Scale

The nominal scale represents the weakest level of measurement. It exists when numbers are used to classify objects, persons, or characteristics. For example, the psychiatric diagnostic system constitutes a nominal scale. With this system patients may be classified as schizophrenic, paranoid, psychoneurotic, or any number of other conditions. The assignment of numbers to psychiatric categories is arbitrary, but patients in different categories receive different numerical labels.

Ordinal Scale

An ordinal scale exists when the categories of a nominal scale can be ranked from most to least on some dimension. Or, alternatively, a sample of subjects can be rank ordered from most to least. For example, 20 psychiatric patients could be ranked from most to least disturbed. The numbers assigned to persons or categories that are ranked do not reflect magnitude, only relative position.

Interval Scale

When the distances between any two numbers on a scale are of known size and the scale points are ordered, an interval scale is achieved. Thus, an interval scale requires a unit of measurement. However, neither the unit of measurement nor the scale points possess absolute magnitude. Intelligence and aptitude tests and some rating scales approach an interval scale of measurement, i.e., the distance between scores of 47 and 42 is approximately the same as the distance between scores of 35 and 30.

Ratio Scale

A ratio scale possesses all of the characteristics of an interval scale and in addition has a true zero point as its origin. Few measurement procedures in the social and behavioral science yield ratio scales; for example, zero intelligence cannot be meaningfully defined. Measurement procedures in the social sciences usually assume an arbitrary anchor point, which is generally the *mean*. Scale values (scores) are then described in terms of distance above or below the mean.

WHAT IS A TEST SCORE?

A test score is usually the simple sum of keyed responses to a set of items that sample the aptitude, skill, or personality trait being measured, e.g., the number of arithmetic problems solved correctly, the number of items checked that are indicative of interest in mechanical activities, etc. In this section the composition of two test scores is illustrated using a test of clerical ability and a self-report personality inventory.

Minnesota Clerical Test

The Minnesota Clerical Test (MCT) (Andrew, Paterson, and Longstaff, 1933) is a test of accuracy in performing tasks related to clerical work. It has been found useful for selecting clerical employees and for advising persons who wish to seek training in the clerical field.

The MCT consists of two parts: Number Checking and Name Checking. Each part consists of 200 items: 100 identical pairs and 100 dissimilar pairs. The examinee is instructed to check the identical pairs. Sample items from the MCT are presented in Table 1. Separate time limits are used for the two parts; the total testing time is 15 minutes.

The MCT Manual (Psychological Corp., 1959) contains detailed instructions for administering and scoring procedures, as well as reliability and validity data and norm tables for a variety of groups. Each examinee's performance is summarized in two scores, one each for Number Checking and Name Checking. The *raw scores* are obtained by subtracting the number of wrong items from the number of correct items. Thus, the scores reflect both speed and accuracy. The interpretation of raw scores on the MCT is discussed in the following section.

Sixteen Personality Factor Questionnaire (Form E)

The Sixteen Personality Factor Questionnaire (16 PF) (Form E) (Institute for Personality and Ability Tests, 1967) is an objective inventory of personality traits that is based on more than 25 years of factor analytic research. As the title indicates, the inventory assesses the examinee's status on 16 relatively independent dimensions of personality. Form E was designed for use with persons of limited education and cultural background and, thus, may be especially applicable in rehabilitation settings.

Table 1. Sample items from the Minnesota Clerical Test[1]

Number Checking

81.	527–529
82.	172438291026–172438291026
83.	7253829142–725382942
84.	836287–836289
85.	62435162839–62435162839

Name Checking

81.	A. Stein & Company–A. Stien & Company
82.	Robert Courtney–Robert S. Courtney
83.	Leonard Music Co.–Leonard Music Co.
84.	George Morgan–George Morgen
85.	Paulson's Cafe–Paulson's Cafe

[1] Reproduced with permission from the *Minnesota Clerical Test*. Copyright 1933, renewed 1961 by the Psychological Corporation, New York.

To illustrate the composition of a typical personality inventory score, the eight items that comprise the Dominance Scale of 16 PF (Form E) are paraphrased in Table 2. The raw score is calculated by counting one point for each response in the keyed direction. Thus, total raw scores on Dominance may range from zero to eight. Higher scores are believed to reflect an assertive, independent, aggressive, stubborn personal disposition, while lower scores are characteristic of a humble, accommodating, conforming, submissive person.

The reader may wonder how the eight items in Table 2 were selected and what evidence supports the interpretation of the total score as a measure of the construct of dominance. These complex, interrelated questions are beyond the scope of this chapter. An overview of strategies of personality inventory construction is presented in Chapter 6. The reader is referred to Nunnally (1967) for a thorough review of the principles and procedures of test construction.

INTERPRETATION OF SCORES

Raw scores derived from psychological tests and inventories are seldom useful for any purpose without additional information regarding the development of the instrument or the performance of representative samples of

Table 2. Eight items that comprise the Dominance Scale of the Sixteen Personality Factor Questionnaire (Form E)[1]

Do you ever tell a lie for the fun of it	or	is that wrong
Do you usually "play it safe"	or	take a risk
Do you sometimes argue with your parents	or	is that wrong
Have you sometimes put a waiter to a lot of extra trouble	or	is that part of his job
Are you very careful not to hurt people's feelings	or	do you sometimes say harsh things
Can you tell a lie to someone's face	or	do you look away
Would you walk any where you wanted to in a strange city	or	would you stay away from dangerous areas
Do you complain about other people's work	or	are you not like that

[1] Paraphrased with permission from the eight items of the Dominance Scale of *The Sixteen Personality Factor Questionnaire* (Form E). Copyright 1967 by the Institute for Personality and Ability Testing.

persons. Three basic procedures for interpreting test scores can be delineated. First, *Criterion-referenced* tests are designed to sample the knowledge or skills required for a particular responsibility or area of performance. Thus, the interpretation of scores is based on the a priori evaluation by experts of the relevance and adequacy of the content of the test. Academic achievement tests and occupational trade tests are instruments most amenable to criterion-referencing.

Second, the *predictive* or functional interpretation of test scores includes the empirical validation of test performance by assessing the relationship between scores and subsequent success in school or on the job. For example, expectancy tables indicate the probability that an individual who attains a given score will complete a training program in television repair. Various types of predictive interpretation procedures are illustrated in Chapter 5.

Third, the *normative* approach to score interpretation if the method most commonly used. Raw scores are converted to some form of standard scores that indicate relative position in a distribution of scores obtained by a group of persons with defined characteristics (referred to as the *norm group*). The normative interpretation of test scores is illustrated in the next section using the MCT and the 16 PF.

Two Examples of Normative Interpretation

Assume that a female client has expressed an interest in employment in the broadly defined clerical area. The MCT was administered in conjunction with that battery of aptitude tests and vocational inventories that purport to assess relevant skills and interests. The client achieves raw scores of 93 and 76 on Number Checking and Name Checking, respectively. What possible interpretation can the counselor place on this MCT performance? He may ask how these scores compare to scores achieved by representative samples of females who have taken the MCT. One possible comparison would use norms for female applicants for four types of clerical positions that are contained in the MCT Manual (Psychological Corp., 1959). The client's scores of 93 and 76 are observed to be fairly low in comparison to the norm groups. They fall below the 30th percentile for each of the four groups, with the Number Checking score close to the 10th percentile on the average. A percentile score simply indicates a person's rank on an ordinal scale ranging from one to 99. More will be said about percentile scores in a subsequent section.

This hypothetical client ranks low in the particular clerical skill that the MCT measures. Does this mean that she should be discouraged from seeking employment in a clerical occupation? Not necessarily. Only if MCT scores are substantially related to successful performance on the job would such an interpretation be warranted. In other words, the usefulness of a normative interpretation of test data is contingent upon the availability of evidence regarding the validity of the test for a particular purpose.

The MCT Manual includes summaries of several validity studies that used various criteria of successful performance for different clerical occupations. For example, one study of 39 experienced bookkeeping machine operators found correlations of 0.51 to 0.47 between net speed of posting and Numbers and Names, respectively. Another study of 48 department store order fillers found correlations of 0.14 and 0.12 between supervisory ratings and Number and Names. Obviously, the validity of the MCT as a measure of "clerical success" is specific to the particular job and criterion of success.

This example illustrates the normative interpretation of the simple test score, i.e., the conversion of raw MCT scores to percentile equivalents. Normative interpretations convert absolute performance on a test or inventory to relative performance by using an appropriate reference group. The selection of an appropriate reference group may be a crucial step in the utilization of test data, e.g., the MCT Manual provides separate norms for applicants and employees in industrial organizations and for males and females as well. If a male is interested in working in a clerical occupation that is dominated by females, should male or female norms be used to interpret his scores? (Females generally score higher on tests similar to the MCT.) Finally, the normative interpretation of test data in counseling requires that the tests be valid for the intended purpose.

Raw scores on the 16 PF are converted to standard sten (*S*tandard *ten*-point) scores using appropriate norm tables. Sten scores range from one to 10 and are derived on the assumption that the trait is normally distributed (this topic is introduced in the following section). Norm tables (or norms) summarize the performance of a large, carefully defined group of persons. A norm table based on the responses of 146 females to the 16 PF (Form E) is presented in the Manual (Institute for Personality and Ability Testing, 1968). This table was used in the following example.

Assume that the hypothetical female client completed the 16 PF as part of the battery of tests and that she responded to seven of the items on the Dominance Scale in the keyed direction. Thus, her raw score would be 7. Using the female norm table her raw score of 7 can be converted to a sten score of 9. Disregarding the precise interpretation of a sten score of 9 for the moment, it can be said that in comparison to the average female, the client tends to be an assertive, independent person. This is, of course, highly relevant information to the counselor's task of working with the client to develop an appropriate rehabilitation plan and, ultimately, effecting a successful job placement.

The issue of validity is much more complicated with personality inventories than with aptitude and achievement tests. Is a person who responds positively to most of the items comprising the 16 PF Dominance Scale really an assertive, aggressive, independent person? Do scores on the inventory correlate with actual behavior? Few personality inventories are validated against behavioral criteria, primarily because of the complexity and cost of conducting the necessary investigations. The reader is referred to the 16 PF Handbook (Cattell, Eber, and Tatsuoka, 1970) for information regarding the validity and interpretation of 16 PF scores and profiles.

Normal Distribution

The normal distribution, or normal frequency curve, is a mathematical distribution that is pictured in introductory psychology textbooks as a symmetrical, bell-shaped curve. Experience has shown that many variables in psychology tend to follow the normal distribution, i.e., most values cluster around the central point or average with fewer values at greater distances from the average. It should be stressed that the normal frequency curve is not "a fact of nature"; rather, it is a theoretical distribution that serves as a good approximation for many empirically defined variables.

The normal distribution is actually a family of distributions, each with a particular mean and standard deviation. Fortunately, all normal distributions can be converted to one *standard normal distribution,* which has an average value, or mean, of zero and a standard deviation of one. The standard normal distribution, or Z-score distribution, has a very useful property for application to psychological measurement: the relationship between distance from the mean and percentage of cases falling under the curve has been calculated for all values. Thus, a *raw* score distribution can be readily converted to a variety of *standard* score distributions with *percentile* interpretations. However, it should be remembered that this conversion procedure is premised on the assumption that the trait or variable under consideration tends to be normally distributed.[1]

Standard Scores and Percentiles

The universal standard score is the Z-score that is obtained by dividing the difference between any raw score and the mean by the standard deviation (SD) of the particular distribution. Thus, a Z-score indicates how many SD units above or below the mean a raw score lies. This can be seen in Figure 1 by comparing the scale points of the SD scale and the Z-score scale: they coincide. Z-scores are almost never used for reporting the results of test performance. But the Z distribution is easily transformed to other standard distributions, four of which are described below.

T-Scores T-scores are transformed standard scores with a mean of 50 and a SD of 10. Thus, a T-score of 65 is one and one-half SD units above the mean (equivalent to a Z-score of +1.5) and corresponds to a percentile of approximately 93 (Figure 1). In other words, a T-score of 65 exceeds 93 percent of the scores in the distribution.

Deviation IQ Scores Deviation IQ scores are transformed scores with a mean of 100 and a SD of 15. Thus, a deviation IQ of 85 is one SD below the mean and corresponds to a percentile of 16. A percentile score of 16 is exceeded by 84 percent of the scores in the distribution. (Not all deviation IQs are based on a SD of 15; the test user should become

---

[1] Non-normal raw score distributions are often "normalized" using nonlinear transformations. Then the percentile interpretation of standard scores based on the normal distribution is appropriate.

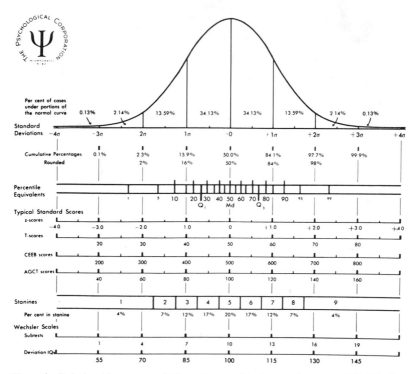

Figure 1. Relationships among different types of test scores in a normal distribution. (From Test Service Bulletin No. 48, 1955, reproduced with permission of the Psychological Corporation.)

familiar with the particular transformed score distribution for every test he uses.)

Stanine Scores   Stanine scores (*Sta*ndard *nine*-point scores) range from one to nine. Each score represents an interval or category that is one-half SD wide (except for the endpoints). The relationship between stanine scores and percentiles is indicated in Figure 1. For example, a stanine score of three is approximately equivalent to a percentile of 17 (the midpoint of the interval). As with T-scores and deviation IQs, the percentile interpretation of stanines assumes a normally distributed trait.

Sten Scores   Sten scores (*Sta*ndard *ten*-point scores) are used in reporting the results of the 16 PF, and they range from one to 10. Like the stanine distribution, the sten distribution results from the partition of the score distribution into categories that are one-half SD wide. The sten distribution differs from the stanine distribution in that the latter has a middle category, while the sten distribution does not. The sten score of nine on Dominance, which was attained by the hypothetical female client, is approximately at the 96th percentile of the distribution.

There are several other standard score systems that are used by various test publishers; for example, the Educational Testing Service uses a scale with a mean of 500 and a SD of 100. Regardless of the particular transformation, all standard score systems can be converted to percentile equivalents for the purpose of reporting the results to clients. Percentiles are the most easily understood scores available for test interpretation. It should be remembered, however, that the percentile distribution con-stitutes an ordinal scale, i.e., the intervals between scale points are not equal throughout the range. This characteristic can be observed in Figure 1 by noting that the percentile scale is compressed at the center and stretched out at the ends. Thus, the difference in ability between two persons at the 80th and 90th percentiles is greater than the difference between two persons at the 50th and 60th percentiles. Standard scores, on the other hand, are much more likely to reflect equivalent units throughout the range of the variable.

Other Normative Systems

Psychological tests that are designed to measure characteristics that develop systematically with age, such as intellectual capacity, psycho-motor skills, scholastic achievement, etc., often summarize performance on age- or grade-equivalent scales. On these scales the client's performance is reported in terms of the performance of the typical 12-year-old male or the average fourth grade pupil, etc. While age and grade scales have some obvious advantages, they are most appropriate for children from middle class home backgrounds. Occasionally, grade-equivalent scores are useful in vocational counseling with an adult, e.g., it would be helpful to know that a client reads as well as the average sixth grader or possesses the arithmetic skills of the typical high school graduate.

Some Cautions

The following brief suggestions and guidelines have been alluded to or discussed earlier in this chapter or in the Introduction (test interpretation is discussed in greater depth in Chapters 4, 5, 8, 9, 14, 15, and 16 of this text):

1. Scores should be interpreted in terms of the specific content of the test from which they are derived. Because test titles may be misleading the counselor may find it helpful to use the scoring key to identify the specific items that contribute to a given score.

2. Test interpretation should include all other relevant information about the client: educational background, motivation, adjustment to disability, etc.

3. Test scores should be interpreted as bands or intervals rather than as single values, thus allowing for the unreliability of the measurement process.

4. Important decisions about clients should not be based on the results of one test or even a single testing session. Only when two or more different instruments suggest the same conclusion should the counselor be ready to make a crucial decision with the client.

5. Test norms should be appropriate to the particular decision that is being made. When selecting a test battery, the psychologist should make sure that adequate normative devices are available.

SUMMARY

The psychological test is a systematic procedure for measuring a sample of a client's behavior. The results of the client's performance are summarized in one or more numerical scores. Raw scores are not useful by themselves because they have no absolute interpretation, as do measures of height and weight. Norms are the bridge for converting raw scores into standard scores and percentiles. Test norms enable the counselor to 1) compare a client's performance to an appropriate reference group, and 2) compare a client's relative performance on several tests. These comparisons assist the counselor in diagnosing a client's strengths and weaknesses in skills, aptitudes, and personal qualities and in predicting success in various educational and vocational areas.

REFERENCES

Andrew, D. M., D. G. Paterson, and H. P. Longstaff. 1933. Minnesota Clerical Test. Psychological Corp., New York.

Angoff, W. H. 1971. Scales, norms, and equivalent scores. In R. L. Thorndike (ed.), Educational Measurement. 2nd Ed. American Council on Education, Washington, D. C.

Cattell, R. B., H. W. Eber, and M. M. Tatsuoka. 1970. Handbook for the Sixteen Personality Factor Questionnaire (16 PF). Institute for Personality and Ability Testing, Champaign, Ill.

Institute for Personality and Ability Testing. 1967. The Sixteen Personality Factor Questionnaire. Form E. IPAT, Champaign, Ill.

Institute for Personality and Ability Testing. 1968. Interim Manual Supplement for Form E, Sixteen Personality Factor Questionnaire. IPAT: Champaign, Ill.

Nunnally, J. 1967. Psychometric Theory. McGraw-Hill, New York.

Psychological Corporation. 1959. Manual for the Minnesota Clerical Test. Rev. Ed. Psychological Corp., New York.

Additional Sources

Anastasi, A. 1968. Psychological Testing. 3rd Ed. ch. 3. Macmillan, New York.

Brown, F. C. 1970. Principles of Educational and Psychological Testing. Ch. 7. Dryden, Hinsdale, Ill.

Cronbach, L. J. 1970. Essentials of Psychological Testing. 3rd Ed. Ch. 4. Harper & Row, New York.

Nunnally, J. 1970. Psychometric Theory. Ch. 8. McGraw-Hill, New York.

2 | Reliability

ROBERT M. THORNDIKE

Whenever measurements of anything are made it may be assumed that there is some purpose to which the measures will be put. In the area of rehabilitation the purposes of measurement range from research to diagnosis to prognosis, but there are certain qualities that any measure must have before it can be put to use, regardless of the nature of the measurement or its application. Two of these qualities that have received considerable attention in the psychometric literature over the years are reliability and validity. In this chapter the basic principles of reliability theory and their application to practical measurement problems are discussed. A similar discussion of validity is presented in the next chapter.

DEFINITIONS OF RELIABILITY

Reliability refers to a class of procedures and ideas dealing with the behavior displayed by persons on measuring devices. A distinction may be made between notions of reliability and notions of validity in terms of the area of concern about the measure. In general, it is fair to say that the study of reliability refers to the evaluation of the relationship of a measuring device to itself, while the term validity refers to the study of the relations of a measuring device to things other than itself. Although this distinction is not perfect (some indices of reliability yield evidence from which validity may be inferred), it is of sufficient generality to serve as a framework for this discussion.

Most of the widely used notions of reliability involve an index of correlation, often a product moment correlation. The correlation of a set of measures obtained from a group of people at one point in time with a second set of measures using the same instrument and the same group at a later time is one form of reliability, often called a coefficient of stability. When the correlation is computed between scores on one set of items and a different set designed to measure the same thing, the result is information about the generality of the instrument, that is, whether the performance of tested persons is specific to a particular set of items. On the other hand, the relationship between performance on a set of items and outcomes from rehabilitation counseling is evidence of the validity of the measure, as is the relationship between the instrument and the theoretical construct that it is designed to measure.

Another way to think about this distinction is to consider what it is that one may wish to make statements about. In a sense, the reliability of an instrument is its ability to predict itself, while its validity is its ability to predict something else. Both of these topics involve the quality of measurement obtained from an instrument, but reliability refers to quality in an isolated sense, while validity involves the usefulness of the instrument for other purposes. As shall be discussed in more detail later, there are several ways to evaluate reliability, each appropriate to some practical situations. A measuring instrument must show some form of internal quality (reliability) before it can be expected to have external utility (validity).

THE CLASSICAL MODEL OF TEST THEORY

Early in the history of psychological measurement investigators of human differences became aware that they were dealing with a rather difficult subject population. It seems to be part of the perverse nature of the human animal that he is inconsistent in his performance. In fact, human behavior is so tremendously variable that the infant science of psychology quickly found itself dealing with types of measurement problems that the older, more mature sciences had not yet needed to confront. Astronomers, chemists, and physicists had not had to be deeply concerned about consistency of measurement because the phenomena that they studied occurred in such regular fashion that subtle inconsistencies were not detected by their measuring devices. The reliability of observation was almost taken for granted, and results could be replicated quite easily because it was assumed that the act of measurement did not alter the object being measured. Also, successive observations of new samples showed high degrees of consistency.

Prototypic psychological measures, such as those of Binet, were very coarse and inaccurate, in an absolute sense, compared to those of the other sciences. However, the variability of human performance, both between groups at one time and within an individual person over time, is so great that even the unrefined instruments of 70 years ago detected this variation. Thus, in a relative sense it is possible to claim that psychological instruments were more sensitive than those of the "hard sciences" because their units of measurement were smaller than the units of variability in the entities studied. Psychologists became acutely aware of variability in performance and developed the study of instability of observations, to be followed a few years later by their hard science counterparts when the latter had developed instruments that detected the subtle variations in their observations. Today, all of the sciences are concerned with the reliability of their measures, but the problems are still most acute for psychology because the magnitude of variation relative to units of measure is still greatest in the study of human behavior.

Repeated Measures and True Scores

Two constructs form the cornerstones of the classical model of reliability. The first of these cornerstones is that each person has some amount of the attribute to be measured. The representation of a person's amount of the attribute as reflected by a given instrument is called his *true score* on that instrument. People differ in their true scores on a measure, but the true score for a person is assumed to be constant across successive administrations of the same or equivalent instruments. For example, if a test of general intelligence were given to the same person on several occasions, it is assumed that some underlying and constant level of intelligence would enter his score on every occasion that he takes the test. (It should be emphasized that this is an assumption. There are times when this assumption is not met, and there are times when it may be inappropriate.)

Error of Measurement

The second cornerstone of the classical reliability model is that each observation includes some component of error, called an *error of measurement.* There is an error of measurement associated with each observation of each person. It is assumed in classical test theory that each occurrence of an error of measurement is independent of (uncorrelated with) all other errors of measurement. Furthermore, it is assumed that the errors for any person are random deviations from his true score (which means that they have a mean of zero and their distribution is normal in shape). Thus, the *observed score* for any person is composed of his true score plus an error of measurement, according to the classical model.

An intimate perspective on the way that the classical model of reliability functions may be obtained by constructing a simplified example. Suppose the golfing ability of John Duffer is being measured, and the particular aspect of John's game under study at the moment is how far he can hit the ball with his driver. The first time John hits the ball he drives it 225 yards off the tee. It may be assumed that this is John's "score" on the driving test, but any experienced duffer knows that any particular shot is some combination of true ability and error. The second shot, even under the same conditions, will never precisely replicate the first. To get a better estimate of John's true ability he hits another shot, then another and another until he has a fairway (and perhaps the rough) littered with golf balls. Each time John hits the ball, the distance of his drive is measured and recorded, so that a sheet of paper is eventually covered with numbers, each of which is an independent estimate of John's ability. (Some assumptions are being made here, for example, that John has been making the same effort on each shot, that no learning has been taking place, and that fatigue has not set in.)

How should this subject's performance be summarized? From a practical point of view, the summary statement of John's ability should predict his future performance as accurately as possible. That is, the next time John steps up to the tee a reasonably accurate prediction could be made about how far he will hit the ball. A large number of observations showing substantial intrapersonal variation have been recorded. Assuming that the data collected so far cover the range of possible outcomes and that John's behavior conforms to the classical model, the best guess about the next drive will be the mean of the distribution of recorded scores. The distribution of lengths of drives will be normal in shape, fitting the model, and the mean may be taken as John's true score. In fact, true score may be operationally defined as the mean of a distribution of scores obtained on successive testings using the same or equivalent measures. It has the additional advantage of permitting the prediction of future performance with the least average error.

Standard Error of Measurement

The distribution of scores earned by John Duffer on the test of golfing ability has another important property in addition to its mean as a definition of true score. This other important property is the variation in scores. True score has been defined as the mean of a series of repeated measures, but each observed score has also been defined as a combination of true scores and some random error of measurement component. That is,

$$X_{oi} = T_i + e_{oi} \tag{1}$$

the observed score of individual i on occasion $o(X_{oi})$ is the sum of his constant true score (T_i) and the error of measurement (e_{oi}) associated with this observation of him. Since the true score is the mean of the distribution, the standard deviation of the distribution of scores is also the standard deviation of the errors of measurement. A special term, standard error of measurement (SEM), has been given to this standard deviation of errors of measurement, and it is defined as the standard deviation of the distribution of errors of measurement.

An important alteration in the definition has now been made. The situation described for John Duffer resulted in the SEM being the standard deviation of observed scores on repeated independent measures of the same subject. This is a valid definition, and an important one, but there are very few situations where a large number of independent repeated measures can be taken. Not only are humans obnoxiously variable as scientific subjects, but they also have this nasty habit of remembering what they did in the test situation the last time. This problem is present to some degree in the golfing example, but it presents particular difficulties when it comes to performance on psychological tests. In fact, the only place where the classical model can be expected to be reasonably appropriate for individual human performance is in those situations where fine discriminations are required and there is no feedback to the subject about his success or failure. Some problems in classical psychophysics are of this kind.

Now, take another look at the revised definition: The standard error of measurement is the standard deviation of the distribution of errors of measurement. Stated in this way, the definition permits the use of a number of subjects, each measured once. (It will be necessary shortly to introduce a second measure on these people.) Each subject has an observed score (X_i), which is composed of his true score and a random error component as shown in formula (1). It may be reasonably assumed that the subjects in this sample will show some variation in their observed scores on the measure, and also that they vary in their true scores and that each one has been measured with some (random) error. Since the errors are independent of the true scores (by assumption!), the variance (squared standard deviation) of observed scores can be represented as the sum of the variance in true scores and the variance of errors, or

$$S_x^2 = S_T^2 + S_e^2$$

from which it can be seen that

$$S_e^2 = S_x^2 - S_T^2 \qquad (2)$$

The distribution of the errors of measurement for the group will be normal in shape with a mean of zero and a variance of S_e^2. Since the objective in measuring someone is to obtain as accurate an estimate as possible of his true score, it will be profitable to reduce S_e^2 relative to S_x^2 in any way that can be done.

Definition of Reliability

The problem with the foregoing definition of the SEM is that it is a verbal definition only. In any given observation or set of observations that portion of performance that is the result of true score cannot be separated from that which is the result of error. There is no way of estimating e_i, and hence no way of computing S_e^2. This problem may be overcome in the following manner.

Assume thet there are two equivalent measures of a characteristic to be measured. (Tests are defined as equivalent if they are designed to measure the same characteristic, have equal means and standard deviations, and have equal standard errors of measurement (Gulliksen, 1950).) Using the deviation score formula for the product moment correlation between two variables it can be shown that

$$r_{x_1 x_2} = S_T^2 / S_x^2 \tag{3}$$

That is, the correlation between equivalent forms of a test is equal to the ratio of the variance of true scores divided by the variance of observed scores.

The result obtained in equation (3) is very important for several reasons. First, it provides the basic definition of reliability as an index of the accuracy or consistency of measurement. Since true scores are constant from one administration of a test to another and across equivalent forms of the same test, *reliability* is defined as:

1. That portion of observed score variance among subjects that is the result of variation in true scores, or
2. that portion of a subject's performance that will remain constant over time.

The second aspect of this definition of reliability will be discussed later. Now, some other implications of equation (3) as they are reflected in the first aspect of the definition will be considered.

An operational definition of reliability as the correlation between two equivalent measures has been established. These measures may be obtained in a variety of ways, which will be discussed shortly. For the present, the definition in equation (3) is sufficient.

Simple manipulation of equation (3) permits an expression for the standard error of measurement to be written in terms of obtainable quantities

$$S_e = S_x\sqrt{1 - r_{x_1 x_2}} \qquad (4)$$

Standard Error of Measurement Revisited

Now that a means of estimating the SEM has been established, it is appropriate to re-examine and extend its interpretations and uses. The value obtained from equation (4) is an estimate of the standard deviation of errors of measurement for a group of subjects, but it is also an estimate of what the standard deviation of the distribution of observed scores for repeated measurements of an individual subject would be if such measures could be obtained. In this sense, the standard error of measurement provides an index of the absolute stability of measurement. Variation in a subject's performance is estimated. The reliability coefficient, on the other hand, is an index of relative stability. It is a correlation coefficient, and, as such, it indicates the degree to which each subject maintains his relative position in the group. Although the reliability coefficient is the index most frequently used to compare various measuring devices on their internal quality (as opposed to their power to predict other variables, which is validity), the standard error of measurement is most important for interpreting individual scores. It is very useful to know that an instrument will order the members of a group consistently, but it is vital in areas such as rehabilitation counseling and educational placement to know how much error is likely to be made in using a test score for diagnostic purposes. When the concern is with individual assessment, an index of the absolute consistency of measurement is of prime importance and greatest descriptive value.

First, errors of measurement as random normal deviates will be considered. The distribution of these errors is normal in shape with a mean of zero and a standard deviation of S_e. Given these assumptions, the most probable value for the error on any single observation is the mean of the distribution, zero. Therefore, the observed score of a particular subject can be taken as a best estimate of his true score,[1] but with full knowledge that there is a risk of being wrong by some amount. The standard error of measurement provides a means of estimating how large the error is likely

---

[1] Technically, the best estimate of a subject's true score is obtained by "regressing" his observed score toward the mean. See Lord and Novick (1968, Ch. 7) for a complete discussion.

to be. It permits a confidence band to be placed around an observed score such that one may be certain, with a specified probability, that the range covered by the confidence band includes the subject's true score.

An example will help to clarify both this point and the computations associated with true and error score variances. Suppose there is a test with the following characteristics: $\overline{X} = 110$, $S_x = 14.5$, $r_{x_1 x_2} = 0.80$. From this information, the standard error of measurement is found to be

$$S_e = 14.5 \sqrt{1-0.80} = 14.5 \, (0.4472) = 6.48$$

$$S_e^2 = 41.99$$

and the variance of true scores is

$$S_e^2 = 0.80 \, (210.75) = 168.2$$

Observed score variance may be broken down as

$$210.25 = 168.2 + 41.99$$

$$(S_x^2) \qquad (S_t^2) \qquad (S_e^2)$$

which is correct within a rounding error of 0.06 and which shows that 80 percent of the observed score variance is the result of variation in true scores.

Now, imagine that a client, Betty, has obtained a score of 97 on this test. By using the standard error of measurement, several things can be determined about Betty. Her most probable true score is 97, but the normal curve properties of errors can be used to conclude that the chances are two in three that her true score lies between 90.52 and 103.48 (97 ± 6.48). This band can be extended to any desired level of confidence by using the formula

$$X - Z_p S_e \leqslant X \leqslant X + Z_p S_e$$

where Z_p is the normal deviate associated with the two-tailed probability p. Thus, for the 95 percent confidence band on Betty's score one finds

$$97 - 1.96 \, (6.48) \leqslant X \leqslant 97 + 1.96 \, (6.48)$$

$$84.23 \leqslant X \leqslant 109.70$$

There is a 95 percent certainty that this interval includes Betty's true score.

It might also be useful to determine the probability that Betty's true score is at least as great as some particular value, such as the group's mean. This can be done by the same general procedure as that for finding Z-scores.

$$Z = \frac{97 - 110}{6.48} = \frac{-13}{6.48} = -2.01$$

$$P_Z = 0.022$$

The probability that Betty's true score is at least as great as the group's mean is slightly greater than one in 50.

The foregoing discussion illustrates a feature of psychological measurement that is all too often overlooked by users of psychological tests. Even when a test has a reliability as high as 0.80 (or even 0.95) the variability of human behavior is such that caution must be exercised in interpreting a client's scores. In the last example the range of reasonably possible scores for Betty was 25.47 units wide! With a test as highly respected as the Stanford-Binet the standard error of measurement is about four units. When treatment decisions must be based on test scores, this is an uncomfortably large possible error. Under such conditions it is often wise to evaluate the probability that the decision indicated by the test is wrong and to weigh this probability against the consequences for the client of using one procedure or another.

VARIATION IN TEST SCORES

The classical test theory model permits two types of variation to influence the scores of a group of subjects on a test. There is variation among subjects in their true levels of the trait being measured, and there is variation within each one's performance because of error. During the 1940s several developments occurred that led to a modification and refinement of the classical model and allowed for additional factors to affect test performance. These advances were summarized most completely in two chapters on reliability by Thorndike (1949, 1951). Consideration of these sources of variation allows one to evaluate the information contained in the several varieties of reliability coefficients discussed in the next section.

Sources of Variation

Table 1 presents the sources of variation enumerated by Thorndike (1951). It is assumed that each of these will have some effect on the scores obtained by subjects on a particular administration of a particular test. Some of them appropriately may be considered as contributions to true scores, while others represent errors of measurement.

Table 1. Possible sources of variance in score on a particular test[1]

I. Lasting and general characteristics of the person:
   A. Level of ability on one or more general traits, which operate in a number of tests
   B. General skills and techniques of taking tests
   C. General ability to comprehend instructions

II. Lasting but specific characteristics of the person:
   A. Specific to the test as a whole (and to parallel forms of it)
     1. Individual level of ability on traits required in this test but not in others
     2. Knowledge and skills specific to the particular form of test items
   B. Specific to particular test items
     1. The "chance" element determining whether the person does or does not know a particular fact (sampling variance in a finite number of items, not the probability of his guessing the answer)

III. Temporary but general characteristics of the person (factors affecting performance on many or all tests at a particular time):
   A. Health
   B. Fatigue
   C. Motivation
   D. Emotional strain
   E. General test-wiseness (partly lasting)
   F. Understanding of mechanics of testing
   G. External conditions of heat, light, ventilation, etc.

IV. Temporary and specific characteristics of the person:
   A. Specific to a test as a whole
     1. Comprehension of the specific test task (insofar as this is distinct from I-B)
     2. Specific tricks or techniques of dealing with the particular test materials (insofar as they are distinct from II-A-2)
     3. Level of practice on the specific skills involved (especially in psychomotor tests)
     4. Momentary "set" for a particular test
   B. Specific to particular test items
     1. Fluctuations and idiosyncrasies of human memory
     2. Unpredictable fluctuations in attention or accuracy, superimposed upon the general level of performance characteristic of the individual

---

Continued

V. Systematic or chance factors affecting the administration of the test
    or the appraisal of test performance:
    A. Conditions of testing: adherence to time limits, freedom from
        distractions, clarity of instructions, etc.
    B. Unreliability or bias in subjective rating of traits or perfor-
        mances

VI. Variance not otherwise accounted for (chance):
    A. "Luck" in selection of answers by "guessing"

---

[1] Reproduced with permission from Thorndike, Robert L., 1951, Reliability. *In* E.
F. Lindquist (ed.), Educational Measurement. American Council on Education,
Washington, D.C.

I. Lasting and General Characteristics   The first category of variation
includes those features of the subject that pervade his performance on a
variety of tests. Aspects such as general intelligence and ability in broad
areas such as verbal fluency, number ability, and spatial relations are
included under category I-A in Table 1. General test-taking skills and
personality characteristics related to behavior in testing situations are
found in I-B, and the ability to understand and to follow directions are
placed in I-C. In a sense, each of these three features is a constant for a
particular subject across several tests and over a substantial period of time.

The differences included in the category of general ability or
intelligence compose a large part of what one would ordinarily want to call
true score variance. However, any relatively stable and general characteristic of the subject that affects performance on the test will be inextric-
ably bound to his level of ability. People differ in the amount of
experience they have had with tests, in their attitudes and anxieties about
tests and the testing situation, in their tendency to guess when they do not
know the answer (as contrasted with their success in guessing), and a host
of other factors that may affect test performance. These features may
undergo some change with time, but they will function as constant
characteristics in most efforts to determine reliability, whether we like it
or not.

II. Lasting but Specific Characteristics   Some characteristics of a
person will remain constant over a period of time but will be specific to a
particular test. In the terminology of factor analysis, the sources of
variation in the preceding paragraph contribute to general or group factors,
while sources that affect only one test may be seen as specific factors. The
characteristics that form this category may be broken down into those
characteristics that affect the whole test (II-A) and those that function
only for particular items (II-B). Under the former heading come character-

istics such as ability or knowledge on the trait that is unique to the test, perhaps including aspects of performance such as those found in single cells of Guilford's (1959) structure of intellect model. Also included here are abilities related to particular types of items. If a test is composed of only one type of item, such as multiple choice, matching, essay, or short answer, differences in ability with that item will appear as consistent features of the subject. When a variety of item types are present in the test, abilities of this kind may have a smaller effect in creating true score differences between subjects.

There are times in the measurement of human abilities when a person will possess a particular piece of information that enables him to answer correctly and without guessing an unusually difficult item. This is likely to happen particularly with a test of knowledge of specific facts, such as a spelling test, but it may also occur in tests of general intelligence or scholastic aptitude. Some isolated aspect of the subject's experience has caused him to learn the meaning or spelling of an obscure term so that he gets a very difficult item correct while missing easier ones. This is a chance event in the sense that the sampling of material for the test happened to include that item rather than some other item of equal difficulty but to which the subject does not know the answer. This item will increase his true score on the test somewhat erroneously. Variation because of this phenomenon is included in section II-B of Table 1.

III. Temporary but General Characteristics It is common to hear students complain that they would have received a better score on a test if they had felt better that day. Most comments of this nature are excuses for lack of study or inadequate preparation; however, a certain amount of variation in test performance may be attributed to relatively short-term fluctuations in items such as those listed in category III of Table 1. The variables included here are considered to be relatively short-term deviations from a subject's normal level of functioning, lasting up to a few days. Factors in this category will affect performance on all tests taken at a particular time but generally will have changed by the time the person is retested.

We may include in this category the demand characteristics of the testing situation when these are subject to change. Some people may approach a testing situation in a very different manner when they are told that the test results will be used for personal guidance or for admission to a program, and this may be reflected in their performance. The way one views an evaluation, as either threatening or supportive, can be particularly important for those who have had repeated unpleasant experiences with testing or who have feelings of inferiority. The effect of this variable on test performance can be minimized by attempting to give a consistently positive, nonthreatening set to all those being tested.

IV. Temporary and Specific Characteristics In addition to those temporary features that affect a whole range of test performances, there are characteristics of the subject that are temporary and reflected in performance only on one test or a part of a test. These features (category IV) include variations in the comprehension of the test instructions or item contents caused by fluctuations in attention, tricks, or insights about the test that are discovered in the course of testing, and random events that occur in the testing situation and affect performance on a few items. For example, consider the response of the student who is concentrating on a final course examination when, without warning, a construction crew attacks the wall directly behind him with a jackhammer. To put it mildly, his concentration is broken. This is admittedly an extreme example, but dropping one's pencil or glasses (or crib sheet) would have a similar effect.

V. Administration and Appraisal of Test Performance The fifth category of sources of variation in the results of measurement includes the qualities of the measurement operation itself. Different test administrators vary in the way in which they read and explain test directions, in the amount of help and encouragement they give, and in the care with which they maintain a standardized environment. If one tester pays close attention to time limits, ensures that everyone has the necessary test materials, etc., and another tester does not, the result may be differences in test performance that are not the result of differences in ability. Also included here are variations because of lack of standardization in the evaluation of performance by graders or raters. The subjectivity involved in evaluating the quality of answers to essay questions is a source of variation in test scores. Halo or other biases in the ratings of behavior provide another example of variation of this sort. If, as is usually the case, it is desired to eliminate these sources of variation, steps must be taken to improve the standardization of evaluation procedures. Making multiple evaluations and using an average of several of them are also beneficial.

VI. Chance Variance Whatever variation is left in test scores is put into category VI, chance and random effects. The most obvious contributor here is the increase in score obtained from being lucky in guessing the correct answer when knowledge is not present. Another source of variation of this type is the chance mismarking of an answer sheet. This may be done either by the person taking a test or by the one evaluating it, as when the subject gives the correct answer to a question on an individual intelligence test but the examiner records the answer in the wrong place. Variation of this type is specific to a particular item on a particular occasion and, as such, represents a close approximation of pure error. The only way to reduce its effect is to take a larger sample of behavior.

Strategies of Data Collection

The variety of ways in which scores on tests can be affected by different aspects of tests and testing situations provides ample evidence that there is no single, true, and correct reliability for any test. Before the value of a statement that the reliability of test X is 0.85 can be judged, there must be some idea of the test author's definition of true and error scores. Different ways of collecting data for a realiability study assign the sources of variation outlined in Table 1 to true and error scores differently. A test that is reported to have a high reliability may be unsuitable for certain purposes if the method used to estimate reliability is inappropriate for the use to which the test is to be put. This section will review the experimental designs for obtaining reliability data and then examine them in terms of the sources of variation assigned to true and error scores by each.

The experimental designs used most frequently for collecting information about the reliability of a test can be described in terms of two dimensions. First, one may inquire whether the study involved a single form of the test or whether multiple equivalent forms (two or more) were administered; second, whether there was a time interval between the first and second testing, and if so, how long it was. The various possibilities under this scheme are outlined in Table 2. Each of these procedures provides a means of obtaining two scores for each subject so that a correlation may be computed. The method by which data are obtained for the designs in the top four cells of the table is straightforward. In the first column the same set of items is administered twice, with or without a time delay, while in the second column two different sets of items are used.

The split-half procedure has some of the features of both columns, although it is properly labeled an immediate equivalent forms method. When only one form of a test exists and it is unfeasible or unwise to administer it twice, two sets of scores may be obtained by dividing the test in half and scoring each half separately. The division may be done before testing to ensure that the two halves are equivalent, or it may be done after testing by scoring odd-numbered items as one test and even-numbered items as another. In either case, two different sets of items are used to obtain the two sets of scores, but there is generally no time interval between the tests.

Restrictions on the Use of Half-test Designs If it is necessary to estimate reliability with a split-half procedure, several important restrictions must be kept in mind. Where items differ markedly in content or difficulty, care must be taken to ensure that these features are equated in

Table 2.   Experimental designs for assessing test
reliability

	Single form	Multiple forms
Interval between testings	Delayed test-retest	Delayed equivalent forms
No interval between testings	Immediate test-retest	Immediate equivalent forms
	Split-half	

the resulting scores. This may require that items be assigned to halves of the test by blocks rather than by random division.

When speed of response is a major component of test score, as is the case with many clerical tests, a split-half procedure is generally not appropriate as an index of reliability. In a pure speed test where all items are very easy and scores generally equal the number of items attempted, an odd-even split of the items will result in each subject obtaining almost identical scores on both halves of the test, yielding an inflated estimate of the test's reliability. The only way to overcome this restriction for speeded tests is to time two halves of the test separately. Otherwise, a test-retest procedure must be used.

A third aspect of the split-half design that restricts its value is the fact that scores are based on relatively few items. The reliability of a test score is dependent to some extent on the number of observations on which it is based. Correlations between half-test scores, therefore, will tend to be lower than would be correlations between scores based on twice as many items, which means that reliability may be underestimated for split-half designs when speed of performance is not a factor. It is possible to overcome this problem by correcting for the reduction in length using the Spearman-Brown formula, which estimates what the correlation would be between two full length equivalent forms of the test. For a more thorough discussion of the use of the Spearman-Brown formula and of the benefits and dangers of split-half reliability estimates, see Thorndike (1951).

Internal Consistency Coefficients There is another problem with the use of split-half methods for estimating reliability, one that is not necessarily of direct concern to test administrators, but which has drawn the attention of measurement theorists. Any particular way of dividing the test in half is only one of a multitude of possible ways. Because there is no necessarily correct way of obtaining two equivalent halves and because different ways of splitting the test will ordinarily yield different estimates of the test's reliability, it is not possible to obtain a unique reliability estimate using split-half procedures. When different splits yield quite different reliability estimates, as may sometimes happen when the test is short, it is desirable to be able to obtain a single index that reflects consistency of measurement for the test as a whole, regardless of variabilities that might be the result of using one split or another.

This problem was first attacked by Kuder and Richardson (1937), and their results have been extended by Hoyt (1941) and Cronbach (1951). Each of these procedures uses the logic of analysis of variance among the items to obtain a reliability coefficient that is a function of the ratio of error variation to the variation among subjects, although different names are applied to the results.

The approach proposed by Kuder and Richardson (1937) assumed that items were dichotomously scored (p = the proportion of subjects getting the item right; $q = 1 - p$, or the proportion of incorrect responses). By adding a number of additional assumptions, namely that all items in the test 1) have the same true score variance and observed score variance, 2) have equal correlations with all other items, and 3) measure the same thing, it is possible to derive a formula that provides a unique estimate of the reliability of a test from a single administration of that test. This is "formula 20" from Kuder and Richardson, which has come to be known and loved as KR 20 reliability. An additional simplifying assumption, that all items in the test are of the same difficulty, leads to Kuder and Richardson's "formula 21." It is the simplest form to which this derivation can lead and requires that only the mean and standard deviation of observed scores be computed.

Kuder and Richardson's approach was generalized to the case of multicategory response items by Hoyt (1941), using analysis of variance directly. Each item is considered as a level of the treatment condition and each subject is observed at all levels, yielding a treatment by subjects or one within design. First, the treatment (item), subject, and total sums of squares are computed and the residual sum of squares is found by subtraction. Second, the mean square for subjects (variance among individual persons) and the mean square error (error variance) are found. Then, these values are substituted in the appropriate formula, and the value that results is a reliability estimate.

Hoyt's procedure is based on the same general assumptions that underlie KR 20 and will yield identical results for the same data. This is also true of Cronbach's coefficient α, as has been shown by Stanley (1971). All three are measures of the extent to which the items in the test are consistent in their "ordering" of the subjects, and for this reason, all three are referred to as *internal consistency coefficients.* They provide statistical indices of the *homogeneity* of the test.

Like the split-half procedures that preceded them, the internal consistency estimates of reliability cannot be used with speeded tests because the coefficients will be inflated when some items have been attempted by few subjects. The problem can be most clearly seen in the Hoyt procedure because unattempted items appear as missing data. That is, the internal consistency methods require that all subjects respond to all items. In addition, it is assumed that the test is completely homogeneous in content. Failure of this second assumption generally will mean that the reliability estimate obtained by one of these internal consistency procedures will be too low. Note that the split-half, test-retest, and parallel forms designs do not require homogeneous tests, merely equivalence of content. For a thorough but difficult discussion of these procedures, their assumptions, and restrictions, see Stanley (1971).

Reliable Sources of Variance

Each of the research designs discussed above yields an estimate of the reliability of measurement provided by the test, but the different designs result in different estimates. The sources of variation outlined in Table 1 may be used to see why this variation in reliability estimates occurs. The main feature of this approach is that some of the sources of variation can be seen as functioning as consistent or systematic variance in some designs and as inconsistent or error variance in others. The allocation of each of the sources to systematic or error variance for each of the designs is summarized in Table 3. The summary provided in this table may not be precisely accurate for a given test using a particular design, but it can serve as a guide for what to expect in the most situations.

The parallel form approach to reliability estimation requires two equivalent forms of the test. If the forms are truly equivalent, they will measure the same general abilities and will require the same test-taking skills. However, care must be taken in their construction so that they are sufficiently similar to measure the same specific abilities or factors but not so similar in their items that they require the same pieces of information. That is, properly prepared parallel forms of a test should have sources I and II-A functioning in a systematic manner, but source II-B should not provide consistent variation among subjects. When there is an interval separating the administration of the forms the temporary factors influencing performance on the whole test (III and IV-A) should vary randomly from subject to subject, while these same factors will result in consistent differences between subjects when there is no delay between testings. In either case, sources resulting from particular items or groups of items

Table 3. Sources of variances for the reliability designs[1]

Sources	Parallel Forms		Test-Retest		Split half	Internal consistency
	Interval	No interval	Interval	No interval		
I	S	S	S	S	S	S
II A	S	S	S	S	S	S
B	E	E	S	S	E	E(?)
III	E	S	E	S	S	S
IV A	E	S	E	S	S	S
B	E	E	E	E	E(?)	E(?)
V	E	E	E	E	–	--
VI	E	E	E	E	E	E

[1] The sources in this table are the sources of variation outlined in Table 1. "S" indicates that variation from the source indicated is systematic and contributes to "true score" variance for this design for data collection; "E" indicates that the listed source contributes to error of measurement or error variance for this design. Where the effect of a source of variation is uncertain, its contribution is followed by a question mark.

(IV-B) and to chance factors (VI) will function as error or inconsistent variation. The effect of administrative factors (V) depends upon the skill of the test administrator in providing a consistent testing environment and in carefully adhering to the time limits and administrative conditions. Differences in administration from one occasion to another may create a substantial systematic effect on test performance. Careful attention to the details of test administration can eliminate this source of variance by making it essentially constant for all subjects on all occasions.

When the two equivalent forms of the test are identical to the extent that they have the same items, we have a test-retest design. Obviously, sources I and II-A will function as systematic sources of variance and contribute to true score variance, but repetition of items means that factors specific to particular test items will also appear as consistent variation. Thus, source II-B will be added to the consistent component of variance and be reflected as true score variation. It is the addition of this knowledge-of-particular-items factor (which is confounded with memory for the response chosen the last time the test was taken) that causes test-retest estimates of reliability to be generally higher than those obtained with a comparable parallel form administration. Of course, when no time interval occurs between administrations, the temporary factors influence consistency of performance in much the same way that they influence performance on parallel forms. However, the potential effect of memory for items on an immediate retest is also much greater than when the retest is delayed, so the use of a test-retest design with no time interval generally should be restricted to tests in which memory cannot play a significant role, for example, in tests of motor performance after a warm-up period.

The split-half and internal consistency designs are quite similar in the way that they allocate the sources of variation to systematic and error components. They both include sources I and II-A as consistent components and, because both use a single administration of the test (no time interval), the temporary sources (III and IV-A) are also treated as systematic. The function of temporary factors affecting less than the whole test is somewhat unclear because effects on single items result in error variance but effects on groups of items may contribute to systematic variation in performance. The split-half procedure will generally treat variation in category II-B as error, while the homogeneity restriction on internal consistency designs may result in some systematic variance arising from this source. The single administration used by either of these designs generally will mean that administration factors (V) are constant and do not affect the reliability estimate, while chance factors (VI) are considered error.

The magnitude of the reliability coefficient obtained for a particular test will be related to the number of sources of variation that can be considered to yield consistent or systematic differences among people. It may be seen from Table 3 that the parallel forms design with a time interval has the fewest sources that are classified as systematic, which means that with other things (such as care in administration) being equal, this design will yield the lowest or most conservative estimate of the test's reliability. A somewhat higher estimate will be obtained with no interval or with a test-delayed retest, the relative magnitude of these two depending on the length of the delay and the potency of the temporary and memory factors. The other designs generally will yield higher estimates of reliability, with the exception that the internal consistency methods are sensitive to violations of the homogeniety assumption. When this assumption is not at least approximately satisfied, an internal consistency coefficient may seriously underestimate the reliability of the test as it might be found by other means. Thus, caution must be exercised in selecting the design for a reliability study and in interpreting the results of such studies.

FACTORS AFFECTING RELIABILITY INTERPRETATION

The proper interpretation of reliability coefficients requires more information than just the magnitude of the coefficient and the design used to obtain it. Various aspects of the distribution of test scores and the relationship of the test to other variables must also be considered when evaluating reliability. In addition, the use to which the test is to be put will affect the relative importance of one or another type of information about the quality of measurement.

Logical Factors

Several designs for obtaining data on the reliability of a test have been presented above. Each of them provides information that is valuable for some testing situations but not for others. Three basic considerations are involved: The breadth of coverage of the test, the assumed nature of the trait that the test is to measure, and the way the test is to be used (concurrently or predictively). A test may appear to have very promising reliability for some situations, but the necessary information to justify its use in others may be absent.

Breadth of Coverage Breadth of coverage refers primarily to the homogeniety that the test has been designed to have. When the score resulting from measurement is claimed to reflect a narrow range of behavior, such as a single factor of ability, one may reasonably require that the internal consistency of the test be high. A low value would indicate that the test might be measuring a complex composite of several dimensions. This inference would be supported if the test were found to have substantial temporal stability as measured by a delayed retest. On the other hand, high internal consistency would be inappropriate in a test that has been designed to measure a complex trait. One might rightfully be suspicious of a test claiming to measure "general psychomotor performance" in a single score and showing high internal consistency because previous research has shown abilities of this type to be only moderately correlated. A test is not necessarily damned by the fact that it may show low to moderate internal consistency. The design may be inappropriate for the particular situation.

Nature of Measured Trait Most tests are designed to measure traits that are relatively stable features of behavior. When the characteristic that the test is assumed to measure can be considered to change relatively little over time it is appropriate and desirable to evaluate the *temporal stability* of test scores by employing a delay between one administration and another. The temporal stability of measurement is so central to most notions of reliability that it may be argued that internal consistency procedures do not estimate reliability at all and should not be assumed to result in reliability coefficients. This view is somewhat narrow and restrictive because it is possible to conceive of traits that fluctuate over time but are highly consistent at one point in time. For example, a measure of hypomania might yield very low temporal stability for a group of cyclic manic-depressives but be highly internally consistent and a valid indicator of current status at any given point in time. Thus, there may be occasions when the conventional notion of reliability as temporal stability is inappropriate. Perhaps a better definition of reliability would be consistency of measurement under appropriate temporal conditions. Regardless of the way reliability is defined, the evaluation of a particular measuring device requires information about consistency of test scores that is appropriate for the assumed nature of the trait.

Uses of the Test   Another aspect of the stability issue involves the way in which the test is to be used. If the test is used to forecast behavior it is essential that the test be able to forecast itself. A test that is to act as a predictor must have temporal stability as shown by a delayed retest or delayed parallel forms design. Otherwise, there is no assurance that anything other than temporary states of individual subjects are being measured. On the other hand, when a test is developed to act as an indicator of current status of the trait, as when a test is used in place of a more costly and time-consuming evaluation procedure, assurances of temporal stability may not be necessary. It may generally be assumed that a test which is stable over the long term will also yield stable evaluations for immediate use, but evidence of short-term consistency is not a substitute for studies of long-term stability.

Consideration of the three factors discussed above leads to one conclusion: to adequately evaluate the reliability of a test for a particular purpose there must be data from a study (or, better yet, a series of studies) that utilized a design appropriate for that purpose. An internal consistency coefficient yields no information about the stability of measurement and a stability coefficient may be inappropriate for evaluating the quality of measurement of traits that are subject to marked temporal fluctuations.

Statistical Factors

All other things being equal, reliability coefficients are higher in heterogeneous samples. In other words, as observed score variance increases, and assuming that error variance remains relatively constant, the reliability coefficient will rise. Formulas are available for estimating the reliability coefficient for a sample that differs in variability from the one in which the reliability study was performed.

Another way in which statistical considerations connected with group variability affect the interpretation of reliability coefficients occurs when there has been selection of the sample on a related variable. The effects of selection may lead to increased or decreased variability in the group, but the possible presence of this effect should not be overlooked when interpreting reports of reliability studies. If, for example, a reliability study for an intelligence test were performed on a group of 10-year-old children and the test is to be used with 6- to 14-year olds (assuming the test is appropriate for a group this diverse and that age is related to intelligence) one might expect the test to have a higher reliability coefficient in the latter group. One may also estimate reliability in the population when the sample has been selected on the basis of some other test. The necessary formula is given by Thorndike (1951).

The problem of assessing the effects of selection on the reliability of the test is more critical when the selection has greatly increased the variability of scores, so that the reliability coefficient is a rather gross overestimate of what the reliability would probably be in a population of interest. There are, for example, intelligence tests on the market for which claims of near perfect reliability are made. At first glance it would appear that our prayers have been answered, until one reads a little more closely and discovers that the test authors used small samples with age ranges of 40 or 50 years. The reliability coefficient of 0.98 or more that the authors might have found would be perfectly true and accurate for their sample, but it would greatly overestimate the reliability one might realistically expect to obtain in the more homogeneous populations with which test users generally work. Reliability studies of this type are Barnum-like demonstrations of how high a coefficient can be obtained with a particular test, rather than useful contributions to knowledge about the test. To be of maximum value for a particular application of a test, the reliability study should be performed with a group that is as similar as possible to the application or target group. This, of course, also means that care must be exercised in the interpretation of reliability coefficients when the target group is exceptionally high or low in its average level of the trait and the reliability study has been performed on a representative sample of the general population. The reliability of the test for special groups, such as brain-damaged children, generally will be lower than the results from a study of normal subjects would indicate.

The length of the test is another factor that affects reliability. The discussion of split-half designs mentioned the necessity of correcting these coefficients by the Spearman-Brown formula in order to estimate the reliability of the full length test from the correlation between halves. There may be times when it is not possible to give an entire test or when it is desirable to use more than one form of the test to increase the precision of measurement. In such cases, a more general form of the Spearman-Brown formula makes it possible to estimate what the reliability of the reduced or expanded test is likely to be. This formula permits one to determine whether a shorter test will have satisfactory reliability or whether the gain in reliability that will be achieved by lengthening the test is likely to be worth the time and expense involved.

REFERENCES

Cronbach, L. J. 1951. Coefficient alpha and the internal structure of tests. Psychometrika 16:297—334.

Cronbach, L. J. 1970. Essentials of Psychological Testing. 3rd Ed. Harper & Row, New York.

Guilford, J. P. 1959. Three faces of intellect. Amer. Psycho. 14:469.

Gulliksen, H. 1950. Theory of Mental Tests. Wiley, New York.

Hoyt, C. 1941. Test reliability estimated by analysis of variance. Psychometrika 6: 153—160.

Kuder, G. F., and M. Richardson. 1937. The theory of estimation of test reliability. Psychometrika 2:151—160.

Lord, F. M., and M. R. Novick. 1968. Statistical Theories of Mental Test Scores. Addison-Wesley, Reading, Mass.

Stanley, J. 1971. Reliability. In R. L. Thorndike (ed.), Educational Measurement. 2nd Ed. American Council on Education, Washington, D. C.

Thorndike, R. L. 1949. Personnel Selection. Wiley, New York.

Thorndike, R. L. 1951. Reliability. 1951. In E. F. Lindquist (ed.), Educational Measurement. American Council on Education, Washington, D. C.

3 | Validity

NANCY E. BETZ and DAVID J. WEISS

There are many uses for psychological test data.[1] For example, an ability or aptitude test may be used to predict performance in an academic curriculum or success in performing a particular job. An achievement test may be used to determine the extent to which a person has mastered a defined area of content. Personality and interest tests may be used by counselors to help them know more about a client or to help clients know more about themselves. Each of these uses of tests implies a particular interpretation of a given test score. A high score on test X suggests good possibilities for job success; a high score on test Y indicates mastery of the content of a job training program or of seventh grade mathematics; and a low score on test Z indicates little interest in social service occupations. Narrowly considered, validity information concerns the accuracy or soundness of each of these specific interpretations of a test score.

TYPES OF VALIDATION DATA

Specific types of validity are important depending on the intended uses of a test. A committee of the American Psychological Association and related organizations has developed recommendations for the kinds of validity information that should be supplied in the test manual for various suggested uses of the test. These recommendations, contained in the revised

---

[1] For simplicity, the authors refer to tests or test scores throughout this chapter. The necessity for validation and the techniques used to determine validity, however, apply to all systematic methods of gathering psychological data, whether they are tests, inventories, ratings, questionnaires, or behavioral observations.

Standards for Educational and Psychological Tests (American Psychological Association, 1974), distinguish three types of validity: content validity, criterion-related validity, and construct validity. Content validity is the standard of evaluation most frequently applied to achievement tests. Criterion-related validity is important when the test is to be used as a predictive device to aid in making practical decisions about people. Construct validity is essential when the psychologist wishes to interpret test scores as indicants of some psychological variable or trait. However, as will be discussed in the following sections, both content and criterion-related validity bear a close relationship to construct validity and are important in establishing construct validity. Because of this close relationship, construct validity will not be discussed in a separate section. A fourth kind of validity, face validity, is of concern when it is necessary to justify or to convey the appropriateness of the test to potential users or testees who are not familiar with the principles and procedures of psychological measurement.

Content Validity

Content validity refers to how well the particular sampling of behaviors of items used to measure a trait or characteristic reflects performance or standing on the whole domain of behaviors that constitutes that trait. That is, a test administrator may be interested in the behavior of a person as expressed in a variety of situations or toward a universe of possible items. If anxiety were being measured, for example, it would be impossibly time consuming to ask the testee about every possible situation that might be anxiety producing. If a person's level of achievement in an American history course were being quantified, it would be impossible to ask him or her questions about every event in the history of America. As a result, a sampling of these behaviors is taken and an attempt to generalize to or make inferences about the testee's level of anxiety or knowledge of American history is made.

Thus, in establishing content validity, items should be chosen from a well defined behavioral domain. Furthermore, the sampling from that domain should be sufficiently broad and representative to allow direct inferences to it.

The achievement test situation, where there is a defined body of knowledge to be learned, provides the most obvious application of the principles of content validity. The test items should be taken from that body of knowledge and not from some other, and the items should be taken systematically from each segment of the subject area so that specific gaps or emphases in the knowledge of any one person will not have a disproportionate effect on the assessment of his or her knowledge. The more precisely the instructor has clarified and organized the relevant subject matter, the easier it will be to construct a test that adequately samples from that subject matter.

However, these principles are important in the construction of any psychological measuring instrument because content validity is directly related to the conceptualization and definition of a construct. For example, in defining the construct of anxiety, it is necessary to specify what behaviors may indicate anxiety (e.g., increased heart rate, sweaty palms, or simply the person's report of feeling anxious) and to specify a universe of situations in which anxiety might be felt. Some people may feel anxious in social situations, some in academic or job situations, some while driving a car or grocery shopping, and some may become anxious in all of these situations. If an estimate of a person's overall tendency toward becoming anxious (the trait or construct) is to be obtained, it is important to sample from the entire range of situations in which the behavior could be exhibited. Thus, as in the achievement test situation, the more precisely the construct-related behaviors are clarified and organized, the better able one will be to make generalizations to it from a sampling of those behaviors.

Evidence in Support of Content Validity

Subjective Judgment   The most usual kind of evidence presented in support of content validity is the subjective judgment of those who construct the test or of other "experts" familiar with the subject area or trait definition. This kind of evidence is usually qualitative and should be accompanied by a detailed definition of the behavioral domain of interest and by a clear specification of the sampling methods used. These judgments can be quantified by having judges rate the appropriateness of each behavior sample or test item as a member of the domain and then calculating indices of inter-judge agreement (Tinsley and Weiss, 1975) on the ratings of each item.

Internal Consistency   Content validity can be indirectly evaluated through the degree to which the test shows high internal consistency reliability or homogeneity. A test is internally consistent if its items show relatively high interrelationships with each other and, thus, with total test score (see Chapter 2 of this text or Ghiselli, 1964). A high internal consistency reliability coefficient indicates that each of the items reflects the same behavioral domain as is implied by the total test score. What is still lacking, however, is the demonstration that the total score reflects the domain as a whole. For example, it would be possible to construct a highly internally consistent test of "mathematics achievement" that was composed only of addition items. All of the items could be highly related to total score, but this total score would certainly not have great generalizability to the domain of mathematics achievement and would not have content validity relative to that domain.

Thus, high internal consistency reveals that all of the items measure the same variable. It provides some evidence that a single domain of content is being sampled. But it remains for other methods, notably construct validation procedures, to establish that this single domain of behavior represents the intended construct faithfully and completely.

Factor Analysis Factor analysis (Harman, 1967; Rummel, 1970; Weiss, 1970, 1971) is a method that can also provide some evidence supporting the content validity of a measuring instrument. The results of a factor analysis of the intercorrelations of test items yield information about how many dimensions or traits are needed to summarize or explain test performance. If a test is constructed to measure one trait and if items are sampled only from behaviors reflecting that trait, a factor analysis yielding a single large "general" factor is evidence that test performance can be explained in terms of that one trait. On the other hand, if the factor analysis yields several factors, the conclusion must be that the test measures more than one trait. Conversely, factor analysis of the items of a test designed to measure several variables (e.g., anxiety, dependence, sociability) should result in factors identifiable as these variables, if the test is to have demonstrated content validity. Again, however, it remains for other validation methods to establish that the factors obtained are accurate and complete representations of the relevant constructs.

Summary Content validation is an essential first step in the establishment of construct validity; to interpret and to attribute psychological meaning to test scores requires knowledge of what behavioral domain the test items reflect. It is perhaps more straightforward to evaluate content validity in achievement tests because the domain consists of stated instructional goals within a defined body of content or knowledge. However, cognizance of the content validity of nonachievement constructs is valuable because it forces careful definition of the behaviors relevant to that construct. Furthermore, the content validity focus requires a specification of the means by which a sampling of those behaviors will permit generalizations or conclusions about some broad explanatory construct or charac-
‣teristic of behavior.

Evidence regarding internal consistency reliability or the factor composition of a measure is important in indicating the extent to which the test items are all samples from the same domain of items or behaviors.

Lack of internal consistency, or a multifactor structure in an instrument assumed to measure a single variable, indicates that something besides the behavioral content of interest influences performance or test score. Regarding internal consistency, factors such as poorly standardized testing conditions, errors in scoring, response sets (e.g., acquiescence or social desirability), or fatigue or sickness of the person being measured may all act to reduce the reliability of the test. And just as they reduce reliability, these factors are also unrelated to the content aims and reduce the content validity of the test. When the factorial evidence is inconsistent with test construction goals of unidimensionality, it may result from poor test construction procedures that placed insufficient weight on the dimensionality of the instrument.

Internal consistency reliability and content validity are really the same thing if it is assumed that test score is an adequate representation of "domain" score. Items that correlate highly with each other and with domain score contribute to high internal consistency reliability and also allow the inference that the items are appropriate samples of domain behavior, thus leading to content validity.

Criterion-related Validity

Criterion-related validity usually refers to the extent to which a measure of a trait demonstrates an association with some independent or external measure of the same trait. This external measure, called the criterion, represents the behavior one is actually interested in, and test scores or other measurements are used to *predict* status or performance on the criterion. For example, scholastic aptitude tests are used to predict success in completing a college curriculum. Success in college is the behavior of interest, and the magnitude of the correlation between test scores and success is an important index of the applied usefulness of the test.

There are two kinds of criterion-related validity. *Predictive* validity is studied when the criterion is measured some time after scores are obtained on the predictor. How present status on the test predicts future status on the criterion variable is of primary interest here. Thus, the correlation between the aptitude test scores of high school seniors and their grades as college juniors would be a predictive validity coefficient.

Concurrent validity is studied when both the predictor and the criterion scores are obtained at the same time. The relationship between present status on the test and present status on the criterion is of primary interest here. The observed relationship between scores on scales of the Minnesota Multiphasic Personality Inventory and present psychiatric status would be concurrent validity data. Similarly, correlations between ability test scores and present performance in school or on the job are examples of concurrent validity coefficients.

In a broader sense, criterion-related validity refers to the direction and extent of the observed relationships between a measure of a trait and other measures or variables that may or may not reflect the same trait. It is in this sense that criterion-related validity may be seen as an integral step in the establishment of the construct validity of a trait measure. Part of the process of establishing the construct validity of a measuring instrument involves showing that scores on the instrument relate to the behaviors it is intended to measure. School performance was originally considered an observable index of the intelligence of children, and it was necessary to show that a test of intelligence correlated with or predicted school performance. Similarly, it should be shown that self-report measures of the traits of anxiety or extroversion are related to other indices of these traits, such as ratings by psychologists or peers.

In addition, however, in the process of elaborating the theory of a construct or trait, hypotheses are made about the variables or traits that should show *no* relationship to scores on a given measuring instrument. For example, in elaborating the theory of the construct of anxiety, it may be hypothesized that it should be independent of measured intelligence because there is no reason to expect that more anxious people should be more intelligent or less so. While intelligence is certainly not a "criterion" of anxiety, a demonstration that measured anxiety does not predict intelligence is consistent with a criterion-related validity approach.

Thus, two kinds of evidence are necessary for the demonstration of criterion-related validity. First, there should be a high relationship shown between a measured variable and other measured variables which that variable ought to predict (i.e., a criterion), and second, to ensure that the measuring instrument does not measure other variables that it ought not to predict, scores on the test should not be related to variables that are not appropriate criteria. Since these potential relationships are best determined by appropriate theory, criterion-related validity becomes a special way of investigating the construct validity of a measuring instrument.

Evidence Supporting Criterion-related Validity The basic kind of evidence in support of criterion-related validity is that of a relationship or an association between two variables. The two variables are the predictor (the operational definition of a central construct) and the criterion (the operational definition of another construct of theoretical or practical interest). The nature and magnitude of the relationship between the two variables is specified in the theory of the central construct.

The idea of a relationship between two variables implies a variety of statistical procedures designed to describe the relationship or association. It is generally suggested (Cronbach and Meehl, 1955; Dunnette, 1966), however, that two different types of statistical data are relevant to establishing criterion-related validity. These include data on mean differences between groups and correlational data. While these two general classes of statistical methods do yield data relevant to criterion-related validity, the distinction between them is artificial. Both mean differences data and correlational data can be construed as measures of relationship or association. Both methods of analysis, then, are consistent with the contention that criterion-related validity is a special case of evidence for demonstrating construct validity. Criterion-related validity investigates a restricted range of hypotheses of association as specified by the theory of the construct being measured.

Score Differences among Groups   One way of establishing criterion-related validity involves the extent to which the test or measuring instrument can differentiate groups of people. In applied situations, one may wish to use test scores to predict success or failure in a job or training program, to separate psychotics from neurotics, or to predict membership in a particular occupation. Or, the hypotheses about the nature of a construct may suggest that different groups of people should perform differently on measures of that construct. For example, an instrument constructed to measure extroversion might be expected to yield higher extroversion scores for a group of successful salesmen than for a group of successful research scientists. In thinking of score differences among groups as an indicator of association it is important to note that there are two variables involved in each of the above situations: test scores and group membership.

It is useful to express the relationship of the predictor measure to group membership by calculating the mean predictor score obtained by people in each group or category. The direction and significance of the difference between these mean scores can provide evidence of criterion-related validity. Thus, if people successful in a job have higher average scores on a test meant to predict job success than do people judged unsuccessful on that job, there is some evidence for the criterion-related validity of the test.

Figure 1 presents hypothetical data on the mean test score differences between groups of successful and unsuccessful employees; three possible results from the analysis of group differences in test scores are shown. In these figures, "S" indicates the successful group and "U" indicates the unsuccessful group; scores on the vertical axis are test scores. The plotted

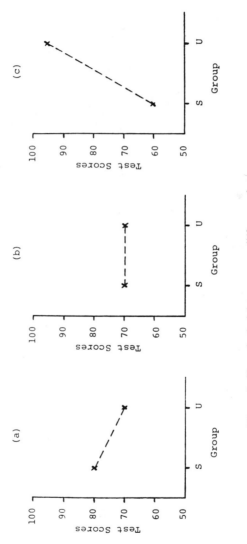

Figure 1. Hypothetical data on mean differences between groups.

points (X) are group mean or average scores. Figure 1a illustrates a case where the "S" group has a higher mean test score (80) than the "U" group (70). If the test score measured a variable hypothesized to be related to success in this fashion, these data might be taken as positive evidence for criterion-related validity.

In Figure 1b, both the successful and unsuccessful groups obtain the same average score of 70. There is, in these data, no association between group classification and test score. The lack of association is reflected by the horizontal line connecting the means of the two groups. Figure 1c shows data where the unsuccessful group obtains a higher mean score on the test (95) than the successful group (60). Because the line joining the two means is not horizontal, there is an association between the two variables (group membership and test score), but whether these data represent validity data depends on the nature of the trait and its nomological net. If the test score represents number of errors made in a clerical test, for example, and the groups are successful and unsuccessful clerks, the data in Figure 1c would be taken as evidence for criterion-related validity. On the other hand, if the test scores are number of words typed accurately in a typing test, the data would be contrary to the hypothesized relationship and would not be evidence for criterion-related validity.

Thus, criterion-related validity does not rest solely on the demonstration of group differences or association. Rather, the data must be in support of an hypothesis derived from the nomological net of the trait being measured.

In addition to meeting the criteria of theoretical relevance, criterion-related validity data must also satisfy the criteria of statistical significance and practical utility. The demonstration of statistical significance involves showing that the observed mean difference between two groups is not likely the result of chance factors. Thus, in Figure 1a, under certain circumstances it is possible that the 10-point difference in group means (80 − 70) could easily have arisen by chance. It could then be concluded that the difference is not important or, in the language of inferential statistics, it is not "statistically significant." On the other hand, a 10-point difference might be very unlikely to occur solely by chance. If this is true, the difference is probably the result of nonchance factors and is labeled "statistically significant." The search for "statistically significant" results is, therefore, one of determining whether the observed mean difference is likely the result of chance factors or whether it represents a real difference between the groups. The methodology of inferential statistics, or how to determine whether the obtained mean differences are statistically significant, is adequately described in a variety of psychological statistics books (Guilford, 1965; Hays, 1963; McNemar, 1969).

However, even a statistically significant difference between the mean scores of different groups on a test is not always a good indication of how useful the test is in a practical situation; with sufficiently large numbers of people in the groups, a practically unimportant difference between the groups can reach statistical significance. To get an idea of the practical usefulness of the test for making predictions about success based on test scores, it is useful to look at the distributions of scores obtained by the groups. Figure 2 shows two hypothetical situations in which there is an equal difference between the mean scores of the "successful" and "unsuccessful" groups; in both cases, the successful group obtains a mean score of 70, while the unsuccessful group scores 50 on the average.

The shaded portion of Figure 2 indicates the area of the score distributions in which scores of one group are the same as scores of the other group. In Figure 2a, the area of overlap is between scores of 50 and 70; thus, a person obtaining a score within this range could be a member of either the successful or the unsuccessful group. For people obtaining a score of 60, half were from the successful group and half were from the unsuccessful group. As the score approaches 70, more of the testees are members of the successful group. Conversely, scores below 60 are more likely to come from members of the unsuccessful group. Scores above 70 are earned only by members of the successful group, while scores below 50 are characteristic only of the unsuccessful. Thus, in Figure 2a overlap in group scores occurs only between the two means. Within this overlap range, the classification into group membership on the basis of a given test score is not as clear as for scores outside of this range.

In Figure 2b the mean difference between the two groups is the same as in Figure 2a. However, because of characteristics of the two distributions, the area of overlap is considerably different. The successful group obtains scores that range from 60 to 90; scores for the unsuccessful group range from 30 to 90. An unamibguous prediction of "unsuccessful" can be made for those with scores between 20 and 60. It is impossible, however, to make an unambiguous prediction of "successful" because there is complete overlap of the "successful" distribution on the "unsuccessful" distribution. In the score range of 60 to 90, which included all of the "successful" testees, there are also many "unsuccessful" testees. Thus, there is considerably more overlap between the distributions of Figure 2b than those of 2a, even though the mean differences are the same.

It is evident that the first predictor does a better job of separating the groups. With the second predictor, although there is the same mean

(a)

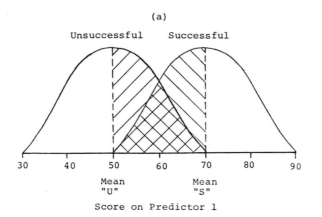

Score on Predictor 1

(b)

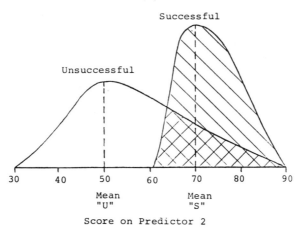

Score on Predictor 2

Figure 2. Hypothetical distributions of scores for two groups on two predictors.

difference, the relationship is not all that clear; some people who failed obtained predictor scores as high as anyone who succeeded. The practical use of these two sets of data will differ according to the nature of the specific applied situation in which they are to be used.

According to Dunnette (1966), if the percentage overlap between the distributions of scores obtained by two different groups, calculated by Tilton's (1937) formula, is greater than 75 percent, the test is not very useful for classification. If the overlap is less than 45 to 50 percent, it suggests that the test can be used as an accurate classificatory device. As an example of the use of Tilton's overlap statistic, most vocational interest scoring keys (such as those of the Strong Vocational Interest Blank) show overlaps of about 35 percent when people in given occupations are compared to people in general (Dunnette, 1966).

Thus, when a difference in the means of two (or more) groups has been found to be statistically significant, it becomes relevant to determine the practical significance of the difference as well. In the case of mean differences, this can be accomplished by an examination of the overlap in the group score distributions or by use of a summary index of overlap, such as Tilton's (1937), to determine the utility of the mean difference for making classifications of group membership based on test scores.

Correlational Data   Correlational data are the other general type of statistical data used to investigate criterion-related validity. Correlations are designed to be indices of relationship or association. The logic of correlation, however, can derive from that of mean differences, as illustrated in Figure 1. As shown there, an association between two variables (group membership and test scores) exists when the means of two groups can be connected by a nonhorizontal line. When the two group means are the same, a horizontal line connects them, indicating that there is no association or relationship between group membership and test scores.

When there are only two categories or groups, such as successful-unsuccessful, the criterion variable is said to be dichotomous. The extent of relationship between test scores and a dichotomous criterion can be summarized by the point-biserial correlation coefficient. The point-biserial can be computed from the data on the mean differences between the two groups or from a product-moment correlation formula (McNemar, 1969). The results of the two formulas are the same, indicating that data on group mean differences can be expressed in terms of a correlation, an index of association, or a relationship. A positive point-biserial correlation would reflect the mean difference shown in Figure 1a. The data in Figure 1c would result in a negative correlation. And, because the means of the two groups in Figure 1b are the same, the point-biserial correlation would be zero, indicating no relationship between group membership and test scores. The values of the point-biserial correlation reflect both the mean difference between the groups and the amount of overlap; a relatively high point-biserial correlation would correspond to greater mean differences and less overlap of the distributions. A point-biserial correlation can vary from +1.0 to −1.0.

The biserial correlation is a measure of relationship much like the point-biserial. It is used when one variable is continuously distributed and the other is dichotomized, or artifically dichotomous. For example, if a distribution of continuous criterion scores (such as scores on a test of job knowledge) were arbitrarily divided at some point and if the top half were designated "successful" and the bottom half "unsuccessful," the biserial correlation would be the appropriate statistic to express the relationship between a set of continuous predictor scores and the dichotomized criterion variable of "successful" versus "unsuccessful" group membership. The biserial is not a product-moment correlation coefficient and, therefore, its interpretation is slightly different from that of many correlation indices. Furthermore, its values tend to be higher than those obtained with the point-biserial and in some cases may exceed ±1.0.

The Pearson product-moment correlation coefficient (r) is the most frequently used index of association. The use of r presumes the existence of two continuous variables. Thus, in contrast to the earlier examples, where one variable was group membership, r assumes that both variables are scores on some kind of measuring instrument or continuous variable. For example, r might be computed to predict from a test score to a measured criterion of success on a job. This criterion could be the degree of job success as indicated by the test of job knowledge mentioned above (but without dividing the score distribution into "successful" and "unsuccessful" groups). Or job success might be measured by a rating scale on which a supervisor of a group of employees rates each employee according to his/her degree of success. Assuming a five-point rating scale, these data might be depicted as in Figure 3.

In Figure 3, the "very successful" group (rated one) had an average test score of 25, while the "very successful" group (rated five) had a mean test score of 65. Connecting the means for the five groups results in an approximately straight line. When the means of a large number of such groups (e.g., for each raw score point on a rating scale with many values) fall on an approximately straight line, it is appropriate to summarize the relationship between the two variables by computing the Pearson product-moment correlation coefficient. Just as the point-biserial correlation summarizes the relationship between group membership on a two-category variable and a continuous variable, r summarizes the degree and direction of relationship between one continuous (i.e., multicategory) variable and another continuous variable.

A positive correlation indicates that higher scores on one variable tend to be associated with higher scores on the other. An r of zero indicates that there is no association between the two variables. In the case of a zero product-moment correlation, just as in the biserial correlation, a straight line drawn to fit the means on one of the variables based on levels of the other will be horizontal. However, when the means themselves do not

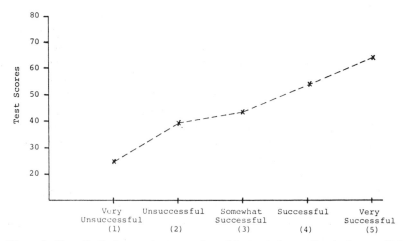

Figure 3. Hypothetical mean test scores for subjects rated according to degree of job success.

approximate a straight line, the Pearson product-moment correlation coefficient will not accurately reflect the relationship that does exist. In this case it is necessary to use the general case of that coefficient, called the eta coefficient or the correlation ratio (Hays, 1963; McNemar, 1969), which indicates the amount of relationship between two variables regardless of whether or not the means fall on a straight line.

It is important to note that correlation (or the related case of mean differences) does not imply causation. Correlation indicates association between two variables; it means that the variables vary together. To demonstrate that one variable *causes* another requires an experimental design in which one variable is systematically manipulated while the other is free to vary. If the second variable can be shown to be experimentally dependent upon the other variable and if it can be shown that there are no other variables that account for this observed dependency, causation might be inferred. Correlational data, however, do not demonstrate experimental dependence and cannot, therefore, be interpreted in a causal framework.

Since correlational data and mean differences data are closely related, correlations between variables must also meet the tests of statistical significance and practical utility. Correlations based on very small samples tend to be considerably higher than they would be if sample sizes were larger. Thus, small sample results can lead to a false conclusion that there is a high relationship between two variables. It is necessary, therefore, for computed correlations to be tested for statistical significance (Guilford, 1965; Hays, 1963; McNemar, 1969), to determine if they are substantially different from zero. On the other hand, very large sample sizes will result in very small correlations that are statistically different from zero. Thus, correlational results must be examined for practical utility.

In addition to providing a summary index of relationship, correlation coefficients permit the researcher to predict from one variable to the other. Such prediction involves estimation of an individual's probable score on one variable given his observed score on the other. For example, if the correlations were known between clerical test score and job performance, the probable job performance level of a new employee can be estimated from knowledge of his/her clerical ability test score. Predictions of this type involve the use of a two-variable regression equation to obtain a predicted score on the criterion variable from a testee's predictor score. Once the predicted score is obtained, the psychologist can obtain an estimate of the amount of error in that prediction for a given practical application by examining the distribution of actual criterion scores around the predicted criterion score. That distribution can be summarized by a quantity called the standard error of estimate. This quantity gives an estimate of the reduction in errors of prediction from knowledge of the correlation between the two variables in comparison to predictions that would be made if the correlation were not known (Hays, 1963). This information can be used to determine the utility of an observed correlation for making predictions about individual persons.

The demonstration of criterion-related validity is not based solely on significant mean differences or significant correlations. Virtually any statistical method of investigating an hypothesis of relationship can be used in the investigation of construct validity. These include, but are not limited to, chi-square analysis (Glass and Stanley, 1970; Siegel, 1956), other methods of computing correlations (McNemar, 1969), the powerful techniques of experimental design (Winer, 1971), and a variety of methods for the analysis of multivariate data (Weiss, in press).

Some Special Problems in Criterion-related Validity

Multiple Variables Criterion variables to be predicted in applied validity studies are frequently complex, or multiple, variables. For example, job performance is frequently predicted from ability tests. But, because of the variety of factors that go into successful performance on a job, adequate validation of predictor tests requires the use of multiple predictor variables to predict a single criterion.

There are a variety of ways of combining data from several test scores in making a single prediction (Weiss, in press). The most common of these combinations, used when the predictors and the criterion are all continuous variables, is multiple correlation or multiple regression. Predictor scores are first weighted according to how well each one predicts the criterion and then are summed to obtain a predicted criterion score. This predicted criterion score is a weighted sum of the predictor scores and can be expressed by the formula $\hat{y} = \beta_1 x_1 + \beta_2 x_2 + \cdots + \beta_n x_n$. In this formula the βs (called beta weights) are the weights attached to each predictor, x, and $\hat{y}$ is the predicted criterion score, or "variate." A variate can be defined as an artificial score constructed from some combination (in this case, a weighted sum) of two or more other scores. The multiple correlation coefficient, R, is the Pearson product-moment correlation between the variate, $\hat{y}$, and the actually obtained criterion scores. The weights (βs) for each predictor variable are determined mathematically in such a way as to maximize the multiple correlation coefficient, R.

The multiple correlation coefficient, derived from the multiple regression equation, describes the relationship between the single criterion variable (e.g., job performance) and a set of predictor variables (e.g., an ability test battery). The magnitude of this correlation and the magnitudes of the beta weights for specific predictor variables can contribute to an interpretation of the criterion-related validity of specific predictors.

Cross-validation   Regression equations are developed within a group where both predictor scores and criterion scores are known, but they are used in groups where only the predictor score is known. That is, if the criterion score for a given subject is already known there is no need to predict it. Regression equations are influenced by sample-specific characteristics of the development group. That is, the correlation between the observed and predicted scores is higher than it should be because of factors unique to a given sample of persons. Consequently, it is always important to make sure that the regression or prediction equation will yield a similar correlation between predicted and actual criterion scores in other groups of persons. This is done by using a procedure called cross-validation, which involves applying the regression equation derived from one group of subjects to the predictor scores of another group. If the predicted criterion scores obtained in this way show a similar degree of relationship to the actual criterion scores of persons in the new group, then there is some assurance that the equation will have more general predictive usefulness. The correlation between the predicted criterion (or variate) scores obtained in this way and the new group's actual criterion scores is called the cross-validated multiple correlation coefficient. This cross-validated correlation gives a more realistic estimate of the degree of relationship between the predictors and the criterion because the inflation resulting from sample-specific error has been eliminated.

Moderator Variables   Another important problem in the demonstration of criterion-related validity results from the fact that some groups or types of people are more or less "predictable" than are other groups. That is, the predictive validity of a test or battery of tests may differ depending on the composition of the group from which the validity coefficient is obtained. For example, Seashore (1961) summarized data showing that the school grades of women in both high school and college are more predictable than are those of men; there is a higher correlation between scholastic aptitude and scholastic achievement in groups of women. Grooms and Endler (1960) found that the grades of anxious college students were more predictable ($r = 0.63$) from aptitude and achievement test data than were those of nonanxious students ($r = 0.19$).

Any variable, such as sex or anxiety, that is not related to the predictor or to the criterion (e.g., both sexes perform equally well on both the predictor and the criterion) but that does influence the degree of relationship between the predictor and the criterion can be called a moderator variable. Moderator variables seem to work by dividing a group of persons into subgroups who are more alike or homogeneous in some characteristic that affects the predictor-criterion relationship.

The discovery of moderator variables is important for several reasons. First, knowing how well a prediction can be made for a person may influence the types of decisions that are made about him or her. Second, if it is known that the prediction for some person is less likely to be accurate, one may wish to gather other types of information about him. Furthermore, it may be found that one test is optimally predictive for one group but that a different test is optimally predictive of the same criterion for others. The efficiency and accuracy of using test scores in prediction can thus be maximized by making use of this information. Finally, the types of moderator variables that are found have implications for the theoretical network of the constructs involved. Certainly, the higher predictability of anxious students suggests something about the construct of an aptitude and its relationship to performance on relevant criteria.

A number of ways have been proposed for discovering which variables are moderators of a given predictor-criterion relationship. One way to discover moderator variables is to examine the composition of the sample or population of interest and hypothesize whether or not there are individual difference variables that might be related to differential predictability among individuals. Sex is an obvious candidate for a moderator variable. But the theory of the construct may suggest others, such as anxiety level, abilities, age, or education. After subgrouping the total sample according to status on the hypothesized moderator variable, separate validity coefficients are calculated for each group. The significance of the difference between the resulting subgroup coefficients indicates the usefulness of the moderator.

Moderator variables can also be found empirically by examining those variables that differentiate persons whose actual criterion scores were close to their predicted criterion scores from those whose actual scores were further from those predicted for them. However, moderator variables found in this way capitalize on sample-specific characteristics and thus need to be cross-validated before they can be assumed to have more general predictive usefulness. In this case, cross-validation involves determining whether or not the moderator variable results in differential predictability in another similar sample.

More information concerning various approaches to discovering and using moderator variables is contained in a recent review of the topic by Zedeck (1971).

Face Validity

Face validity concerns the extent to which the instrument appears to or "looks like" it measures what it is intended to measure. Probably the major reason for having a test with face validity is to ensure that it is acceptable to potential users and test takers. For example, if a test used to predict job performance has no obvious relationship to the job itself, personnel departments may be less likely to use it, and job applicants may see the test as irrelevant and/or unfair.

Face validity is not the same thing as content validity, even though there is some similarity in their definitions. Face validity concerns judgments about a test *after* it has been constructed. Content validity, on the other hand, is the concern *while* the test is being constructed that the test's items are a reflection or an adequate sampling of a defined domain of content thought to bear a relationship to the trait being measured. Some tests may have content validity but not face validity if the relationship of item content to the underlying trait is subtle or indirect.

Face validity is also irrelevant to criterion-related validity, in which empirical relationships are the important factor. Thus, there are instances in which a test looks like it should correlate with a criterion but it does not, and there are instances of instruments that bear no obvious relationship to a criterion but actually correlate well with it. Face validity might be helpful in formulating hypotheses about instruments that might predict a certain criterion, such as a test of job performance that actually included elements of the job. But these hypotheses will be useful only if the test-criterion relationships are actually observed.

Because the construct validity of a measuring instrument is based on the evaluation of all the empirical data available on an instrument, face validity also has no relationship to construct validity. Consequently, face validity is not an appropriate kind of evidence for the evaluation of the validity of a measuring instrument. An instrument is not valid simply because it appears to be valid. Face validity is relevent to a test only as it establishes "rapport" between test taker and test administrator or ensures that the test will be used; it has no other influence in determining the validity of a measuring instrument.

VALIDITY OF MEASUREMENT AND PRACTICAL VALIDITY

Establishing the validity of psychological tests is essential to ensure their usefulness in applied situations and to contribute to the theoretical understanding of the important variables or constructs underlying the behavior of individual persons. The issues and methods relevant to these two overall aims are somewhat different and, in some cases, contradictory.

Validity Evidence in Applied Situations

The major requirement for the usefulness of psychological tests in applied situations is the demonstration of their ability to predict to some criterion measure or to predict membership in a defined group of people. In this situation, there is no necessary requirement that the test bear a common sense relationship to that which it predicts, nor that there be a solid basis for interpreting the meaning of the test scores. In practical applications, the test does not need to measure anything but only to *predict* something.

But practical criterion-related validity coefficients tend to lack generalizability across situations. A lack of a logical, common sense or theory-based rationale for the obtained predictor-criterion relationship may lead to relationships that are based on characteristics or factors quite specific to the group involved. That is, finding that test X predicts job success in company Y does not necessarily mean that it will predict success in the same job in company Z. Each predictor must be validated in that situation and with that group of people with whom it is to be used. Thus, constructing tests to predict specific criteria without regard to considerations of the test's meaning or interpretability tends to be a somewhat wasteful and inefficient endeavor.

The Utility of Psychological Tests Cronbach and Gleser (1965) stress that the applied usefulness of a psychological test depends not on the absolute size of the criterion-related validity coefficient but rather on the test's ability to aid in making correct decisions concerning the selection or placement of persons. The utility of a test refers to its overall usefulness in decision-making. This approach requires cognizance of the accuracy and importance of the decisions made. It also requires consideration of the costs involved both in constructing and in using the test and of the effects of erroneous decisions.

According to Cronbach and Gleser (1965), in the use of the typical criterion-related validity coefficient all errors of prediction are considered equal. For example, the error of underestimating the performance of one person is weighted equally with the error of overestimating the performance of another. With the concept of utility, however, some errors may be evaluated as more serious (i.e., costly) than others. And a test that leads to more errors, but errors of a less serious nature, may be considered to have higher utility than a test that leads to fewer, but more costly, errors in decision-making.

Another factor influencing the utility of a psychological measure concerns its "incremental validity," a term introduced by Sechrest (1963). Incremental validity concerns the extent to which the test improves upon the accuracy of decision-making that is possible using already available and perhaps less expensive methods. For example, constructing a test to have a predictive validity of r = 0.90 will not have much utility if some already available measure does nearly as good a job in prediction. On the other hand, even a test with a low predictive validity may have utility if there are no other bases upon which to make the necessary decision.

The importance of decision-making also leads to the use of data concerning mean score differences between groups and the overlap of their distributions, rather than on computation of simple correlation coefficients. This is so because much decision-making involves an accept-reject decision, and the extent to which a test can differentiate "successes" from "failures" is directly expressed by the overlap of their test score distributions.

Other factors that must be taken into account in evaluating the utility of a test in a particular situation are the base rates and the selection ratio. Base rates (Meehl and Rosen, 1955) are the expected a priori proportions of people who will fall into a given classification (i.e., success or failure on a job). The selection ratio, on the other hand, is the proportion of available applicants that must be selected to fulfill the needs of a given organization. Further variables and details involved in the evaluation of the utility of psychological tests may be found in Cronbach and Gleser (1965). Their discussion emphasizes the need to consider a broad base of information in the evaluation of the applied usefulness of psychological tests.

Validity of Trait Measurement

The scientific aims of psychology, as opposed to its practical applications, indicate the necessity for adequate psychological theories and theory-based research. The existence of appropriate theory leads to the measurement of constructs and the understanding of behavior in terms of these broad explanatory constructs. Not only do the procedures of construct validation lead to a better understanding and basis of interpretation of a measurement itself, but they help to elucidate the nature and action of the important constructs of behavior. Following the rationale of construct validation, tests that have been shown to reflect meaningful psychological variables will be more generalizable to a variety of applied predictive needs. For example, a theoretical network describing the factors relevant to success or status on any particular criterion variable should make it possible to select those tests or predictors that, through construct validation procedures, have been shown to reflect precisely those factors. A construct-oriented approach to the selection of valid predictor instruments should be more efficient than an approach that is based on a trial-and-error search to identify those predictors that predict a criterion in a given applied situation.

SUMMARY

The approach taken in this chapter stresses the overriding importance of theory-based measurement and construct validation procedures. If a measuring instrument is constructed to measure some important psychological variable rather than just to predict a specific criterion, both its scientific and practical usefulness should be greatly enhanced.

REFERENCES

American Psychological Association. 1974. Standards for Educational and Psychological Tests. American Psychological Association, Washington, D.C.

Cronbach, L. J., and G. Gleser. 1965. Psychological Tests and Personnel Decisions. University of Illinois Press, Urbana.

Cronbach, L. J., and P. E. Meehl. 1955. Construct validity in psychological tests. Psych. Bull. 52:281–302.

Dunnette, M. D. 1966. Personnel Selection and Placement. Brooks/Cole, Belmont, Calif.

Ghiselli, E. E. 1964. Theory of Psychological Measurement. McGraw-Hill, New York.

Glass, G. V., and J. C. Stanley. 1970. Statistical Methods in Education and Psychology. Prentice-Hall, Englewood Cliffs, N.J.

Grooms, R. R., and N. S. Endler. 1960. The effect of anxiety on academic achievement. J. Ed. Psych. 51:299–304.

Guilford, J. P. 1965. Fundamental Statistics in Psychology and Education. 4th Ed. McGraw-Hill, New York.

Harman, H. H. 1967. Modern Factor Analysis. Rev. Ed. University of Chicago Press, Chicago.

Hays, W. 1963. Statistics for Psychologists. Holt, Rinehart and Winston, New York.

McNemar, Q. 1969. Psychological Statistics. 4th Ed. Wiley, New York.

Meehl, P. E., and A. Rosen. 1955. Antecedent probability and the efficiency of psychometric signs, patterns, or cutting scores. Psych. Bull. 52:194–216.

Rummel, R. J. 1970. Applied Factor Analysis. Northwestern University Press, Evanston, Ill.

Seashore, H. G. 1961. Women are more predictable than men. Presidential address, Division 17, American Psychological Association Annual Convention, September, New York.

Sechrest, L. 1963. Incremental validity. Ed. Psych. Meas. 23:153–158.

Siegel, S. 1956. Nonparametric Statistics for the Behavioral Sciences. McGraw-Hill, New York.

Tilton, J. W. 1937. The measurement of overlapping. J. Ed. Psych. 28:656–662.

Tinsley, H. E. A., and D. J. Weiss. 1975. Interrater reliability and agreement of subjective judgments. J. Counsel. Psych. 22:358–376.

Weiss, D. J. 1970. Factor analysis and counseling research. J. Counsel. Psych. 17:477–485.

Weiss, D. J. 1971. Further considerations in applications of factor analysis. J. Counsel. Psych. 18:85–92.

Weiss, D. J. Multivariate procedures. In M. D. Dunnette (ed.), Handbook of Industrial and Organizational Psychology. Rand McNally, New York. (In press.)

Winer, B. J. 1971. Statistical Principles in Experimental Design. 2nd Ed. McGraw-Hill, New York.

Zedeck, S. 1971. Problems with the use of "moderator" variables. Psych. Bull. 76:295–310.

II
REVIEW
OF INSTRUMENTS

4 | Intelligence Tests

GREGORY A. MILLER

There is no better way to introduce the subject of intelligence testing than to briefly review the history of its development. Considerable evidence exists showing that systematic evaluation procedures were utilized thousands of years before the birth of Christ. However, the measurement of basic mental faculties probably did not occur before the latter years of the nineteenth century, during which time a very important group of tests designed to measure intelligence were developed.

An early leader in this field was Sir Francis Galton, an English biologist, who applied the principles of variation and selection that had been set forth by Charles Darwin, his cousin, to the measurement of physical and mental traits. It was, however, Dr. James McKeen Cattell, an American, who introduced the term mental test in the late nineteenth century. The tests of Galton and Cattell were primarily measures of sensory discrimination processes, such as reaction time, perception of pitch, judgment of time intervals, judgment of weights, etc. The tests, however, turned out to be unrelated to one another and to any practical criteria of intellectual functioning or educational achievement.

While Cattell was conducting his work in America, Alfred Binet in France had been challenged by a practical problem in public education to develop methods for diagnosing below normal intelligence levels. He constructed scales of intelligence that have dominated the field ever since. The practical tests used today really owe their origin to Binet because he used a clinical approach and focused on developing tests as diagnostic tools.

From rudimentary beginnings nearly 100 years ago, tests have grown into big business in the United States, and millions of tests are administered annually. Americans may well be more analyzed and tested than any other people in the world. Perhaps tests would not have lasted as long as they have if it were not that, unlike most other assessment procedures, tests are open to review, re-evaluation, and constant scrutiny from the scientific community. In fact, it is this very objectivity that has enabled mental testing to make a significant contribution to the public welfare.

DEFINITIONS OF INTELLIGENCE

It is surprising that with this wide acceptance of tests and, more specifically, intelligence tests, no one seems to have a very clear idea of what intelligence is. A symposium was held more than 50 years ago at which prominent psychologists were asked to give their ideas regarding the nature of intelligence. They gave an amazing variety of answers, not one of which was very specific. Certainly a similar survey today would not reveal substantially different results.

Binet was obviously interested in the ability to learn, i.e., to success-fully perform school work. It was this ability that he was trying to detect with his early tests. It appears that most of the better known tests today attempt to get at this ability; hence, the term scholastic aptitude is often used interchangeably with mental ability, intelligence, and IQ in test titles. Most characterizations of intelligence by noted authorities include the ability to reason, to solve problems and to use "higher mental processes," to do original thinking, and to adapt to novel situations. All of these are included in the ability to "succeed" in school. As the vast majority of Americans are subjected to school, this may suffice as a definition of intelligence.

Some prominent psychologists who developed mental ability tests defined intelligence as follows: Binet (1916) regarded intelligence as pri-marily a "collection of faculties." i.e., practical sense, initiative, judgment, and the ability to adapt oneself to circumstances. Wechsler (1958) defined intelligence as the "aggregate or global capacity of the individual to act purposefully, to think rationally, and to deal effectively with his environ-ment." Terman (1916) defined it as the "ability to think in terms of abstract ideas." Goddard (1946) characterized intelligence as "the degree of availability of one's experiences for the solution of immediate problems and the anticipation of future ones."

This author feels that intelligence is a function of the total personal-ity. An understanding of intelligence cannot be achieved by analyzing it element by element. It is too intrinsically interrelated with emotional feelings, attitudes, moods, well-being, and experiences. It cannot live an independent life; it can only be defined and, of course, measured, as a functioning part of a unit called the person. Perhaps, with apologies to Robert Frost, intelligence can be said to be undefinable but unmistakable; we know it when we see it.

No final distinction between intelligence and aptitude has been made. These two terms are often used interchangeably, yet some authors do distinguish between them. There have been attempts to differentiate between the two, but difficulties arise when specific intelligence tests are considered. Perhaps the best solution is to follow the general nomenclature used by the authors of various tests. Lyman (1963) states that "for most purposes, intelligence tests may be thought of as tests of general aptitude or scholastic aptitude. When so regarded they are most typically used in predicting achievement in school, college, or training programs."

A thorough discussion of the above material may be found in a variety of texts and more recently in books by Dubois (1970), Edwards (1971, 1972), Jackson and Messick (1967), Lyman (1963), and Mehrens and Lehmann (1975).

USE OF INTELLIGENCE TESTS IN REHABILITATION COUNSELING

The rehabilitation counselor does not need to be trained in the administration of intelligence tests, but he should be familiar with the major tests in use, and especially with their strengths and deficiencies for various purposes. He must be able to read and to interpret psychological reports and to converse intelligently with the clinical psychologist with whom he contracts to evaluate his clients. Basic knowledge of the field is essential because intelligence test results come to the counselor from sources other than his own efforts or those purchased from a consultant. For example, intelligence test results may accompany material forwarded by a referral source such as an employment agency, a correctional facility, or a mental health center. Because rehabilitation counselors usually do not select the tests that are administered to their clients they must be able to specify the purpose for which the client is being tested. This should be sufficient guidance for most testing consultants.

The trained clinician who administers tests should be able to make judgments about the validity of scores with regard to the socio-economic background of the client, his handicaps, particular motivation, emotional state, and other variables in the testing process. These considerations are perhaps as important, if not more so, than the scores themselves. After all, in an individualized, standardized, psychological examination the clinician is given the opportunity to examine and to observe another person in a most unique and special way. Testing someone for clinical purposes is not simple measuring; rather, it is the observation of a person in action in an attempt to understand and to empathize with the ways in which his responses come about. The examiner is more than simply a machine, an automaton, who goes through the mechanics of administering a test. He presents the client with a variety of challenging situations to see how he copes with them. For example, when a client squirms in his chair and avoids color on a Rorschach card, or avoids responding to a particular vocabulary word on the WAIS, he provides important clinical data, some of which is reflected in test scores and some not. The scores that are used are an essential aid in identifying with greater precision some of the characteristics of a response. There are other aspects of a response that go unscored but should not go unnoticed or unused. Ideally, all of the qualitative features of a response should be included in the test protocol. The examiner should make an exact record of what transpires between himself and the client, including the client's verbatim responses to test items proper, some indication of the direction of the examiner's inquiries, and the client's attitudinal and emotional expressions, such as sighing, exclamations, manner, tone of voice, and so forth. Pauses are usually significant and should be noted with some identifying adjective, such as "thoughtful," "hesitant," "vague," "confused," "guarded," "reluctant."

The question of the relative weight to be placed upon "clinical" observations and formal scores in assembling a picture of a particular client's personality structure demands the constant consideration of the developing psychological examiner. With increasing experience, the examiner comes to appreciate more profoundly the wealth of clinical information contained in test responses. The rehabilitation counselor must demand this expertise from his psychological consultant.

DESCRIPTION OF SELECTED TESTS

From the approximately 120 mental ability tests listed in *The Seventh Mental Measurements Yearbook* (Buros, 1972) several individual and group tests were selected as most useful to the rehabilitation counselor in client planning. In addition to the *Yearbook,* there are several other sources of information about psychological tests: *Tests in Print II* (Buros, 1974) is a comprehensive bibliography of more than 2,500 tests; catalogs distributed by test publishers describe new and recently revised tests; and professional journals publish reviews of new tests.

The differences between individual and group intelligence tests are both obvious and important. While the test administrator has little actual interaction with examinees taking a group test, the individual test requires constant interaction between the examiner and the examinee. Because of the high amount of interaction, observation of test behavior can be accomplished that can not be done in a group test situation. Even though scores on individual and group tests correlate substantially, group tests remain their best at mid-range. In rehabilitation counseling decisions are often made with clients who scores fall outside the normal range, which suggests that individual tests should predominate in psychological examinations conducted for rehabilitation counselors.

Individual Tests

The most commonly used individual tests of mental ability are those in the Wechsler series, specifically, the Wechsler Adult Intelligence Scale (WAIS) and the Wechsler Intelligence Scale for Children—Revised (WISC-R).

The Wechsler Adult Intelligence Scale (WAIS) The WAIS was published in 1955 and is used with clients 16 years of age and older. It is generally regarded as the best single instrument available for the measurement of adult intelligence, and it requires approximately 45 minutes to administer under normal conditions. The WAIS and its predecessors have been used and studied so widely that an enormous body of literature has been accumulated (see Buros, 1972, for a lengthy but only partial list). But the interest here is in briefly discussing the reliability of the test and its validity for the prediction of on-the-job success.

As stated above, Wechsler (1958) defined intelligence as "the aggregate or global capacity of the individual to act purposefully, to think rationally, and to deal effectively with his environment." The WAIS is a test of general intelligence that provides three IQ scores (Verbal IQ, Performance IQ, and Full Scale IQ) from six verbal and five performance subtests. Counselors should not confuse the 11 subtests with factors or special aptitudes that add up to general intelligence. The subtests were devised to make the WAIS a clinical, diagnostic instrument. The original Wechsler studies were conducted on patient populations at the Bellevue Hospital in New York City. The accumulated evidence supports the WAIS as a sensitive measure of intellectual functioning, but it provides little support for the WAIS as a tool for differential diagnosis except as individual clinicians personally validate it for that purpose.

Assessment of reliability of the WAIS is a complex subject. Split-half reliability of the WAIS is high, and test-retest reliability over intervening periods of several weeks to several years is also high. Wechsler (1958) summarizes the reliability of the WAIS as follows: "A difference of five IQ points between retests will ordinarily include about 50% of the cases; a difference of ten points, 75% or more of the cases, and so on. In terms of prediction, the chances are one in two that a subject's IQ on retest will not differ by more than five points, one in four that it will not differ by more than ten points, and one in twenty that it will not differ by more than fifteen points."

Clinicians often do pattern analysis of WAIS subscales. In fact, the front page of the record form suggests it, even though a "disclaimer" is printed. A common practice is to note and interpret differences between Verbal and Performance IQ scores. Even though Verbal and Performance Scale IQs are highly correlated with each other, they are almost never in perfect agreement. One wonders then what magnitude of difference between Verbal and Performance scores is large enough to base a conclusion on it. Wechsler suggests that differences of 10 or more points will be found in less than 32 cases in 100; differences of 15 or more points in 13 cases in 100; and differences of 20 points or more only twice in 100. He also suggests that differences may be associated with normal factors such as educational and vocational history of client, present occupation, cultural, and possible racial differences. One study suggests that "acting out" youths characteristically have large elevations of performance scores over verbal scores. Since few studies support the interpretation of Verbal/Performance differences, and fewer yet provide clues about diagnostic significance, rehabilitation counselors probably should not attempt to interpret or to use such differences.

For the rehabilitation counselor the question is: "Can we use WAIS results to predict educational or vocational success?" The answer is a qualified "yes" to the question of educational success because low and moderate correlations with grades in high school and college have been reported. However, published works relating IQ scores to occupational success are very limited and uncertain. Super and Crites (1962) conclude that "the use of more than the total or verbal score as a rough index of the educational and occupational level which the person in question may attain is unwarranted, and for most persons, this can be done at least as well and more economically by means of paper-and-pencil tests."

The Wechsler Intelligence Scale for Children—Revised The Wechsler Intelligence Scale for Children—Revised (Wechsler, 1974) is mentioned primarily because it is a new test that has been available only since April of 1974 and is used with clients less than 17 years of age, which is one more year than its predecessor, the Wechsler Intelligence Scale for Children. Because some rehabilitation clients are in that age group and also because this is a new test with new norms, it is worthy of mention. The WISC-R consists of the same 12 tests that constituted the original 1949 WISC, with the exception of the modification or elimination of items felt by some test users to be ambiguous, obsolete, or unfair to particular groups of children.

Wechsler (1974) states that "at least half of the items from the other test, except Picture Arrangement, were retained intact or with slight modifications. Picture Arrangement was substantially altered." The changes in the standardization of the battery, such as the inclusion of a proportionally representative sample of non-whites taken from the 1970 U.S. census, make this a desirable test to use if the client is less than 17 years of age.

The Revised Stanford-Binet Intelligence Scale Form L-M The Revised Stanford-Binet Intelligence Scale Form L-M, 1960 Edition, is briefly mentioned here. While it is primarily a scale for children, for the few times that this test might be given in a rehabilitation setting, a careful note should be made to use the 1972 norms, which substantially lower IQs compared to the 1960 norms.

The Peabody Picture Vocabulary Test The Peabody Picture Vocabulary Test is an individual wide-range picture vocabulary test using a graduated series of 150 plates, each containing four pictures. It is advertised as being especially appropriate for speech impaired, cerebral palsied, withdrawn, distractable, mentally retarded, and remedial reading cases. Also, it only takes about 15 minutes to administer and to score, and it requires no verbal response.

The Wechsler Memory Scale The Wechsler Memory Scale may be used for the individual examination of adults with special defects, such as aphasia, senility, and organic brain damage, and it can be given in about 15 minutes. It may not properly be called an intelligence test, but it yields a Memory Quotient and is standardized on a group appropriate to the field of rehabilitation counseling.

Intelligence Test Modifications on Handicapped and Nonhandicapped Children Brief mention should be made of a recently issued final report, *Final Report: Intelligence Test Modifications on Handicapped and Nonhandicapped Children*[1] by Sattler (1972), which indicates some success in adequately modifying Binet and WISC (1949) items for handicapped children less than 15 years of age.

Group Tests

Selected group tests that can be administered either to a group of clients or to individual clients and are appropriate for rehabilitation fields are discussed below.

Otis Mental Ability Tests Otis mental ability tests have enjoyed wide-spread use at all levels of the educational system for the past 50 years. The Otis Group Intelligence Scale, published in 1918, was one of

---

[1]Copies of this report may be obtained from Dr. Sattler at San Diego State University, San Diego, California.

the first group tests of mental ability and the first to be used in American schools. During the 1920s various forms of the Otis Self-Administering Tests of Mental Ability were published. The third revision of the Otis test resulted in the preparation of the Otis Quick-Scoring Mental Ability Test published in the mid-1930s. The Otis-Lennon Mental Ability Test published in 1960 constitutes the fourth major revision in the Otis series. The Otis is a paper-and-pencil general intelligence test, which requires that the examinee be able to read reasonably well. It is considered an "omnibus" measure of intelligence that provides one global score. With 75 or 80 items, it is designed to cover the three areas basic to most general intelligence tests: verbal reasoning, arithmetic reasoning, and spatial relations. The items are arranged within the test in ascending order of difficulty. Forms are available for students of all grade levels and for adults. It can be given with either 20- or 30-minute time limits (40 minutes for the Otis-Lennon test). Counselors using Otis results should be sure to ascertain the form and time limit upon which a client's score is based.

The Otis is reviewed here because scores often are available from student's school records; it is a quick test that can be administered by a nonprofessional person, and it is inexpensive. It can also be used as a screening device for selecting training level. Of course, if local norms are established, its predictive efficiency might be much greater for particular jobs, plants, or industries.

The Army General Classification Test (AGCT) The next test to be discussed is the Army General Classification Test, First Civilian Edition (AGCT). Designed for persons with a tenth grade education, it measures general ability and aptitude for learning jobs. It is a revision of the World War II test given to all army inductees. The test takes about 1 hour to administer and requires a minimal level of reading ability. Although newer and longer (150 items), the AGCT is very similar to the Otis; that is, it is a one score test composed of items of increasing difficulty. It is used as an IQ measure by many correctional facilities. However, the deficiencies of the AGCT are greater than those of the Otis. It is based on the first of four forms developed in 1940 and 1941 for classifying draftees. The last two forms of the AGCT were administered to millions of service personnel of World War II. The first form, which was used relatively little, is referred to as the "civilian edition" by the publishers, suggesting that validity data applying to the later forms are equally applicable to the first form. The norms are based on a sample of young, mostly male, relatively physically and mentally normal subjects, which is not the typical description of most clients seen by the rehabilitation counselor. Also, many of the items are so out of date as to be distracting to the test taker, e.g., "cigarettes—two packs for a quarter," "milk—nine cents a quart." The AGCT results probably should not be used by rehabilitation counselors unless the client's AGCT score is high on the norm for a military specialty with rather direct transferability to a civilian occupation or if it merely lends support to conclusions based on other, more reliable data.

The Chicago Nonverbal Examination The Chicago Nonverbal Examination is designed specifically for children. However, it can be used with adults who are handicapped in the use of the English language, such as the deaf, clients with a reading difficulty, or clients who have been brought up in a foreign language environment. Pantomime directions are available; the test takes about 25 minutes to administer.

The Raven Progressive Matrices The Raven Progressive Matrices is a nonverbal test series constructed to aid in assessing intellectual ability by requiring the examinee to solve problems presented in abstract figures and designs. A revision titled the Coloured Progressive Matrices, in which the designs are presented in several colors, is designed for use with young children and with older persons who are mentally subnormal or impaired; it would be especially applicable with rehabilitation clients. Both tests take between 15 and 45 minutes to administer.

The Beta Examination The revised Beta Examination is a well known revision of the earlier World War I Army Beta test that provides a measure of mental ability without requiring the subject to read. Standardization permits securing a basic IQ that is similar in statistical meaning to the Wechsler IQ. It contains six subtests, takes 30 minutes to administer, and is standardized through age 59.

TEST INTERPRETATION

As Goldman (1971) points out, there are questions of fundamental concern both to clients and to society in general that cannot be dealt with through even the most sophisticated statistical approaches.[2] For a brief example, stop for a moment and think of the meanings that can be attached to the word "success" as applied to careers. The success issue is not a measurement question; rather, it is a question of values and one that the counselor must raise with each client he serves. To paraphrase Goldman, the statistical bases for interpretation offer hope mainly for the

---

[2] The author is indebted to the Iowa series, "Studies in Continuing Education for Rehabilitation Counselors (SCERC)" for much of the information on test interpretation. The complete Studies on tape or in manuscript form are available from the Materials Development Center, Department of Rehabilitation and Manpower Services, School of Education, University of Wisconsin—Stout, Menomonie, Wisconsin 54751.

future, and not for immediately usable methods. Instead of a well developed, statistically supported arsenal of tests, there is a collection of odds and ends. At this point, it is apparent that success, broadly defined, can be achieved in most occupations with a variety of abilities, behaviors, and other characteristics. Thus, the counselor should be aware of the severe limitations of the present imperfect data. As he always has, he must in large measure fall back upon a logical, inductive process in which a theory of the individual client is developed. From this model the counselor draws inferences about how the client will behave in yet untried situations, such as training or employment.

This inferential process is often referred to as a clinical process, in contrast to a statistical process. The counselor develops a dynamic model of his client through the collection of data inferences drawn from the data itself, further data, further inferences, and finally, hypotheses tested. In this process, the counselor is constantly seeking to fill out the model, or picture, of his client so that the data about the client assists him in more accurately predicting future behavior.

The counselor is cautioned when developing this individual model of the client to let it develop from the facts, the inferences from the facts, and the results of hypothesis testing about the facts, and not from some preconception or stereotype based on a rigid theory that does not allow for individual differences.

It has also been suggested that counselors, if they had time, might wish to use the same inductive process to build a model of the other side of the picture, the typical or perhaps ideal student of a particular training program, or ideal machinist, or perhaps, ideal machinist in a particular plant or firm. If such model building could, indeed, be accomplished, counselors then could seek to match individual clients with the typical or ideal models for particular companies, jobs, or educational programs.

Obviously, this method would be extremely time consuming and very tentative, but it should be tried. In fact, it is done, although not necessarily in a planned fashion. For example, whenever a plan is written for a client and supporting evidence is written into the plan, the counselor predicts client success and, perhaps, even satisfaction in a training program and/or an occupation. The prediction is based upon a whole series of steps in which the counselor collected data, drew inferences from it, sought support for his inferences by collecting more data, made further inferences, and finally, upon the basis of a pattern of such data-to-inferences-to-data-to-inferences steps, established some hypotheses about the client's future behavior. The plan is merely a formal promulgation of the counselor's hypotheses about his client. In another way, counselors often place in case records predictive statements and supporting evidence prior to the development of a rehabilitation plan. These may constitute the inferences that precede the establishment of hypotheses. So, the method is used; the point is to improve upon it.

It is especially important that the process be a conscious one. It should be expected to take time. In fact, it can only be accomplished where the counselor and client expect to have a number of interviews covering a period of months, at the least. It has been suggested that the tentative interpretations—the inferences that precede hypothesis development and testing—should be shared with clients as a safeguard against serious errors of logic on the part of the counselor.

Goldman (1971) suggests five ways of improving the effectiveness of the clinical interpretive methods. 1) The counselor must know his tests as a mechanic knows his tools. This includes specific knowledge of the dependability of scores, the types of valid applications, and the norms and what they mean in terms of the people with whom he deals. 2) If the counselor is to use tests and other data to build a model of his clients, the counselor must know a great deal about people, their personalities, and individual differences. 3) Successful use of the clinical process seems to require two major skills: creative skill in producing likely hypotheses, and an inclination toward scientific rigor and reasonable cautiousness. This latter skill is exemplified by a willingness to modify or to reject a hypothesis in the light of new data. 4) The counselor should be familiar with the educational and employment situations about which he is going to make inferences. Knowledge about such situations should be constantly sought and updated. The use of published resources, as well as personal contacts, field trips to factories, observation of people at work, etc., should be as natural to a counselor as eating. Finally, the clients themselves are often a reliable and interesting source of information about various occupations. 5) Perhaps most important of all, a counselor must study his own performance as an interpreter of tests and other data. He should constantly check himself for evidence of biases that blind him to alternative interpretations. Perhaps the counselor should first study his own values. Maybe the beginning point for such examination would be to set forth in rank order his own criteria of success; perhaps he should even try to attach weights to the various criteria. Then the counselor might study these carefully so that, when interacting with a client, he can constantly check himself to determine that he is not imposing his own values upon the client.

The counselor should be interested in his hit rate—the accuracy with which he is able to assist a client in predicting success. Rehabilitation counselors usually have no systematic method of getting client feedback that would help them to determine a client's success over a period of time. Lack of feedback is a major obstacle to further development of the counselor as a clinical interpreter.

The research on communicating test results is rather sparse. The major conclusion based upon the research is that different counselors probably achieve equal success using different methods. Thus, competent counselors using Method A of test interpretation get good results, while incompetent counselors using the same method get poor results and, if there is an approximate balance of competence and incompetence in the sample, the seeming outcome will be no advantage for Method A. Most of the published studies are open to criticism on the basis of lack of differentiation of counselor ability or preference for method.

However, some expert advice can be given on how to report test results effectively to clients. Super and Crites (1962) list five rules. 1) Give the client simple statistical predictions based on test data. For example, say "Eighty out of 100 students with scores like yours on this test succeed in drafting." 2) Allow the client to evaluate the prediction as it applies to himself. Pause for a long time if necessary in order to let the client react to the facts. 3) Remain neutral toward the test data and the client's reactions. Express no opinions, give no advice, listen warmly and respectfully; in short, provide acceptance, not agreement. 4) Facilitate the client's self-evaluation and subsequent decisions by recognizing and reflecting client feelings and attitudes. For example, say "You expected this but it is hard to take." Thus, the counselor facilitates the client's further exploration of feelings, releases related tensions, and permits the viewing of data and implications more objectively. 5) Avoid persuasive methods; do not impose artificial motivation upon the client.

Concerning the sequence of reporting test scores, there are good arguments in individual cases for presenting either interest or ability results before IQ results. The same is true of the choice between presentation of high or low scores first, if such there be. The type of scores used in reporting should also be considered. Although the standard score is statistically preferable, percentile scores seem to be more widely understood and more readily comprehensible and probably should be used in preference to all others. The counselor should keep in mind that differences between percentile scores represent varying differences in raw scores, depending upon where such differences occur in the distribution. There is no valid basis for interpreting client responses to individual test items unless the counselor suspects a mismarked answer sheet on a group test.

The counselor should encourage the client to relate test data to other information. The client should be assured that there are no unknown interests, that there is no real self to be revealed by tests that was unknown to the client. The client should openly attempt to relate his preferences, interests, and self-assessment of his abilities to test data. In this way, he will see and understand that test data are really secondary in importance to nontest data and that a rational combination of the two best facilitates appropriate decisions.

SUMMARY

To summarize this section several specific suggestions to aid the counselor in utilizing test information are paraphrased from Lyman (1963). 1) Test interpretation is most effective if it is an integral aspect of the total counseling situation. 2) The counselor should be very careful with the words he uses because clients will remember much of what he says, including careless remarks and any distortions he may inadvertently give. 3) The counselor should be sure to specify the norm group with which the client is being compared. 4) It is, of course, much more difficult to interpret low scores than high ones, but low scores will be more easily accepted if stated in objective terms, e.g., "Only 5 percent of people with scores like yours have successfully completed this training program." 5) The counselor must never make an absolute prediction by stating that a given score indicates that the client can or cannot do this or that. 6) The counselor must not assume that the client will remember everything he is told and expect him to repeat some of the things that he understands. 7) The client should be the one to decide what he is going to do; the counselor makes suggestions, but not decisions. The tests cannot give directions, they can only point the way down the road more clearly. 8) An interpretation must not be forced on the client. If the client does not want to know the results, at least at this time, the counselor should leave him alone until he is ready, rather than wasting the client's time and his own. 9) The counselor should know what he is doing and then it will be more natural and effective. The client should be assured that demonstrated achievement is more conclusive evidence than a score on a test intended to predict achievement.

REFERENCES

Army General Classification Test. 1947. Science Research Associates, Chicago.

Binet, A., and T. Simon. 1916. The Development of Intelligence in Children. Training School Publication #11. Vineland, N.J.

Brown, A. W. 1936. Chicago Non-Verbal Examination. Psychological Corp., New York.

Buros, O. K., ed. 1972. The Seventh Mental Measurement Yearbook. Gryphon Press, Highland Park, N.J.

Buros, O. K. 1974. Tests in Print II. Gryphon Press, Highland Park, N.J.

Dubois, P. H. 1970. A History of Psychological Testing. Allyn and Bacon, Inc., Boston.

Dunn, L. M. 1964. Peabody Picture Vocabulary Test. American Guidance Service, Inc., Circle Pines, Minn.

Edwards, A. J. 1971. Individual Mental Testing. Part I. Intext Educational Pub., Scranton.

Edwards, A. J. 1972. Individual Mental Testing. Part II. Intext Educational Pub., Scranton.

Goddard, H. H. 1946. What is intelligence? J. Soc. Psych. 24:51–69.

Goldman, L. 1971. Using Tests in Counseling. 2nd Ed. Prentice-Hall, Englewood Cliffs, N.J.

Jackson, D. N., and S. Messick. 1967. Problems in Human Assessment. McGraw-Hill, New York.

Kellogg, D. E., and Morton, N. W. 1946. Revised Beta Examination. Psychological Corp., New York.

Lyman, H. B. 1963. Test Scores and What They Mean. Prentice-Hall, Englewood Cliffs, N.J.

Mehrens, W. A., and I. J. Lehmann. 1975. Standardized Tests in Education. 2nd Ed. Holt, Rinehart and Winston, New York.

Otis Mental Abilities Tests. 1960. Harcourt, Brace, Jovanovich, Inc., New York.

Raven, J. C. 1938/1947. Raven Progressive Matrices. Psychological Corp., New York.

Sattler, J. M. 1972. Final Report: Intelligence Test Modifications on Handicapped and Nonhandicapped Children. Project No. 15-P-55277/9-02. Research Grant from the Division of Research and Demonstration Grants, Social and Rehabilitation Service, Dept. of Health, Education, and Welfare, Washington, D.C.

Sattler, J. M. 1974. Assessment of Children's Intelligence. W. B. Saunders, Philadelphia.

Super, D. E., and J. O. Crites. 1962. Appraising Vocational Fitness by Means of Psychological Tests. Rev. Ed. Harper & Row, New York.

Terman, L. M. 1916. The Measurement of Intelligence. Houghton Mifflin, Boston.

Terman, L. M., and M. A. Merrill. 1960. Stanford-Binet Intelligence Scale. Houghton Mifflin, Boston.

Wechsler, D. 1945/1947. Wechsler Memory Scale. Psychological Corp., New York.

Wechsler, D. 1955. Wechsler Adult Intelligence Scale. Psychological Corp., New York.

Wechsler, D. 1958. The Measurement of Adult Intelligence. Fourth ed. Williams & Wilkins, Baltimore.

Wechsler, D. 1974. Wechsler Intelligence Scale for Children–Revised. Psychological Corp., New York.

Aptitude and Achievement Tests

RANDALL M. PARKER and CARL E. HANSEN

Aptitude and achievement tests have come to assume primary importance in the evaluative, counseling, planning, and job placement activities performed by personnel in rehabilitation settings. With few exceptions no other types of psychometric instruments have the practical utility that aptitude and achievement tests possess in determining a person's level of performance in both academic and vocational pursuits. In addition, few other types of tests are able to match the high levels of reliability and validity typically obtained for well standardized aptitude and achievement instruments. These instruments, when carefully selected, administered, and interpreted, have unrivaled potential in facilitating the attainment of academic and vocational goals by persons with handicapping conditions.

This chapter will present general considerations and background information about both aptitude and achievement tests and will give a general description and evaluation of these tests; it will introduce strategies for interpretation of test results, identify and elucidate several critical issues in aptitude and achievement testing; and, finally, it will describe and evaluate selected aptitude and achievement tests that may prove useful in rehabilitation settings. The overall focus of the chapter will be global in that aptitude and achievement test batteries, as opposed to specialized tests (e.g. of musical aptitudes), will be emphasized.

The assistance of Jim Daniels in preparing this chapter is gratefully acknowledged.

GENERAL CONSIDERATION OF
APTITUDE AND ACHIEVEMENT TESTS

Aptitude and achievement tests paradoxically appear to have both marked differences and striking similarities. Aptitude tests are intended to measure a person's capacity to learn or to develop proficiency in a particular endeavor, assuming that appropriate training is provided. In contrast, achievement tests are intended to measure how much a person has learned in both information and skills from some training efforts. Inspection of the items of both types of tests would reveal differences in content between most aptitude and achievement tests. Aptitude items frequently consist of tasks similar to those in many intelligence tests, that is, tasks emphasizing problem-solving ability as opposed to tasks requiring reproduction or integration of learned information. Items in achievement tests, in contrast, would typically focus on the ability to demonstrate previously learned material, thus tending to emphasize memory rather than problem-solving ability. In addition, scores obtained on aptitude tests are usually determined in terms of specific ability areas, such as mechanical and

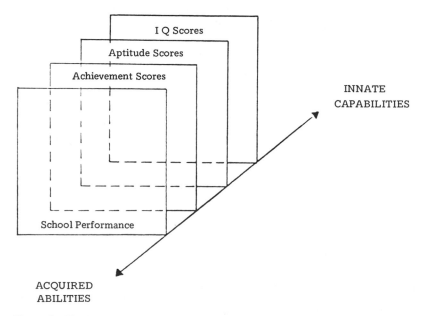

Figure 1. The interrelationship and overlap of measured intelligence, aptitude, and achievement with academic performance depicted along a continuum of level of learning versus inheritance.

spatial abilities. Achievement tests are frequently scored in course content areas, such as science and social studies. Historically, psychometricians have regarded aptitude and achievement tests as basically divergent in that aptitude tests tend to measure innate aspects of ability while achievement tests attempt to assess the level of acquired abilities.

More recently experts have regarded these differences as mostly illusory (Anastasi, 1968). Research has demonstrated that intelligence, aptitude, and achievement tests intercorrelate very highly, suggesting that they all measure mostly the same construct. Therefore, there is a tendency to refer to all of the above types of tests as "academic aptitude tests," signifying the fact that they all correlate highly with academic performance. Figure 1 displays this interrelationship.

EVALUATION OF APTITUDE AND ACHIEVEMENT TESTS

Although the topics of reliability and validity are covered in depth in other chapters of this text, a review of the essentials as they relate to aptitude and achievement tests are covered in this section. These two topics are of paramount importance in test evaluation, and they are especially important in the present context. The relatively high degree of both reliability and validity constitutes one of the major distinguishing characteristics of aptitude and achievement tests.

Reliability of Aptitude and Achievement Tests

Siebel (1968) has provided a sampling of reliability coefficients typical of well standardized aptitude and achievement tests. He reports the reliability of 16 subtests sampled from six major achievement and aptitude batteries including subtests from the California Achievement Test, Differential Aptitude Test, School and College Ability Test, Sequential Tests of Educational Progress, SRA Achievement Series, and the Stanford Achievement Test. The coefficients ranged from 0.83 to 0.94 for the various subtests. To take a specific example, a reliability coefficient of 0.94 was obtained for 12th grade males on the Space Relations subtest of the Differential Aptitude Test. This level of reliability means that a score obtained on this test would be fairly consistent from one test adminstration to another because the reported coefficient in this case is a test-retest coefficient. Moreover, in general terms, a high degree of reliability reflects the fact that there is little random error in determining the score.

Helmstadter (1964) surveyed 183 well known psychometric instruments to investigate their reliabilities. He found that the median reliabilities of achievement batteries, scholastic ability tests, and aptitude batteries are 0.92, 0.90, and 0.88, respectively. Objective personality tests, interest inventories, and attitude scales have somewhat lower median reliabilities: 0.85, 0.84, and 0.79, respectively. The results of this survey could be summarized by stating that the reliabilities for aptitude, achievement, and ability tests tend to cluster in the high 80s and low 90s. On the other hand, reliabilities for personality, interest, and attitude measures tend to fall in the high 70s and low 80s. This comprehensive picture supports the assertion that the reliabilities of aptitude and achievement tests are superior to most other kinds of tests.

Validity of Aptitude and Achievement Tests

When compared to other kinds of tests, the validity of aptitude and achievement tests, generally speaking, is relatively high. Considering the fact that validity is usually regarded as the single most important aspect of a test, aptitude and achievement tests should be regarded as possessing high potential for use in rehabilitation and other settings.

To evaluate the general validity of a category of tests, e.g., aptitude or achievement tests, the procedure followed is to review the obtained validity indices reported in the test manuals and in the research literature. The types of validity indices usually dealt with are those of predictive and concurrent validity because they do not involve a person's judgment and are roughly comparable from one study to another. Siebel (1968) reported that validity coefficients for achievement and aptitude tests usually range from 0.30 to 0.60, although some (particularly concurrent indices) reach 0.80! Siebel reviewed the test manuals for the California Achievement Tests, Differential Aptitude Tests, School and College Ability Tests, Sequential Tests of Educational Progress, and SRA Achievement Series. Concurrent and predictive validity indices ranged from 0.40 to 0.80 for these well known and well established tests. For example, scores on the Abstract Reasoning subtest of the Differential Aptitude Tests (DAT) for 225 ninth grade boys correlated 0.40 with grades in mathematics. Scores for 510 ninth grade students on the Science subtest of the SRA Achievement Series correlated 0.80 with scores on the Science Background subtest of the Iowa Tests of Educational Development. As in the latter case, it is not unusual to find concurrent validity indices that approach the level of the reliability coefficients for the tests. In fact, when the tests are very similar, the concurrent validity coefficient may represent an equivalent forms reliability coefficient. As such, they are probably overestimates of true validity.

In 1966 Ghiselli published a landmark study that assessed the general level of validity of occupational aptitude tests. Professional literature published from 1919 to 1964 was systematically searched for relevant studies. In order to report the data systematically, Ghiselli grouped jobs according to both the *Dictionary of Occupational Titles* and the *General Occupational Classification System.* He also grouped tests into those of intellectual abilities, spatial and mechanical abilities, perceptual accuracy, motor abilities, and personality traits. A serious methodological problem was to define and to set standards for acceptable criteria of occupational success. Two broad categories of criteria were identified. The first category, training criteria, included things such as grades in occupational training courses. The second category, proficiency criteria, included supervisor's ratings of job performance, measures of production, dollar volume of sales, and frequency of accidents. Finally, Ghiselli had to deal with the statistical enigma of combining validity coefficients over a series of studies in a meaningful way. To accomplish this, validity coefficients were averaged after Fisher's Z transformation was employed. Because of the statistical error involved in averaging coefficients of tests with widely varying reliabilities, the reader was cautioned that the average validity coefficients presented were most likely underestimates of the true coefficient.

Table 1 provides a summary of much of the data presented by Ghiselli. Each validity coefficient represents a transformed average for all occupational groups and test categories for which data were available. Each individual coefficient making up the average was based on a sample of 100 persons or more. Inspection of the data presented yields the overall conclusion that the average validity coefficients for training criteria are on the order of 0.10 higher than those for proficiency criteria, the average overall coefficient for training being 0.30 and for proficiency, 0.19. A number of reasons could be postulated to explain this finding, including the fact that training criteria tend to be more reliable than proficiency criteria. Furthermore, the total average coefficient for tests of intellectual ability and of spatial and mechanical ability are approximately 0.15 greater for training than proficiency criteria. On the other hand, coefficients for perceptual accuracy and motor ability tests appear to be about the same for both categories of criteria. Only two pairs of coefficients were available for personality tests, and therefore any general conclusions should be reserved.

For clerical, protective, service, trades and crafts, and industrial occupations trainability is predicted rather well by tests of intellectual abilities, spatial and mechanical abilities, and perceptual accuracy. Predic-

Table 1. Average validity coefficients for four classes of tests over eight occupational groups[1]

Occupational	Tests					
	Intellectual Abilities	Spatial and Mechanical Abilities	Perceptual Accuracy	Motor Abilities	Personality Traits	Total
Managerial						
Training	0.25	0.23	0.19		0.17	
Proficiency						
Clerical						
Training	0.47	0.33	0.40	0.15	0.17	0.35
Proficiency	0.27	0.20	0.27	0.15	0.23	0.23
Sales						
Training	0.18	0.07	-0.02		0.30	
Proficiency						
Protective						
Training	0.35	0.34	0.30		-0.13	0.28
Proficiency	0.23	0.16	0.17	0.19	0.21	0.15
Service						
Training	0.54	0.42	-0.10	-0.05	0.16	0.55
Proficiency	0.03					-0.02
Vehicle Operation						
Training	0.15	0.30	0.08			0.23
Proficiency	0.14	0.20	0.36	0.30	0.26	0.13
Trades and Crafts						
Training	0.41	0.41	0.31	0.17	0.16	0.27
Proficiency	0.19	0.23	0.22	0.19	0.25	0.19
Industrial						
Training	0.40	0.39	0.22	0.34		0.27
Proficiency	0.16	0.16	0.18	0.17	0.26	0.17
Total						
Training	0.35	0.36	0.26	0.18	0.05	0.30
Proficiency	0.19	0.20	0.23	0.17	0.08	0.19

[1] Adapted from Ghiselli (1966).

tion of job proficiency for the occupational groups is much more tenuous. There seems to be little differential among the various kinds of tests in predicting job proficiency; most of the coefficients are on the order of 0.20. This generalization, however, breaks down, particularly for sales and service occupations, where personality tests appear to predict job proficiency with a greater validity than do the other tests.

Average validity coefficients are rather unsatisfying indices of the predictive power of tests because the validity of tests would obviously vary tremendously. Ghiselli concludes his study by computing more meaningful maximal validity coefficients that represent the highest average coefficient over tests, occupations, and criteria. Ghiselli (1966) concludes his book with the following evaluative statement:

> The average of the maximal validity coefficients is .47 for training criteria, and .33 for proficiency criteria. Taking all jobs as a whole, then, it can be said that by and large the maximal power of tests to predict success in training is of the order of .50 and to predict success on the job itself is of the order of .35. . . . The highest of the maximal coefficients for training criteria is .59, which is for intelligence tests applied in the protective occupations; and the highest coefficient for proficiency criteria is .46, which is for perceptual speed tests used in the selection of computing clerks. Another statement of the maximal predictive power of tests might be of the order of .60 for training criteria, and .45 for proficiency criteria. The highest validity found in any of the single studies reviewed for this summary, studies in which more than 100 workers were used, were .77 for training criteria and .66 for proficiency criteria. In both of these investigations the coefficients were for intelligence tests applied in the trades and crafts. Therefore a final statement of the maximal predictive power of tests, based upon experience with them, is a validity coefficient of the order of .75 for trainability and .65 for job proficiency. . . . One can choose among these three descriptions of the maximal predictive power of tests, depending upon one's degree of enthusiasm for tests. . . . It is apparent that even the most optimistic supporter of tests cannot claim that they predict occupational success with what might be termed a high degree of accuracy. Nevertheless in most situations tests can have a sufficiently high degree of predictive power to be of considerable practical value in a selection of personnel (pp. 125–127).

INTERPRETATION OF TEST RESULTS

The interpretation of aptitude and achievement test results may serve many purposes. The client, the counselor, and the rehabilitation agency all have varying interests in the information gleaned from the administration of a psychometric battery. Nevertheless, the focal point of interest is the client. Goldman (1961) presents a comprehensive list of the purposes that testing may serve in general counseling situations:

1. Precounseling diagnostic information—to determine the nature and extent of the client's problem as well as the treatment and services from which he may benefit
2. Information for the process of counseling—to delineate the client's abilities, interests, needs, etc., to aid in structuring the counseling relationship
3. Information to aid the client in decision-making—to provide information to the client himself so that he may determine future directions in the vocational, personal, social, etc., areas of his life
4. Information to stimulate client's discussion of areas not previously considered—to give the client information about himself of which he was unaware to act as a catalyst in self-exploration
5. Laying the groundwork for later counseling and decision-making—to involve the client in selection and interpretation of tests that will lead to a better understanding of the counseling process and its decision-making nature
6. Research—to provide the counselor or other researchers with experimental data

Although psychological testing may serve many valuable purposes as an integral part of the counseling process, a number of pitfalls await the unsuspecting counselor. The manner in which the tests are selected, administered, and interpreted may serve to structure the whole tone of the counseling process. An aggressive counselor who employs his expertise in selecting, administering, and interpreting tests with little client participation may force the client to assume a passive role. He may expect the counselor to continue his active behavior to an extreme, including making decisions that only the client can responsibly make. A positive, growth-producing counseling relationship no longer exists when either the client or the counselor does not participate.

The counselor must continue to be sensitive to the client's feelings while interpreting test results. While interpreting tests counselors frequently assume the role of a knowledgeable technician who is describing findings to an objective and unbiased observer. The fact is that many clients will respond irrationally to much of the information provided by the testing data. For instance, when faced with a client's questioning of the accuracy of a score that does not meet his unrealistically positive expectations of himself, how should a counselor respond? Should the counselor cite validity studies in support of the results, or discuss the fallibility of test scores, thus siding with the client? In most cases both of these kinds of counselor reactions are destructive to client growth. Client's feelings must be explored, and the client must be given an opportunity to work through his feelings. The counselor must not only avoid assuming the role of the technical psychometric expert, he must also avoid subjective value judgements. Referring to test scores as "very high," "average," etc., communicates the counselor's values which, in turn, may adversely affect counseling. The *client's* reactions and value judgements regarding test scores are the more appropriate topics to be dealt with. The counselor must take care to function as a facilitative agent in this phase of counseling (Bordin, 1968).

There are a number of technical aids to help the counselor present testing data cogently to clients without becoming overly subjective. These aids may be divided into two groups, descriptive and predictive interpretative devices. Norms and test profiles are included under the descriptive heading. They present information regarding the client's standing relative to the performance of other similar individuals. The counselor must extrapolate, or make an educated guess, to come up with any statements of what the results mean in terms of the client's future. Predictive devices, on the other hand, allow the counselor to attach probability statements regarding the success of a client's future plans. Such predictive devices include expectancy tables, multiple cut-off procedures, and regression and discriminant equations.

Descriptive Interpretive Devices

Norms Norms are the most basic kind of interpretative aid at the descriptive level. They allow the counselor to describe the client's level of performance relative to an appropriate comparison group. Raw scores, usually taken as the number of items answered correctly, are totally meaningless in and of themselves. Knowing that a client answered 50 items correctly on a verbal ability test gives no information whatsoever about his relative level of performance. If, however, it had been previously established that a raw score of 50 on this particular test was equivalent to the average performance of college graduates, the score than becomes meaningful. Tables of norms allow one to convert raw scores to more meaningful derived scores, such as percentiles. Percentile scores refer to the percentage of people in the standardization sample who obtained lower raw scores, and they are the most often reported and the most easily understood derived scores. Considerable judgement must be exercised frequently in selecting the proper table of norms when several are available. One question that often arises in rehabilitation settings is, "When interpreting the test scores of a handicapped client, should norms based on nonhandicapped or handicapped groups be used?" This and other related questions will be discussed in more detail in a later section.

Profiles A profile is a graphic, comparative representation of a number of test scores. Profiling test scores can provide the client with an extremely meaningful picture of his relative performance on a series of tests. However, profiles not meeting the following three basic requirements may be extremely misleading. The first requirement is that the subtests reported on a profile must be similar in content and nature. Profiling scores from both aptitude and interest tests side by side may be very confusing for both client and counselor. The second assumption is that the scale units must be the same across the whole profile; the whole profile should be plotted in terms of the same derived score, e.g., percentiles. Third, the standardization samples upon which the derived scores are based must be identical, or at least very similar, from test to test. Once these requirements are met, test score profiles are a most useful tool in the counselors repertoire of interpretive aids.

Predictive Interpretive Devices

Multiple Cut-off Procedures One of the basic modes of prediction of success based on test scores is the multiple cut-off approach. Test authors, researchers, local institutions and agencies, etc., will frequently develop cutting scores for use in their selection procedures. For example, colleges frequently develop cutting scores on tests of scholastic aptitude for use in the selection of student applicants. To develop cutting scores one should first determine which measures of a set are more important in the performance of a job or other criterion task. Then, for each of the selected measures a cut-off score is statistically computed so that there is maximal differentiation between successful and unsuccessful workers. Each cutting score, therefore, represents the least amount of each important characteristic a person needs to succeed in a particular endeavor.

The General Aptitude Test Battery (GATB), which is covered extensively in Chapter 11 of this text, employs the multiple cut-off procedure. According to research by the U.S. Employment Service three aptitudes are essential for a Counselor II, namely, general intelligence, verbal aptitude, and clerical perception. To be minimally equipped to handle the job, an applicant is expected to score at the 60th percentile or above on each of the three aptitudes. If an applicant scored substantially above the 60th percentile cut-off on two aptitudes but fell below the required level on one, he would be regarded as not meeting the minimal aptitude qualifications of the job. The multiple cut-off approach, thus, assumes that a superior aptitude in one area does not compensate for a substandard aptitude in another important area. This assumption has been disputed without any final resolution.

Expectancy Tables The expectancy table is a simple and easily constructed device that can be used to interpret test results to clients in terms of probable future outcomes. A simple expectancy table depicts the relationship between one predictor variable and a criterion variable, e.g., IQ (predictor) versus grades in college (criterion). Table 2 demonstrates the relationship between scores on the College Qualification Tests (CQT) and grade point average (GPA). Inspection of Table 2 reveals that for this sample of men those receiving high CQT scores tended to get A and B grades (39 percent), while those with low CQT scores tended to obtain D and F grades. For similar samples one could generalize these results. That is, for a man who received a high CQT score, one could estimate that his chances of getting an A or B average would be approximately 39 out of 100.

Counselors can easily construct their own tables when they possess both the initial test score and eventual outcome data for a group of clients. The first step in constructing an expectancy table is to categorize both the predictor and the criterion variables into meaningful units; for example, one could categorize verbal reasoning scores into high, middle, and low groups. The final step is to fill in the cells of the expectancy table with the data that has been gathered both in raw frequencies and in percentages.

Table 2. Relationship between CQT total score and college GPA in a sample of men (N = 1,340)[1]

	Grade point average (GPA)			
CQT total	D and F (%)	C (%)	A and B (%)	
High	16	45	39	100
Middle	43	50	7	100
Low	80	19	1	100

Note: High designations indicate one fell in the 70th to 99th percentile range; middle, in the 30th to 69th percentile range; and low, in the 0 to 29th percentile range.

[1] From Wesman, A. 1966. Double-entry expectancy tables. *Test Service Bulletin* No. 56, May. The Psychological Corporation, New York.

These tables represent a significant extension of a norm's table to include the relationship of the test score to later outcome.

Regression and Discriminant Equations Particularly since the advent of computer technology, sophisticated statistical techniques have become available as aids in test interpretation. Two of the most frequently discussed statistical techniques are multiple linear regression and discriminant analysis. Regression analysis is a method allowing one to compute weights of the importance of predictor variables as they relate to a criterion. For instance, this technique could be employed to determine weights to be applied to measures of verbal and numerical aptitude in predicting success as an accountant. One may develop the weights so that when each weight is multiplied by its respective predictor score and summed the result will be scaled in terms of the criterion of interest. Utilizing such weights with the verbal and numerical aptitude measures mentioned, one could obtain a predicted criterion score on the same scale on which it was originally measured. Thus, if the criterion of success as an accountant was a supervisor's rating of success on a five-point scale, the result of the regression equation would be expected to fall on the same one to five scale.

Discriminant equations are very similar in nature, although their ultimate purpose in interpretation is somewhat different. Such equations may be used to determine one's similarity and differences from several other groups using a number of test scores. In contrast to the regression equation that yields a predicted criterion score, the discriminant equation would yield a score that could then be compared with discriminant scores of other groups. Similar discriminant scores between an individual and a group would indicate similarity in the criteria of interest. The interested reader may wish to refer to Goldman (1961) for a more detailed, but nontechnical, discussion of regression and discriminant methods.

ISSUES IN APTITUDE AND ACHIEVEMENT TESTING

General Versus Special Norms

A frequent and troublesome question encountered by rehabilitation personnel is, "Should general norms be used with handicapped or culturally different clients, or should special norms be developed that compare clients only to those with similar disabilities or cultural backgrounds?" On one side of this issue are those who proclaim that general norms should be used because the handicapped client will have to compete with the nonhandicapped population in obtaining employment. Those on the other side, however, state emphatically that the use of general norms discriminate unfairly against handicapped persons. This issue is most confusing until one analyzes the question in terms of concepts introduced earlier in this chapter.

Previously, both descriptive and predictive interpretive devices were discussed. Descriptive devices, including norms, merely serve to locate the client's performance within some reference group. But by using norms one might determine that a particular client scored at the 75th percentile in mechanical aptitude, i.e., he scored better than 75 percent of the comparison group. If the reference group in this case were successful auto mechanics, one might predict that this client would also be successful as an auto mechanic. However, this kind of prediction would involve subjective judgement, assuming there is no research evidence that a score at the 75th percentile ensures a high probability of success in auto mechanics.

If, on the other hand, all the relevant variables in auto mechanic performance had been identified and a predictive device had been developed, e.g., a regression equation, the client's chances for success in auto mechanics could be directly determined with a specified degree of statistical certainty. This latter procedure would require little or no subjectivity in making the prediction. The above two predicting modes are frequently referred to as clinical, or subjective, prediction and statistical, or actuarial, prediction. These two forms of prediction will be discussed in greater detail in the next section.

In any particular instance the same test scores could be used to describe and to make predictions about a client's behavior. However, rehabilitation personnel frequently fail to make a conceptual separation between descriptions and predictions, and this is a major cause for the confusion surrounding the general versus the special norms controversy. For descriptive purposes one may easily decide to use either or both handicapped and nonhandicapped norms to ascertain a client's standing within the selected norm group. It is within the realm of prediction that the issue becomes most confused. Predictions based solely on scores derived from norms involve armchair speculation, or what has been referred to as clinical judgement. A number of authors (e.g., Meehl, 1954) have pointed out the precariousness of making clinical judgements. If possible, predictive devices should be employed in making predictions; in this way one can be aware of one's chances of making a correct prediction. The general versus special norms issue dissipates when considering prediction because norms are not predictive devices. When one wishes to use norms in a descriptive fashion, there should be no difficulty in selecting either or both general and specific norms, assuming both are available.

Clinical Versus Statistical Prediction

The history of science is replete with examples of human observational and judgemental error. Human error is particularly pervasive in the behavioral sciences. Psychiatric diagnoses, for example, are subject to tremendous variations. In summarizing six studies Zubin (1967) found that agreement among psychiatrists on diagnosing mental patients ranged from 38 to 84 percent. In diagnosing general conditions, such as psychosis, neurosis, or organic brain damage, agreement ranged from 64 to 84 percent. However, in diagnosing more specific forms of psychiatric disorder, agreement ranged from 38 to 66 percent. These and other similar studies lead to the serious questioning of professional judgements based primarily on experience and intuition. Meehl (1954), motivated by such concerns, sought to determine the relative accuracy of clinical judgement when compared to statistical prediction. Reviewing the literature, Meehl located 19 relevant and unambiguous studies relating to this issue. Of the studies, 10 indicated no difference between the two methods of prediction, and nine found differences in favor of statistical prediction. In an effort to answer criticisms of Meehl's work by Gough (1962), Holt (1958), and others, Sawyer (1966) sought to replicate and extend Meehl's earlier investigation. Sawyer reviewed 45 studies that allowed for a comparison of the accuracy of clinical versus statistical prediction on dimensions of both data collection and data integration. The results were strongly supportive of Meehl's study; statistical prediction was clearly equal or superior to clinical prediction, regardless of the mode of data collection.

Similar concerns are extant in rehabilitation counseling. Two studies are of particular interest. Roehlke (1965) compared statistical prediction with the clinical predictions of rehabilitation counselors regarding the outcome of rehabilitation programs for a sample of psychiatrically disabled clients. Statistical predictions based on demographic, psychological, and vocational variables yielded an averaged predictive accuracy of about 80 percent. The most effective counselors reached a 55 percent level of predictive accuracy, while many others did much worse.

Bolton (1968) compared statistical and counselor clinical assessments of the feasability of rehabilitation clients for services in a state rehabilitation program. As with previous studies, statistical predictions were generally more accurate than clinical predictions. Of 28 counselors who closed at least 35 cases, however, two exceeded the statistical formula in predictive accuracy. Although there was a wide variability in counselor predictive accuracy, no relationship was found between accuracy and either education or experience of the counselor.

In spite of the fact that only a few selected studies relating to this issue have been reviewed here, more extensive reviews have led to the same conclusion: statistical prediction employing what were earlier referred to as predictive interpretive devices are, with few exceptions, equally as accurate as or more accurate than the professional judgement of psychiatrists, psychologists, counselors, etc. These conclusions may place the rehabilitation counselor in a quandry, because predictive interpretive devices, i.e., statistical modes of prediction, are unavailable to him. Therefore, the counselor must continue to use his intuition in decision-making. Nevertheless, counselors should be constantly aware of the fallability of their intuitive judgements and might, in addition, keep records of the various judgements they are required to make so that they may determine their accuracy in predicting client outcome. Perhaps through keeping such records, counselors could identify and correct recurrent errors they make.

The Criterion Problem

One of the most trying difficulties faced by test developers and users alike is obtaining good criteria that may be employed in validating or evaluating tests. Indices of predictive validity, obviously, are useless unless the criterion employed is itself reliable, valid, and relevant. Because they are relatively easy to obtain, ratings are very frequently used as criteria. Ratings, however, are often particularly troublesome because of their characteristic lack of reliability and validity. Other criterion measures frequently used include rate of work, quality of work, number of absences, safety record, etc.

Some rehabilitation workers tend to ignore this issue because they believe state rehabilitation agencies have found the "ultimate" criterion—the case closure. It is unquestionably true that with this criterion one can determine a client's employment status with nearly perfect reliability. There is, however, a question regarding the validity of this measurement. Referring back to earlier discussions in this chapter, validity attempts to determine whether a test measures what it purports to measure. A valid criterion for measuring the success of a client's rehabilitation should provide a global assessment of his ability to function successfully. Certainly, success in a rehabilitation program cannot be measured solely by whether a person obtains employment. Undeniably there are other more humanistic aspects involved in rehabilitation; for instance, a measure of the client's level of psychological adjustment to his disability. It is the humanistic, as well as the economic, justification of the rehabilitation program that has engendered general support for the program. Suffice it to say, the criterion problem in rehabilitation will most likely remain a central issue for some time.

Ethical Issues in Testing

Judicious use of tests, test scores, and psychological reports is a paramount ethical responsibility of the rehabilitation counselor (NRCA Ethics Subcommittee, 1972). The principle of confidentiality must be observed in handling information obtained from psychological tests. Informed consent of the client should be obtained by counselors who wish to communicate testing information to persons outside their agency. Among the several other ethical principles that have relevance to testing and test information, the principles of responsibility, competence, and client welfare also bear mention. Rehabilitation personnel without training or supervised experience in test administration and interpretation should refrain from these activities. The client's welfare can be seriously jeopardized by irresponsible and incompetent handling of psychological material. Material obtained from aptitude and achievement tests, and particularly from intelligence and personality tests, can have pronounced positive as well as negative effects on a client's self-understanding and self-esteem. Faulty or careless interpretation can have disastrous and irreversible effects on a client. Allowing a client to read a psychological test report that was prepared for the counselor is an example of an extremely questionable practice. A counselor who is untrained in this area should consider obtaining the services of a competent professional, and thus avoid any potential harm to the client or to the counselor-client relationship. Knowledge and practice of ethical principles is the ultimate criterion of professionalism.

DESCRIPTION AND EVALUATION
OF SELECTED APTITUDE AND ACHIEVEMENT TESTS

In order to familiarize the reader with a number of aptitude and achievement tests that may prove useful in rehabilitation settings, the following list of tests was prepared. In compiling such a listing the authors relied heavily on Buros' *The Seventh Mental Measurements Yearbook* (1972), which presents descriptions and critical reviews of 1,157 published tests. The organization of the *Yearbook* (MMY) includes a classification of tests into 15 major categories. The 15 categories in the order of the numbers of tests in each are: vocational, personality, miscellaneous, intelligence, reading, mathematics, science, foreign language, English, social studies, speech and hearing, achievement, sensory-motor, fine arts, and multi-aptitude tests. There are a total of 10 published multi-aptitude and 36 published achievement batteries, according to Buros. Together they comprise about 4 percent of the total number of tests. Inspection of these 46 tests resulted in the identification of six achievement batteries and seven multi-aptitude batteries that would most likely be appropriate for adult testing in rehabilitation settings. The greatest number of tests were eliminated because they were intended primarily for use with children in school settings. Others were eliminated because the tests were outdated or extremely limited in terms of reliability and validity data. Each of these 13 tests will be described and evaluated according to a five-point outline.

Achievement Batteries

Adult Basic Learning Examination (ABLE) 1967–71. B. Karlson, R. Madden, and E. Gardner. Harcourt, Brace, Jovanovich, New York.

A) Groups to which applicable: Adults
B) Constructs scored: Vocabulary, reading, spelling, arithmetic (computations, and problem solving), and total
C) Test type, forms available, and format: Group test with three levels available, including level one—adults with achievement levels grades 1 to 4; level two—adults with achievement levels grades 5 to 8; and level three—adults with achievement levels grades 9 to 12. Two forms are available for each level
D) Time requires: Level one—145 minutes; level two—145 minutes; level three—250 minutes
E) Critical comments: The primary purpose of this battery is to determine the educational levels of adults who have not completed eight grades of formal education. Split-half reliability coefficients are generally in the 0.80s and 0.90s and concurrent validity indices with subtests of the Stanford Achievement Test are generally in the 0.70s. The reviewer in Buros suggested that this test has promise, but that other more thoroughly developed tests can accomplish the same goals.

Peabody Individual Achievement Test (PIAT) L. M. Dunn and F. C. Markwardt. American Guidance Service, Circle Pines, Minn.

A) Groups to which applicable: Kindergarten to 12th grade
B) Constructs scored: Mathematics, reading recognition, reading comprehension, spelling, general information, and total
C) Test type, forms available, and format: Individual test with one form, using test plates in two volumes with separate manual
D) Time required: 30 to 40 minutes

E) Critical comments: This test was designed to provide a quick test of educational level for a broad range of ages. Test-retest reliability is reported in the 0.80s for the total test and scores on the individual subtests range from 0.60s to the 0.80s. Correlation between the PIAT total scores and the PPVT IQs has a median of 0.68. According to the Buros reviewer the test has promise because of its short administration time, attractive packaging, and broad range of usage potential; however, the lack of subtests in science and social studies, plus the lower validity and reliability scores as compared to group test competitors, seems to point to the need for more research and revision.

SRA Reading and Arithmetic Indexes **(SRA-RAI)** 1968. Science Research Associates, Chicago.

A) Groups to which applicable: Age 14 years and older
B) Constructs scored: Reading and arithmetic
C) Test type, forms available, and format: Two self-scored individual or group tests with one form each. Arithmetic has four levels: computation of whole numbers, fractions, decimals, and percentages. Reading has five levels: picture work association, word decoding, comprehension of words, phrases, and sentences
D) Time required: 50 to 60 minutes
E) Critical comments: The purpose of this test is to assess basic reading and computational skills of persons with poor educational backgrounds. The KR 20 reliability estimate is reported as 0.87 on reading and 0.91 to 0.95 on arithmetic. The reviewer in Buros feels that validity has not been established and, though the test may be useful in some situations, caution by the user is recommended.

Tests of Adult Basic Education **(TABE)** 1957–1967. California Test Bureau/McGraw Hill, Monterey, Calif.

A) Groups to which applicable: Adults
B) Constructs scored: Arithmetic, reading, language, and total
C) Test type, forms available, and format: Group test with three levels, two alternate forms each, locator test. Level E—adults at reading level of grades 2 to 4; level M—adults at reading levels of grades 4 to 6; level D—adults at reading levels of grades 7 to 9; and Locator—to establish level.
D) Time required: Level E—94 minutes in two sessions; level M—158 minutes in three sessions; level D—176 minutes in three sessions; Locator test—30 minutes

E) Critical comments: The purpose of this test is to diagnose basic educational skills levels in adult semiliterates. Reliability and validity scores were not reported for this test but were "inherited" from the California Achievement Test from which this test was adapted. The reviewers in Buros felt that "inheriting" reliability and validity was a somewhat questionable practice in the light of the fact that the CAT was developed for grade school children and the TABE is for adults. However, in a test market with few tests, this test might have usage potential because of the inclusion of a language mechanics test.

Tests of General Educational Development (GED) 1944–1970. General Educational Development Testing Service of the American Council on Education, Washington, D.C.

A) Groups to which applicable: Adults
B) Constructs scores: Interpretation of reading materials from the social studies, natural sciences, and literature, general mathematical ability, and correctness and effectiveness of expression
C) Test type, forms available, and format: Individual or group test in booklet format with separate answer sheets. Several different forms are available from different years as well as special editions for blind or partially sighted
D) Time required: 120 minutes per test
E) Critical comments: This test was designed for candidates for high school equivalency certificates.

Wide Range Achievement Test, Revised Edition (WRAT) 1940–1965. J. R. Jastak, S. R. Jastak, and S. W. Gijou. Guidance Associates, Pleasantville, N.Y.

A) Groups to which applicable: Age five to adult
B) Constructs scored: Spelling, arithmetic, and reading
C) Test type, forms available, and format: Individual test with one form; two levels: ages 5 to 12, age 12 and older. Verbal form available for those who find the regular test too difficult
D) Time required: 20 to 30 minutes
E) Critical comments: This brief test was designed as a rough indicator of educational achievement in three areas. Reliability is reported in the high 0.90s, a fact that draws some skepticism from the reviewers in Buros. No conventional validity scores are available, the authors preferring internal consistency as a measure of validity. The reviewers suggest that the most effective use for this test is in a clinical setting as a broad screening device.

Aptitude Batteries

Differential Aptitude Tests (DAT) 1947–1969. G. K. Bennett, H. G. Seashore, and A. G. Wesman. Psychological Corporation, New York.

A) Groups to which applicable: Grades 8 to 12 and adults
B) Constructs scores: Booklet 1—verbal reasoning, numerical ability, total, abstract reasoning, and clerical speed and accuracy; Booklet 2—mechanical reasoning, space relations, spelling, and grammar
C) Test type, forms available, and format: Individual or group test in booklet format with separate answer sheets. Two equivalent forms, also two original forms available
D) Time required: 181 minutes in two or more sessions
E) Critical comments: The purpose of the DAT is to provide an in-depth assessment of aptitudes possessed by an individual. Reliability coefficients are reported for each test, sex, and grade. Validity seems effectively established with correlations reported between the DAT and school grades, other aptitude tests, and vocational success. The test is not completely successful as a differential instrument but is a very successful predictor of future performance. The VR + NA composite is a good measure of general academic ability.

Flanagan Aptitude Classification Tests (FACT) 1951–1960. J. C. Flanagan. Science Research Associates, Chicago.

A) Groups to which applicable: Grades 9 to 12 and adults
B) Constructs scored: Inspection, coding, memory, precision, assembly, scales, coordination, judgment and comprehension, arithmetic, patterns, components, tables, mechanics, expression, reasoning, ingenuity, vocabulary, and planning
C) Test type, forms available, and format: Group test with two levels; the 16-test form has separate booklets for tenth grade to adult, and the 19-test edition for grades 9 to 12
D) Time required: 258 minutes in two sessions; individual tests range from 3 to 35 minutes
E) Critical comments: The primary purpose of this test is to provide an accurate vocational predictor by testing a wide range of separate aptitudes. Individual tests do not meet reliability criteria, but they are meant to be used in combination and, when used that way, are high enough for individual prediction. According to the Buros reviewer, predictive validity indices with college progress are relatively good, but are not good with business and clerical performance.

Because of its approach toward predicting vocational success, this test has promise. However, because of the mass of testing materials, greater success may be achieved by an individual administration than by a group testing.

General Aptitude Test Battery **(GATB)** 1946–1970. United States Testing and Employment Service, United States Government Printing Office, Washington, D.C. (See Chapter 11.)

A) Groups to which applicable: Age 16 and older
B) Constructs scored: Intelligence, verbal, numerical, spatial, form perception, clerical perception, motor coordination, finger dexterity, and manual dexterity
C) Test type, forms available, and format: Group test with two forms: One with expendable booklet and the other with separate answer sheets. Also included are a screening exercise and a pretesting orientation exercise for use as test-taking practice for disadvantaged persons
D) Time required: 39 minutes working time; 150 minutes administration time
E) Critical comments: This test was originally designed to determine vocational aptitudes of persons of high school age or older. In comparison with other test batteries, the GATB has high reliability and validity indices. This test should be useful to vocational counselors, but, according to the reviewer in Buros, the test needs to be updated to take into account the change in composition of the work force as well as to avail itself of use of the computer in order to arrive at a more precise prediction model.

Measurement of Skill **(MOS)** 1956–1967. Walter V. Clarke Associates, Inc. AVA Publications, Providence, R.I.

A) Groups to which applicable: Adults
B) Constructs scored: Skill in vocabulary, numbers, shapes, orientation, thinking, and memory; also speed and accuracy and finger skills
C) Test type, forms available, and format: Group test in booklet format with three forms available: English, Italian, and Portugese
D) Time required: 42 minutes working time; 82 minutes administration time
E) Critical comments: The MOS was designed to be a brief battery of placement tests for use in screening in either business, industrial, or educational settings.

National Institute for Personnel Research Intermediate Battery 1964–1969. A. M. Wilcocks. National Institute for Personnel Research, Johannesburg, S.A.

A) Groups to which applicable: Teenagers and adults
B) Constructs scored: Mental alertness, arithmetical problems, computation, spot the error (speed, accuracy), reading comprehension, spelling, and vocabulary
C) Test type, forms available, and format: Group test in booklet format with separate answer sheets. Two forms are available; also, a special Afrikaans edition is available
D) Time required: 165 minutes working time; 210 minutes administration time
E) Critical comments: The purpose of this test is to measure a broad range of aptitudes for use in job or educational screening. No reliability data for the spot the error test is reported, and no validity data for the whole test is presented.

Nonreading Aptitude Test Battery, 1969 Edition **(NATB)** 1965–1970. U.S. Training and Employment Service. U.S. Government Printing Office and National Computer Systems, Washington, D.C. (See Chapter 11.)

A) Groups to which applicable: Grades 9 to 12 and adults
B) Constructs scored: Intelligence, verbal, numerical, spatial, form perception, clerical perception, motor coordination, finger dexterity, and manual dexterity
C) Test type, forms available, and format: Group test with one form available. Includes 10 paper and pencil tests
D) Time required: 190 minutes administration time
Critical comments: This test is a nonreading adaptation of the GATB intended primarily for disadvantaged, semiliterate groups. Norms are the same as for the GATB; this is somewhat questionable in view of the fact that the GATB was designed for a reading population and the NATB was not.

Primary Mental Abilities, 1962 Edition **(PMA)** 1946–1969. L. L. Thurstone and T. G. Thurstone. Science Research Associates, Chicago.

A) Groups to which applicable: Kindergarten to 12th grade and adults
B) Constructs scored: Verbal meaning, spatial relations, perceptual speed, number facility, reasoning, and total
C) Test type, forms available, and format: Group test in booklet with

separate answer sheets. One form available with six levels: kindergarten to first grade, grades 2 to 4, grades 4 to 6, grades 6 to 9, grades 9 to 12, and adult

D) Time required: Grades K–4, 65 to 75 minutes; grades 4–6, 52 minutes; grades 6 and older, 34 minutes

E) Critical comments: The PMA was designed to provide differential measures of aptitudes in a broad range of age groups. Test-retest reliabilities are reported to be in the 0.80s and 0.90s. There is little evidence of differential validity at any level, but the verbal meaning, numerical facility, and total scores correlate highly with school grades. According to the reviewers in Buros, the PMA does not fare well in a comparison of technical aspects with the DAT and other aptitude batteries.

REFERENCES

Anastasi, A. 1968. Psychological Testing. 3rd Ed. Macmillan, New York.

Bolton, B. 1968. Clinical versus statistical prediction in rehabilitation counseling. Unpublished doctoral dissertation, University of Wisconsin, Madison.

Bordin, E. 1968. Psychological Counseling. 2nd Ed. Appleton-Century-Crofts, New York.

Buros, O. 1972. The Seventh Mental Measurements Yearbook. Gryphon Press, Highland Park, N.J.

Ghiselli, E. 1966. The Validity of Occupational Aptitude Tests. Wiley, New York.

Goldman, L. 1961. Using Tests in Counseling. Appleton-Century-Crofts, New York.

Gough, H. 1962. Clinical vs. statistical prediction in psychology. In L. Postman (ed.), Psychology in the Making, pp. 526–584. Knopf, New York.

Helmstadter, G. 1964. Principles of Psychological Measurement. Appleton-Century-Crofts, New York.

Holt, R. 1958. Clinical and statistical prediction: A reformulation and some new data. J. Abnorm. Soc. Psych. 56:1–12.

Meehl, P. 1954. Clinical Versus Statistical Prediction. University of Minnesota Press, Minneapolis.

NRCA Ethics Subcommittee. 1972. Ethical standards for rehabilitation counselors. J. Appl. Rehab. Counsel. 3(4):218–228.

Roehlke, H. 1965. Predicting outcome of rehabilitation of psychiatric patients. Unpublished doctoral dissertation, University of Missouri, Columbia.

Sawyer, J. 1966. Measurement and prediction, clinical and statistical. Psych. Bull. 66:178–200.

Siebel, D. 1968. Measurement of aptitude and achievement. In D. Whitla (ed.), Handbook of Measurement and Assessment in Behavioral Sciences, pp. 261–314. Addison-Wesley, Reading, Mass.

Wesman, A. 1966. Double-entry expectancy tables. Test Service Bulletin, No. 56. Psychological Corp., New York.

Zubin, J. 1967. Classification of the behavior disorders. *In* P. Farnsworth (ed.), Annual Review of Psychology 18:373–406. Annual Reviews Inc., Palo Alto, Calif.

Personality and Psychopathology Inventories

$\textcircled{6}$

HERBERT W. EBER

In the early days of the rehabilitation movement, when services emphasized physical restoration, the assessment of personality was (rightly) considered irrelevant in most cases.

A veteran with a history of successful work experience returned from the war with a missing leg. Arrangements were made to provide a prosthesis and training in its use. If his previous work was unsuitable for a man with marginal leg function, a new job, as similar as possible to the old one, was chosen. Training may have been provided, and even placement help in the rare case where this was needed.

Thus, the former truck driver became a dispatcher, the former mechanic a carburetor specialist, the civil engineer a draftsman for other (more mobile) engineers. Serious problems required more comprehensive services. A double amputee may have required two prostheses and possibly a wheelchair as well.

When the movement broadened its base to include nonveterans, little was changed. The basic methods still worked. Clients were selected for feasibility; lack of previous work history was not considered disqualifying, but it did lower the apparent odds for success. An understaffed agency selected few such clients.

When rehabilitation was asked to undertake work with the mentally retarded, the severely disabled, the mentally ill, the alcoholic, and later the socially disadvantaged, counselors fell, by and large, into two groups. One

101

group maintained, with some justification, that the job could not be done. They resisted the "new" clients, convinced that the problems were too severe and the assets too few.

A second, larger group was determined to apply to the new clients the procedures that had succeeded with the old ones. They provided physical restoration, training, placement, and follow-up services. In some cases they succeeded. More complex and difficult cases might not yield the same amount of achievement per rehabilitation dollar spent, might require more and different services, might take longer to achieve less. Still, successes were plentiful, and the movement again seemed to demonstrate its essential competence.

INTRODUCTION OF PERSONALITY ASSESSMENT IN VOCATIONAL REHABILITATION

As more difficult cases were undertaken and the proportion of failures grew, a curious phenomenon appeared. In many cases, the degree and type of disability had little apparent relationship to outcome. Retardates with IQs around 60 did not, apparently, work significantly less successfully than those with IQs around 65. Schizophrenics with similar pathology at acceptance often showed radically different outcomes. Rehabilitation success among alcoholics bore remarkably little relation to degree, duration, etc., of the drinking problem.

Careful evaluation of clients, often in rehabilitation centers, confirmed the impression that the relationship between the disability and the handicap was far from a one-to-one correspondence. Old timers remembered the amputee who never came to rehabilitation therapy. He lost a leg, bought a new one, and went back to work. Perhaps the handicap was not really the direct consequence of the missing leg alone. Perhaps there were other qualities of the person that could amplify or minimize disability. Perhaps some attention to personality would be fruitful.

At about the same time, rehabilitation began to work with clients whose primary problems lay in the area of psychopathology or personality disturbance. Here, the tradition of defining a relevant rehabilitation plan demanded a reasonably precise assessment.

The needs of rehabilitation attracted psychologists whose clinical skills seemed relevant to the task. Slowly at first, but increasingly in the 1960s, psychological practitioners addressed their expertise to rehabilitation problems. The results were not inevitably happy, but seemed generally favorable. The assessment of personality and psychopathology appeared to offer rehabilitation another tool for use with some of the more difficult clients.

As the practice of assessing and considering a client's personality characteristics became more common in vocational rehabilitation, some further advantages appeared. Some personality characteristics are not in themselves either disabling or facilitating. Rather, they predispose the person to function well in some areas and badly in others. That domain of personality usually described as "vocational interests" is the most obvious example, but broader personality characteristics can be equally important. Highly extroverted people are not usually happy when working in isolation, and vice versa. A reasonable degree of matching between a person's temperament and habits and the demands of a job seemed a promising avenue for further exploration.

Questionnaires and Inventories

As personality assessment was used more often, two factors appeared to encourage the use of questionnaires and inventories. One was cost. Large scale use of personality data simply could not be undertaken with existing budgets if the expense of several hours of a clinical psychologist's time had to be met. Many psychologists continued to function in terms of their accustomed clinical roles, but the cost tended to discourage personality assessment except in those cases where it was clearly necessary.

The second factor presented a more serious problem. Beginning in the mid 1950s the literature contained increasing references to the unreliability and lack of validity of expert judgment. Psychologists began by studying themselves, and the results were not encouraging. Meehl (1954) suggested that all the evidence favored the desirability of a good cookbook rather than a skilled practitioner. Goldberg (1968), and later a number of his coworkers at the Oregon Research Institute (1970), repeatedly demonstrated that simple actuarial models showed greater reliability and validity than did experienced clinicians. The studies were broadened to include practitioners in disciplines other than psychology. Physicians were shown to be less than perfect in their judgments (Goldberg, 1968). Stockbrokers, college admissions officers, juvenile judges—all of these appeared to be functioning with greater than zero validity, but all found their judgment improved in effectiveness by simple models based on their past performance.

Objective Assessment Devices

Some efforts were made to objectify data obtained through projective tests and similar methods of personality assessment, but the efforts were difficult and only marginally rewarding. On the other hand, the questionnaires and inventories lent themselves to objective scoring, and the scores provided immediate primary data for analysis by explicit decision rules.

The pioneers in the use of objective assessment devices, primarily inventories and questionnaires, may well have begun practical use of these methods mainly on the basis of cost considerations. However, as experience developed, it was demonstrated that those devices work. They did not work very well then and do not work very well today; however, they work better than any known alternative, and they do produce meaningful data, replicable relationships, and demonstrably valid predictions of human behavior.

CLASSIFICATION OF INSTRUMENTS

The term "personality" has been used in a variety of ways, usually encompassing virtually all of the behavior patterns of a human being, including intelligence, habits, temperament, psychopathology, motivation, preferences, and interests. Such use of the term is certainly appropriate in some contexts, but it leads to classification of virtually any assessment techniques as "personality tests," including chemical tests of the content of the blood, tests of physiological functioning, measures of intelligence and aptitude, and virtually anything else.

A more narrow use of the term personality within the realm of testing has developed and gained widespread acceptance. Such a use limits personality to nonintellective, nonability measures; grossly physiological tests are excluded, but the lines of demarcation become increasingly fuzzy as test development proceeds. Anxiety is clearly a component of what is meant by personality in this context. However, is the determination of blood chemistry to assess anxiety-related biochemical profiles a personality test? Intelligence is not considered a part of personality in this context, but what about the use of the esoteric items of intellectual information as a means of assessing motivation? The term personality becomes both too broad and too narrow, although it must be admitted that the users of tests have worried little about this lack of conceptual clarity.

Personality and Psychopathology

Some years ago this author proposed that it might be worthwhile to use the term "personality test" in a still narrower context. Imbued with the spirit of coauthorship of the Handbook for the Sixteen Personality Factor Questionnaire (Cattell, Eber, and Tatsuoka, 1970), it was suggested that the general area of habit and temperament should be described as that which is measured by personality tests, whereas gross distortions of the person's functioning (to which many personality tests are grossly insensitive) should be more accurately described as "psychopathology." Such usage would mean that tests which focus upon the normal range of variation of habits, temperament, and ways of behaving would be classified as personality tests, while the primarily clinical devices such as the Minnesota Multiphasic Personality Inventory (Hathaway and McKinley, 1951), would be described as *measures of psychopathology* (despite the use of the word personality in test titles).

It is only fair to say that the suggestion for this separation of terms has not been widely accepted, but it is now seen occasionally, and this author continues to suggest it and will use that classification in this chapter.

In keeping with that rather narrow pair of definitions, some instruments that are often considered to be personality tests will not be considered here. The Edwards Personal Preference Schedule (Edwards, 1954), for example, is clearly a measure of preference and motivation, and while one can certainly infer personality variables from it, this is little different from the fact that one can infer personality variables from virtually anything else. The vocational interest tests (Campbell, 1971; Kuder, 1966) similarly can be used to infer personality variables, but they are tests of motivation and preference, and thus do not seem best classified as personality and psychopathology inventories. Obviously, the projective techniques are excluded on a different basis because they are not inventories. Finally, life history methods, which claim to analyze personality in terms of "real data" rather than questionnaires, are here accepted at face value and are thus omitted from consideration. This is done despite the fact that most life history material does not really deal with facts of history but rather with responses to questionnaires about the history.

In terms of classification between psychopathology and personality, it must be admitted that some tests overlap considerably, and all tests overlap to some small degree. The evidence from the Sixteen Personality Factor Questionnaire is that neurosis and anxiety are clearly distortions of normal personality characteristics, and thus psychopathology of a certain type is built into the personality domain. By the same token, empirically based instruments, such as the MMPI and the California Psychological Inventory (CPI) (Gough, 1960), can readily be used in either fashion, although to different degrees of validity. The MMPI can become a personality inventory when someone develops an empirical scale that is primarily of a personality rather than of a psychopathology nature. The CPI inherently has both kinds of scales, and, of course, any test can have such scales if it contains suitable items. Turning back to the 16 PF, it cannot be a good measure of certain kinds of pathology because it does not include the correct items. One cannot discover schizophrenia without asking about hallucinations, delusions, and similar gross pathological disturbances.

Traits and States

There is another classification that is often ignored but that is intuitively utilized by psychologists and others who may well never formally verbalize the distinction. Certain characteristics of the person are relatively stable, change slowly if at all, and are usually described by the term traits. Other characteristics, or other aspects of the same characteristics in some cases, change rapidly and easily, fluctuating in response to factors such as time of day, time of the month, and environmental stimuli of various sorts, or interpersonal situations and perceptions. Such characteristics are usually distinguished from traits by the term states, but it should be abundantly clear that pure measures of a trait or a state are impossible. Fluctuation related to the concept of state will have to take place within a characteristic that exists initially at some level, and if there is a difference between persons in their mean level as well as in the fluctuation, then that is clear evidence that both a state and a trait exist. By the same token, few trait characteristics remain completely stable from situation to situation, even within tolerable errors of measurement. It seems likely that stability and fluctuation are relative matters and that one might more precisely speak of relatively "trait-like" and "state-like" characteristics.

The area of anxiety provides an excellent case in point. There is clear evidence of a characterological trait, "anxiety," emerging repeatedly from various tests, although sometimes given different names by different test authors. Test-retest correlations on this trait are typically quite high, and correlations between measures obtained from different tests, despite different strategies of test construction, are typically in the 70s or 80s. It must be emphasized, however, that items that fluctuate rapidly have been systematically deleted from tests of the anxiety trait. In the past few years, some psychologists have systematically gathered such items, and shown clear evidence for the existence of anxiety as a state also, a finding that is completely in keeping with the judgment of both skilled clinicians and laymen. People obviously become more anxious under pressure, less anxious in situations that offer stability, more or less anxious under the influence of certain biochemical substances, etc. On the other hand, the differences in mean levels between different people are equally clear. It would seem that it is meaningful to think of anxiety as both a trait and a state, and to distinguish between them whenever the occasion makes such distinction appropriate.

As a final word about the concepts of trait and state, it should be emphasized that the ability to measure states is primitive compared to the ability to measure trait characteristics. Perhaps this is so because trait measurement is of more enduring value, making it economically more feasible to concentrate upon these from a standpoint of predicting the future. The personality measurer is rarely asked to predict the behavior of a subject during the next 15 minutes; he is often asked to predict that behavior over a longer span. Clearly trait measurements are more likely to be relevant, and perhaps this accounts for the rather strong emphasis upon trait characteristics in the available measurement tools.

STRATEGIES OF INVENTORY DESIGN

There are essentially three methods by which test items can be selected and gathered into scales, represented symbolically by the armchair, the scoring key, and the mathematical model. All of these strategies can be empirical to varying degrees, utilizing validation procedures of varying adequacy. Large data banks are not the exclusive property of any of these methods, not is their absence an appropriate indication. The differences are matters of philosophy and, while the writer has very clear preferences in this regard, it must be admitted that these are only preferences. Empirically, scales of all three types work. As Goldberg (1972) has shown so clearly, the predictive utility of a set of items is essentially given by the items and the conditions under which they were administered and by the criterion data against which validation is to take place. The different strategies do not typically yield differential validities.

The Armchair Method

The armchair method symbolizes intuitive, rational test construction. The psychologist uses his understanding of human behavior to determine which factors or traits are to be measured and then assembles items to perform the assessment on the basis of that same understanding. Norms are used and empirical validation is undertaken, but the basic concepts originated in the psychologist's head and the use of those concepts will tend to be dictated by that strategy. The term "armchair psychology" has had negative connotations in the history of the science; such connotations seem unwarranted. Jackson (1973) has suggested that a group of under-graduate students, if asked to design a test, would probably not do appreciably worse than the level of competence achieved by some of the other, more "scientific," methods. The critical issue is empirical validation, and when that is done properly, intuitive strategies can develop effective and powerful methods.

The Scoring Key Method

The scoring key and the criteria against which scale construction is undertaken represent what Goldberg has described as external strategies. These are sometimes called "empirical," but that is not necessarily their major distinction from other types of scales. The critical issue is not that empirical data are used, or that those scales that work are selected; rather, the strategy focuses upon empirical data as the only consideration. In its extreme form, concern with rational and intuitive issues is discouraged, and concern with theoretical issues is seen as irrelevant. The term "dust-bowl empiricism" has been disparagingly applied to the practitioners of external strategies. It is unfair criticism. Because they emphasize use of those things that work, they are often much more ready to subject their methods to the test of empirical validation than are the practitioners of other strategies. The fact that the scales work is hardly a criticism.

The Mathematical Model

The mathematical model symbolizes a concern with theoretical issues of the "real" structure of personality. There is the assumption that proper theory must inevitably lead to measurement of relevant characteristics, and that empirical validity will follow when scales are constructed to conform with models of the person's internal reality. In its extreme form, this strategy has been accused of leading to "reification of factors," that is, the tendency to treat abstract concepts as if they were "real things." Cattell, perhaps one of the most extreme advocates of such a strategy, has essentially countered this argument by emphasizing his convictions that there are real things. Less extreme theorists are less concerned about ultimate realities, but prefer to work with the models on an "as if" basis. In any case, the critical issue again is one of empirical validation. Of the making of factor analytic scales there is little end; of the development of cross validated, cross matched instruments, spanning dozens of studies and years of effort, there is too little beginning.

SELF REPORT VERSUS MORE OBJECTIVE MEASURES

Questionnaires are subject to faking and other types of distortion, and because of this, there has been a long-standing hope that more objective measures could be developed. The task is mammoth; the hope that projective tests such as the Rorschach, the various thematic devices, and similar materials would produce the desired result has been, by and large, a futile one. To put it bluntly, a successful objective test device demands that the client not know what he is doing while the psychologist does know; projective tests have generally been instances where neither did.

The monumental nature of the task to be done has not completely discouraged psychologists; several objective batteries have been developed and described in the literature, and some are even quite comprehensive and stable. However, the difficulties of administration have prevented large scale research, and so the literature contains no particularly exciting criterion associations between the test batteries using the gadgets from the psychologist's laboratory and socially relevant behaviors. One wishes it were otherwise, but the practical needs of applied situations continue to dictate that the more convenient questionnaires be used.

GENERAL PURPOSE VERSUS SPECIFIC TRAIT TESTS

It is intuitively obvious, and in fact even true, that special purpose instruments that focus directly upon the behavior whose prediction is desired can ask questions of a very specific nature and, to the degree that valid answers can be obtained, can be more predictive in the short run than can general purpose instruments. This focus and specificity have convinced some practitioners that such special purpose instruments are the ideal.

However, in the long run, specific circumstances change, and the predictions derived from highly specific instruments lose validity very rapidly. General purpose data, on the other hand, become *more* predictive with elapsed time. An instrument designed to predict how well a client will function on a job tomorrow could achieve significant increases in validity by considering the specific environment, the nature of the supervision, the exact task to be done, and even those relatively fluctuating personality variables that approach the nature of states. However, that is rarely the task. Rehabilitation is not as much interested in how this man will do tomorrow morning as they are interested in how he will do during the next 20 years. The tendency for validity to increase with time is a major advantage of the general purpose instruments, and in most situations we should be willing to settle for the lower validities to gain increased hardiness over time and space.

There is a second reason to prefer the basic personality dimensions rather than special purpose scales. When a new situation occurs, a new prediction is to be made, or some similar circumstances develop, basic data can be recombined into the best known equations for the particular new purpose at hand, and a reasonably adequate prediction can be made. Special purpose scales, on the other hand, do not lend themselves to this. The comprehensive nature of the original data has been lost when a purely empirical scale has been keyed. Unless the original items were saved, and a key for the new situation, using those items, is available, the prediction of new behaviors that were not at issue at the time of original testing can proceed only by the thinnest and most tenuous inference. Again, initial specificity is obtained at the price of hardiness.

Finally, there is another reason why this author prefers instruments of broad scope that are well grounded in psychometric theory. When a treatment program, or any type of intervention, is to be designed on the basis of test findings, empirical scales are a poor choice. This author has fantasized about the Army method for treating psychopathy, utilizing, in satire, the Army's well known tendency to deal with any job in terms of manageable segments.

Suppose that an empirical scale has been developed to discriminate between good and bad combat infantry men; then fancy the possibility that the item "I think George Washington was a greater president than Abraham Lincoln" (answered true) is found to be a significant predictor of combat effectiveness. Clearly then combat training must include classes designed to convince the recruits that George Washington was, in fact, a greater president than Abraham Lincoln. If the scale contains 15 items of which the above is one, then logic would dictate that 15 percent of the time spent in preparing people for the psychological conditions of combat should be spent upon such classes.

On the other hand, an example from this author's own experience suggests a less satirical approach. A group of unsuccessful candidates for a rehabilitation program shows a distinctive personality pattern of the 16 PF, a pattern that centers around the presence of unusually high values of the factor M. Various acquaintances are contacted, and in the discussion that ensues a reasonable and logical basis for the relationship is hypothesized. The findings are cross validated successfully, and so a treatment program designed to reduce the M factor in this particular population is described. The program may well be ineffectual, ill conceived, or oriented toward the wrong thing. It is, however, an empirically sound generalization from both findings in that situation and general psychological theory, and its chances of success would seem to be somewhat greater than classes dealing with the relative merits of various United States presidents.

In a sense, this is still a matter of transferability and hardiness, but it is also more. If psychology is to progress beyond the artistic competence of individual practitioners, small progress can be made upon pure empiricism, but one can expect sounder and more rapid eventual progress when that empiricism is utilized along with a developing body of theoretical knowledge.

SOME GENERAL PURPOSE INSTRUMENTS

The nature of this chapter, and the availability of literally hundreds of tests, precludes any reasonable listing or description of questionnaires that could be considered for use in rehabilitation. Fortunately, full lists, descriptions, and critical reviews are readily available (Buros, 1970).

It is appropriate, however, to mention some commonly used instruments and to draw attention to some of their strengths and weaknesses. Nothing approaching comprehensive coverage is intended, and, while this author clearly believes certain approaches to be of superior merit, no objective ratings of quality should be inferred from this discussion.

The Minnesota Multiphasic Personality Inventory Test

Perhaps the most commonly used instrument is the Minnesota Multiphasic Personality Inventory (Hathaway and McKinley, 1951), commonly referred to as the MMPI. Oriented primarily toward psychopathology, the test nevertheless has literally hundreds of scorable scales, many specific to particular questions of importance to rehabilitation, and many that qualify as scales of "personality" within the narrow definition suggested above. Few if any state variables are directly attacked by MMPI item content, but the nature of psychopathology seems "state-like" in some respects, and state patterns do emerge quite clearly upon successive uses of the test.

There is little doubt that the MMPI is the most frequently researched questionnaire in the world. Thousands of articles, books, monographs, etc., preclude even the compilation of a definitive bibiography. Excellent source books are, however, readily available, including Hathaway and Meehl (1951) and Dahlstrom and Welsh (1960).

The outstanding strengths of the MMPI are its ubiquity and its philosophical emphasis on empirical validation. There is hardly an area of human functioning that has not been related to some MMPI scale(s). Entering a new, and to him unfamiliar, area the psychologist has only to consult the literature and some empirically validated approach will be found. The nature of the test has discouraged armchair speculation; the large item pool has made structural modeling difficult (although far from impossible). Hence, MMPI references usually contain directions on "how to do it"; Meehl's "cookbook" realized, at least in part. It may not be a good cookbook, but in many applications the recipes represent the closest approach of psychology to a usable, dependable technology.

The weaknesses of the MMPI are the obverse sides of its strengths. There are too many items; yet fewer items during the formative years would probably have substantially narrowed the availability of useful recipes. Subsets of the item pool are frequently used, but omission from a particular study of items that are considered irrelevant at that moment dilutes the comprehensive coverage that otherwise constitutes a major source of strength.

The emphasis upon empiricism, to the exclusion (until recently) of mathematical or logical models, tends to tie the MMPI to a questionable technology of "code types." An ingenious scheme to reduce overwhelming complexity of data during precomputer days has become something of a trap. One *can* factor analyze MMPI items; one *can* use such model-oriented new scales; one *can* reduce item redundancy, and one *can* develop and use newer, subgroup specific (and therefore fairer?) norms. However, is the result an MMPI? In a very real sense, it is not. Vast quantities of published research become irrelevant when code types based on "standard" norms are abandoned. A new test has been created, and calling it the MMPI may gain political benefits (or liabilities), but does not enhance the clarity of scientific psychology.

The California Psychological Inventory Test

Among many tests used much less frequently than the MMPI, but still used often enough to be considered here, is the California Psychological Inventory (Gough, 1960), usually called CPI. Actually, the two are closely related, siblings in philosophy and no less than cousins in content. CPI contains many MMPI "items"; but the MMPI was itself a compendium of items from many previous tests, so that assigning item ownership to tests is a tenuous matter.

In any case, all standard and most other MMPI scales can be scored, after a fashion, from the CPI pool of 480 items. Adjustment of norms for different numbers of items per scale is necessary, but conversion tables do exist. In addition, CPI's primary scales orient the test more toward the normal personality, using to advantage new items included by Gough. The philosophy of scale development is precisely that of the MMPI, and so both virtues and defects are similar. The CPI literature is of an order of magnitude less than that for the MMPI, but there are transfer and overlap, and there is also an excellent handbook (Megargee, 1972). The psychologist who finds MMPI concepts and philosophy congenial will find the CPI coverage of nonpathological dimensions most helpful.

The MMPI and CPI are tests in the category symbolized above by the scoring key. The symbol of the armchair, rational test development by the unaided but well trained mind, is represented by no major general purpose tests of personality. Rational test construction does appear at its best in some research designs and in some narrow, situation-specific scales. It is also often present, in disguise, as the so-called "criterion" in research and evaluation. Typically, survey items designed to measure opinions, attitudes, morale, group structure, etc., are constructed by rational techniques. Unfortunately, the rigor and discipline of empirical validation are not always undertaken.

The Eysenck Personality Inventory Test

Turning then to model-directed tests, the simplest in common use is the Eysenck Personality Inventory (Eysenck and Eysenck, 1968), or EPI. Grounded in a two-factor theory of personality (extroversion and neurosis), the test has been quite successful in demonstrating meaningful criterion associations. Many of these seem obvious and trivial, but some equally obvious things turn out to be nonexistent or untrue; one could well be happy to know that certain obvious relationships really exist, are stable and dependable, and can be potentially useful.

EPI has shown that receptionists are really more extroverted than key punch operators, that psychiatric patients are really more "neurotic" than normals, that violent delinquents are more extroverted than nonviolent ones, etc. Confirmation of theory derives from such facts; practical use is, in this author's opinion, another matter.

If the rehabilitation decision is one of therapy versus no therapy, receptionist versus key punch operators, etc., then EPI data can certainly add weight to the decision evidence. If, however, more complex issues of intervention are raised, e.g., what kind of therapy, then richer data sources seem necessary. The simplicity of EPI is appealing until prescriptive remediation is demanded.

The Sixteen Personality Factor Questionnaire

A much more complex model-oriented instrument (too complex by some opinion) is the Sixteen Personality Factor Questionnaire (Cattell, Eber, and Tatsuoka, 1970), or 16 PF. This author obviously cannot discuss this instrument objectively, but some strengths and weaknesses can be cited.

Among the former is the solid grounding in 25 years of personality theory building by Cattell, his students, and his coworkers. A substantial body of research also exists in the literature, not so much as with MMPI, but more than with most other tests. New editions of the test, with better factor saturation than earlier versions, are easily obtained and used. Broader (and fewer) scales, derived from second-order factors, are easily calculated, including the two espoused by Eysenck.

A major weakness of 16 PF was, until recently, its failure to cover psychopathology. Strictly speaking, it should have disclaimed such coverage, but it is sensitive to some aspects of pathology, i.e., maladjustment and anxiety, and the distinctions of various pathologies have not been very clear. With the publication of the pathological supplement, Manual for the Clinical Analysis Questionnaire, Part II (Delhees and Cattell, 1971), the 28-factor coverage is quite comprehensive.

A second weakness of the Cattell et al. tests is that, in striving for comprehensive coverage in a reasonable testing time, few items per score (factor) are used. The remedy for this, strongly urged by the test authors, is to combine forms, and norms for the various reasonable combinations of forms are presented. In practice, however, few psychologists use more than one form, and thus reliabilities are often not all that could be desired (although certainly all that could be expected from such brief individual scales).

On the other hand, psychometric wisdom clearly mitigates in favor of measuring 28 relevant dimensions with six to eight items each rather than measuring fewer factors with more intensive coverage. Compromise between the accuracy desired and the fear of exhausting the test taker must remain a matter of professional judgment.

Some New Tests

In the past few years, significant developments in psychometric technology and in its application by electronic computers have resulted in promising new tests. Not enough time has elapsed to permit relating these tests directly to rehabilitation effort or to provide the extensive applied research base that would encourage such use.

When a test author (and his students and coworkers) develop, research, and publish a new instrument, it is "ready to use," but for what purpose? Time must elapse before those who find the test congenial enough for experimental use can publish results and thereby swell the number of additional experimenters.

The Bentler Personality Inventory (Bentler, 1972), and the Comrey Personality Scales (Comrey, 1970) are interesting examples of such new tests. The former is, or was until recently, available for research use only.

The latter is formally published, but not yet well enough known to attract wide-spread application.

SUMMARY

A brief history of personality assessment in rehabilitation has been presented. Also, some classifications of instruments by area of focus, strategy of design, objectivity, and specificity have been listed and discussed. Finally, some examples of general purpose personality questionnaires have been examined.

REFERENCES

Bentler, P. M. 1972. Bentler Personality Inventory. University of California, Los Angeles.

Buros, O. K., ed. 1970. Personality Tests and Reviews. Gryphon Press, Highland Park, N.J.

Campbell, D. P. 1971. Handbook for the Strong Vocational Interest Blank. Stanford University Press, Stanford, Calif.

Cattell, R. B., H. W. Eber, and M. Tatsuoka. 1970. Handbook for the Sixteen Personality Factor Questionnaire. IPAT, Champaign, Ill.

Comrey, W. L. 1970. Comrey Personality Scales. ESI Testing Service, San Diego.

Dahlstrom, W. G., and G. S. Welsh. 1960. Minnesota Multiphasic Personality Inventory Handbook. The University of Minnesota Press, Minneapolis.

Delhees, K. H., and R. B. Cattell. 1971. Manual for the Clinical Analysis Questionnaire (Interim Experimental Edition). IPAT, Champaign, Ill.

Edwards, A. L. 1954. Manual: Edwards Personal Preference Schedule. Psychological Corp., New York.

Eysenck, H., and S. Eysenck. 1968. Manual for the Eysenck Personality Inventory. Educational and Industrial Testing Service, San Diego.

Goldberg, L. R. 1968. Simple models or simple processes? Some research on clinical judgments. Amer. Psychol. 23:483–496.

Goldberg, L. R. 1972. Parameters of personality inventory construction and utilization: A comparison of prediction strategies and tactics. Multivariate Behavioral Research Monographs, 7:72–2.

Gough, H. G. 1960. Manual for the California Psychological Inventory. Rev. Ed. Consulting Psychologist Press, Palo Alto.

Hathaway, S. R., and J. C. McKinley. 1951. The Minnesota Multiphasic Personality Inventory. Psychological Corp., New York.

Hathaway, S. R., and P. E. Meehl. 1951. An Atlas for the Clinical Use of the MMPI. University of Minnesota Press, Minneapolis.

Jackson, D. N. 1973. Informal Discussion at 1973 Meeting, Society for Multivariate Experimental Psychology.

Kuder, G. F. 1966. Occupational Interest Survey General Manual. SRA, Chicago.

Meehl, P. E. 1954. Clinical Versus Statistical Prediction: A Theoretical Analysis and a Review of the Evidence. University of Minnesota Press, Minneapolis.

Megargee, E. I. 1972. The California Psychological Inventory Handbook. Jossey-Bass, San Francisco.

Oregon Research Institute. 1970. The O.R.I. Research Program in Personality Assessment. Summary Progress Report. Eugene, Oregon.

7 | Projective Techniques

JACK M. PLUMMER

The importance of the psychological evaluation becomes more apparent as the rehabilitation caseload increases, both for disability determination and for client readiness evaluation in general. Information for special consideration includes prior behavior patterns, precipitating causes of the disorder, efforts toward recovery, support from family and community, and the client's current levels of personality functioning (Richman, 1964).

Personality has generally been defined as those significant enduring behavioral characteristics of the person. In this regard, personality may be considered as composed of several aspects: intelligence, abilities or achievement, skills and educational levels; motives, or tendencies and efforts to move toward certain goals; aptitudes, predictive abilities for successful performance in skill and academic areas such as pilot training, law, medicine, graduate school; values, the meaningfulness and importance of things and the good or bad aspects of such things, goals or processes; interests, the attractiveness and concern and enjoyable aspects of things, activities and goals, such as the preference and appeal of a job position or status, the job task, or benefits attained; social and interpersonal behaviors; and the person's incorporated aspects of self-identification and personalized actions and reactions in thought content and processes, emotional responsiveness and feelings, such as anxiety and frustration and tension levels.

PERSONALITY APPRAISAL: PSYCHODIAGNOSIS

Because clinical psychology is essentially concerned with the individual person, one of the clinician's tasks and objectives is personality appraisal, or psychodiagnosis, the assessment of the personality in order to provide a description of the person. The purpose of personality appraisal is to provide a description of a person, to understand how he functions or acts and reacts, his mode or pattern of behaviors and identification and use of defense mechanisms, and the characteristic effectiveness of such efforts for adjustment, where and how the person functions effectively, and where and how situations and reactions increase his liabilities. Explanations and predictions of situations that could enhance effective functioning, such as response to psychotherapy or specific environments or relationships, may also be included. Information may be integrated and a conclusion drawn for a diagnostic category (Schafer, 1965).

Biological and physiological factors, interactions with others during one's lifetime, and sociocultural factors are some of the various aspects that may influence personality development. The clinician must, therefore, use a variety of methods to gain information about a particular subject. Methods to gather data may include the case history, biographical sketch using physical, familial, social, educational, and medical data; psychometric testing, objective tests that yield quantitative information about the subject's intellectual functioning, academic achievement levels, specific interests, and inventories or questionnaires concerning typical feelings, relationships, attitudes, actions; the clinical interview, a verbal interchange with the subject to provide direct observations and flexibility of approach utilizing either leading questions or, as the interview progresses, direct questions with or without a predetermined sequence; situational tasks, such as free time or play time with observations of behaviors in the unstructured situation; and projective techniques.

A combination of tests is usually employed for the psychological evaluation. The selection of the set of tests utilized is determined by those most appropriate to meet the needs of the particular subject and the purposes for the evaluation. The test battery usually includes at least an interview, a test of intelligence, an objective personality test, and a projective technique.

PROJECTION

Ego Defenses

Ego defenses are those unconscious devices, methods, and barriers that people use primarily to maintain equilibrium, to deal with inner energies, impulses, affects, and outer stimuli and demands of the world. Defenses are used as barriers and buffers against inner and outer forces that may disintegrate personality functioning or severely damage self-esteem. Listings of ego defenses or defensive mechanisms may be considered as incomplete and as examples of various authors' attempts to classify complex activities that change over time, are often used in combination, overlap, and serve purposes other than the primary ones. Lists of defenses usually include at least the following: compensation, denial, fantasy, identification, introjection, isolation, rationalization, reaction formation, repression, and projection.

As a defense, projection falsifies both inner awareness and perceptions of the outer world, especially other people. Projection is specifically a misbelief and a misperception, because it is the process by which a person attributes to others certain characteristics, such as urges, wishes, or fears, that are his own. This process is usually unknown to or unrecognized by the person. Projection is, therefore, placing outside of oneself and onto others those certain aspects of oneself that would be disturbing or disrupting if consciously recognized.

Various authors have taken issue with the definition of projection as an ego defense, arguing that projective techniques do not tap projection in that limited sense. A treatise of the history, concepts, and philosophy of projective techniques was given by Shneidman (1965).

Projective Techniques

The terms projective and projective techniques refer to certain situations, content, and procedures to gain personal information from someone. Neither the terms nor the information gained is limited to the definition of projection as a defense. Shneidman (1965) illustrated the difficulty in defining projective techniques and located various classifications or descriptions that the techniques have been given. Seven designations for the Rorschach method alone were found. In summary, Shneidman stated:

> It would thus appear that the Rorschach procedure is a perception constitutive diagnostic experimental visual-stimulus interpretive voluntary indirect free-response associative technique. And what is of equal interest is that the different classifiers made different groupings of the same tests . . . (p. 502).

In contrast, with the objective structured test the subject knows what he is expected to do and how he is to do it. The situation is direct and has a definite meaning for all subjects (Cronbach, 1960).

Projective techniques, however, provide the subject with a relatively ambiguous stimulus, an unstructured situation or task, with such little commonly recognized pattern that he may designate almost any meaning that he can and wishes. The subject must use *what* he has in the *manner* available for use. In this way he literally must put himself into his performance. The performance represents who he is, what he has to use, and how he uses it, in other words, his personality structure and function. He must use what he has; he cannot use what he does not have. The projective situation provides the subject with the opportunity to interpret the vague stimulus or situation and thereby to use his personal content and his own ways of seeing, interpreting, and dealing with the world. Thus, the subject reveals much of his own personal characteristics and processes, his individuality of functioning.

Personality *structure* refers to the description of *what* the person has and the organization of those dimensions. Personality *function* may be considered as the *dynamics,* the change and interactions and uses of the structural components. Projective techniques provide the subject with opportunities to expose both personality structure and functioning. The projective setting also allows the expression of aspects, such as perceptual processes, associations, needs, drives, and abilities, that are unknown to or unrecognized by the subject and have no direct verbal channel for expression.

The definitions of projective techniques could include word association procedures, play therapy and art therapy, psychodrama and role-play techniques (Anderson and Anderson, 1964) and performance tasks (Cronbach, 1960). The concern here, however, is with those procedures referred to in the literature as projective techniques, or "tests," and commonly included as part of a test battery for personality appraisal and diagnostic purposes. A multitude of varied methods are used as projective techniques. The following are a few of these diversified methods: the utilization of inkblots, such as Holtzman Inkblot Technique, Howard Ink Blot Test, and Rorschach; drawing tasks, such as Buck's House-Tree-Person and Mackover's Draw-A-Person; responses to pictures, such as the Blacky Pictures, Children's Apperception Test and Thematic Apperception Test, Rosenzweig Picture-Frustration Test, and Szondi Test; and completion of incomplete sentences, such as Rotter Incomplete Sentences Blank.

The literature indicates that the most popular techniques reported in published research and clinical use are the Draw-A-Person, Rorschach, and Thematic Apperception Test. These methods are presented here as representative of the field of projective psychology in personality appraisal.

Draw-A-Person (DAP)   The DAP technique is a rather unstructured situational task that requires the subject to adjust to the situation and produce a graphic product with few guidelines. The administration of the DAP includes the presentation of a regular letter-size sheet of paper and a medium soft lead pencil to the subject with the request to draw-a-person. When this drawing is completed, the examiner removes the paper and presents a second sheet to the subject with the instruction to draw a person of the opposite sex of the first one.

The subject's attitude and approach to the task are noted. Any comments or questions in regard to the situation or task itself are answered with general statements. Questions concerning skills in drawing, hesitations, and reluctance to draw are responded to with reassurances that the ability to draw is not in question, that the examiner is interested in how subjects try to draw a person, and that any way is all right, and/or that the subject should draw the entire human figure. If the subject just draws a head he may be told to now complete the entire figure; if a stick figure is drawn he may be requested to draw a whole person.

In regard to the actual drawing, the examiner is interested in its size, its location on the sheet of paper, heavy, or dim and smooth, or erratic lines, erasures and reinforcements, shading, symmetry, and completion and proportion of parts. The examiner also considers the content of the drawing, such as the postures of the figures, facial and bodily expressions, individual aspects included or omitted, such as body features, clothing, and accessories.

When the drawing task is completed, the examiner often either asks the subject to tell a story about each of the persons he has drawn or the examiner may create this setting and ask specific questions in regard to such aspects of the drawings as activities, age, interpersonal relationships, emotions, wishes, and best and worst parts.

The assumptions that form part of the foundation for the use and interpretation of the DAP are that any behavior has some importance and meaning and may be grist for the examiner's mill and that each drawing reflects the subject's body image or self-concept. In the situational task presented to the subject and during his performance he may be verbally and behaviorally expressive, asking questions, expressing doubt or confidence, frowning or smiling, wrinkling the paper, chewing on the pencil, tapping his finger or shaking his head, finishing his task with a sigh of relief or a request to draw again. Such behaviors may offer additional supportive information for personality diagnosis.

The body is a person's most close and private reference point, and during development different sensations, emotions, attitudes, ideas, and activities have become associated with various parts of the body through personal experiences learned in or through interpersonal, social, and cultural conditions. The drawing of a person provides the subject with an appropriate method for self-expression. The subject must use his entire personal system, verbal and nonverbal, conscious and unconscious, of experiences, values, meanings, and conflicts to produce an organized, objective representation of a human figure. In this manner the subject extends, expresses, projects himself into his performance and graphic product (Freeman, 1959; Levy, 1950; Levy, 1967; Machover, 1964, 1965).

Rorschach   The Rorschach method of personality appraisal consists of a set of 10 cards, each of which has a symmetrical inkblot on one side. Five of the inkblots are achromatic, black and white with variously shaded areas. Two of the blots are black and white with some color, and three are chromatic, composed of various colors. The cards are presented one at a time in series. The instructions to the subject may include some description of the stimulus cards and the manner in which they will be presented. The examiner may mention 1) that the cards will be presented one at a time, each card has an inkblot, and different people see in them different things; 2) there are no right or wrong answers; 3) the interest is in what the subject may see, of what it reminds him, what it makes him think of, or what he thinks it could be. All other responses by the examiner are to be nondirective and noncommittal. If the subject has initial comments or specific questions, the examiner may explain that the topics will be discussed or the questions will be answered after the procedure is completed.

During the first phase of the examination, the examiner notes all of the subject's behaviors: any verbalizations or behaviors of the subject not apparently related to the task; position of the card for each response; time between presentation of each card and first response, time between responses, and total time spent on each card; and as close as possible a verbatim recording of each response.

The second phase of the examination is the *inquiry,* which is conducted to gather that information needed to score the responses. The examiner uses the subject's wording for each response to identify what part of the blot was used, the location, and what features of the blot (the determinants) assisted the subject in producing the response. An *analogy* period may be utilized to further clarify responses and resolve scoring problems not answered during the inquiry. During the analogy period, the ready use of the determinant in one response is checked to see if it had been used in other responses. This phase of the procedure assists the examiner in assessing whether or not the subject used a certain determinant or was hesitant to use, insensitive to, or unable to verbalize the determinant.

A *testing-the-limits procedure* is often used as an additional phase of the examination. This phase offers much assistance in .clarifying and elaborating the subject's functioning. The process is to provide additional framework for the subject in order to gain more information about his personality structure and functioning. For example, if the subject used the entire blot for each response, it may be necessary to find out if he can develop responses to parts of the blots, or, given a particular detail of a blot, can he develop a response, or, given a response made by others, can he fit it to a part of the blot. Also, it may be necessary to check out determinants in this manner: can he find human content or animal content, can he develop responses with color or integrate color and form, is he able to generalize shading from one blot to another or even utilize shading as a determinant? The subject may even be asked to choose the blot he likes best and the one he likes least and to give the reasons for his choices.

Scoring and interpretation of the responses to the Rorschach vary among different systems, such as Beck et al. (1961), Exner (1969), Klopfer et al. (1954), Rappaport, Gill, and Schafer (1968), and Schafer (1965), yet the similarities and agreements far exceed the differences. Standard notations are used for scoring several categories of each response: *location,* the area and amount of the blot utilized, such as the whole blot (W), large parts or details of the blot commonly perceived as the basis for a response (D), unusual areas and small details (Dd), and white spaces (S); *determinants,* those qualities or characteristics of the blot as perceived by the subject and contributing to the response, such as the shape or form of the blot (F), color (C) and how well color is integrated with form and which is dominant in the response (CF or FC), various classifications of form with shading for surface and texture effect (c), depth (K), or an object with three dimensions projected on a two-dimensional plane (k), such as an x-ray response, and responses in which the subject has projected movement or action, such as human movement (M), animal movement (FM), or inanimate movement (m), such as a river running (mf); *content,* or what the subject of the response is, such as human (H), animal (A), man-made object (Obj), and plant (Pl) among others; *popular* (P) responses and *original* (O) responses are rated according to those responses that are commonly given or infrequently occur.

Rather than focusing upon any single notation unit, such as a W or an M or an H, the clinical evaluation of the Rorschach is concerned with responses within each scoring category and relationships of responses from the various categories. Interpretations are based upon the sequence of scoring categories for each blot and between blots, as well as the interrelations of the various categories per response and between responses. An example of the first aspect may be attention to a W location score followed by a response using a D and whether this succession remains the same for all blots or where and how it changes. In the second instance of concern for the interrelations of categories, the examiner may consider the use of certain determinants, such as M, as they occur with certain location scores and content, such as H. Examples of various interrelationships of categories that give rise to different interpretations are a response to the whole blot, W, using color with little form, CF, and content of ice cream, food, or a Dd with CF and explosion as content.

Additional behaviors are noted and influence interpretations, yet they receive no formal "scores." Such responses include rejection of a card, positioning of the card prior to and during response, clarifying, and any additional information gained during the testing-the-limits period.

Thus, interpretations of the subject's performance are based upon molar considerations to provide a global description of his personality, how he experiences and deals with the world through his various dimensions (Beck et al., 1961; Freeman, 1959; Klopfer et al., 1954; Rabin, 1964).

The Rorschach technique is a standardized task that provides the subject with the opportunity to utilize his various aspects in his available manner. The interest of the examiner is in both what is produced and how it is produced. Because personality is a multidimensional functioning unit, its examination is most appropriately conducted with a multidimensional tool. In this regard, the Rorschach method elicits a behavioral sample composed of responses contributed from the conscious intellectual level, emotional reactivity and expression, and fantasy activities, repression, and conflict areas (Beck, 1964a, 1964b; Beck et al., 1961; Lindner, 1950; McArthur, 1972).

Thematic Apperception Test (TAT) The TAT was designed by Henry A. Murray in 1943. This projective method provides more structured stimuli and task than does the DAP or Rorschach. The materials for the TAT include a set of 30 cards with vague pictures and one blank card. Most of the pictures contain one or more persons in an indistinct activity or situation. There are four overlapping series of cards, each of which contains 20 cards for use with either boys, girls, males more than 14 years of age, and females more than 14 years old.

The TAT technique consists of using the appropriate series of 20 cards, which includes the blank card, for the particular subject. The administration of the TAT usually entails two sessions of approximately 1 hour each, with 10 cards presented during each session. The examiner mentions that there are no right or wrong responses, and that this is a test of imagination. One card will be presented at a time; each card depicts a scene, and the subject is to make up a story about each scene. The directions given to the subject are: tell what led up to the scene, what is happening and the feelings of the characters at this time, and what the outcome will be. The subject's responses are recorded as closely as possible to verbatim. The examiner also makes note of behaviors related to the task, such as pauses, variations in speech and voice, comments, and emotional expressions in regard to the task itself, particular pictures, or special topics.

There are a variety of approaches for systematic analysis of the subject's responses to the TAT. Systems for classification, "scoring," and interpretation include those by Bellak (1947, 1950) and Murray (1943). The various "scoring" methods have used checklists to select and tally responses for categories (Bellack, 1954; Tomkins, 1947; Wyatt, 1947) or ratings for intensity (Aron, 1949). The emphasis of Murray's system is upon the identification of the subject's needs, such as achievement, affiliation, acquisition, nurturance, and aggression, and the "presses" of his environment, such as failure, rejection, or punishment. The subject's needs are identified through the *hero* of his stories with whom the subject identifies. The hero is recognized by similarities with the subject's sex, age, and other characteristics, and is often the central figure of the story and most often discussed and subjectively described. The *presses* are those environmental forces that satisfy or frustrate personal needs. Tomkins' (1947) analysis includes four main scoring categories: 1) vectors, or the direction of behaviors, such as toward, against, with; 2) levels of psychological functioning, such as perceptual, thought, behavioral; 3) conditions or states that are not behaviors, such as lack and danger; and 4) qualifiers, such as intensity and causality.

The TAT elicits a comprehensive description of personality in terms of content, the subject's interpersonal relationships, thoughts and fantasies, attitudes and emotional reactions, needs, tensions, and conflicts. The assumption of the method is that an author's creation contains his own meanings, interpretations, experiences, needs, wishes, and values. In essence, the story includes the personality characteristics of the author (Allen, 1969; Bellak, 1950; Fiedler, 1973; Holt, 1964; Krutch, 1972; Rosenthal, 1970; Scott, 1972).

Research

Review of the literature, such as journals and reference materials (the *Journal of Projective Techniques and Personality Assessment;* the *Journal of Consulting and Clinical Psychology;* and Buros' *Mental Measurements Yearbook*) and summaries contained in textbooks offer the following conclusions about the validity and reliability of projective techniques: invalid and valid; unreliable and dependable; negative and positive; should not be used and a necessary part of a test battery; difficult, dull, of questionable utility and acceptable and of promising benefit; superficial and penetrating; inconclusive or contradictory and supportive results.

During the last two decades there has been much emphasis upon both the clinical development of projective techniques and the objective research procedures and results. The clinical development has included the use of projective methods in a variety of settings and with a variety of purposes, with children and adults, and with individuals and groups, such as education, industry, military, prison, hospital, and clinic. The primary use of projective techniques has been for personality evaluation and clinical diagnosis. Development continues unabated with recent elaboration and clarification of scoring and interpretation (Burstein, 1972; Exner, 1969; Klopfer, 1956; Klopfer et al., 1970; Ogdon, 1969) and concern for the stimuli, examiner, and interaction of the examiner and the subject (Dana, 1972; Hammer, 1967).

Objective, experimental research has primarily emphasized such psychometric issues as validity, reliability, and scoring. In this regard, evidence has been meager for placing the projective methods on the threshold of either "test" or "measurement."

Additional research has been urged, not only to be conducted on the techniques but also the clinicians' orientations, biases, abilities, and actions during and following administration, investigation of group differences, and cross validation of studies differentiating groups.

The projective techniques are not tests of single, specific entities (traits) with scores based upon numerical scaling. The methods are standardized procedures to collect a behavioral sample of a person in action, how he experiences the world and the processes he uses to deal with it. The shorthand notations, labels, and categories are for record keeping and indicators of personality processes for interpretations; they are not scores based upon mathematics (Burstein, 1972; Dana, 1972; Harris, 1972; McArthur, 1972). These techniques are tests in the sense of providing a challenge, a trying situation for the subject to attempt to meet with his personal resources. Thus, the projective methods provide opportunities for the subject to demonstrate what resources he has and how he uses them. Such methods are utilized to assess personality, to estimate content, configuration, and functioning of personality. The purpose is to describe and to understand the person. Clinical labels and diagnostic categories are not given directly by these methods (Brown, 1970; McArthur, 1972; Piotrowski, 1965).

In essence, Shneidman (1965) stated that in spite of their equivocal validity status, psychologists in clinical settings use projective techniques because they are influenced by the concept of unconscious motivation and the need to use other than a direct approach to personality appraisal; their interest in a holistic approach, emphasis upon personality functioning and personality as a process, a way of "organizing and patterning the life situation" so that unstructured techniques may tap the person's "private world"; and the critique that objective tests may tap structure or what is there or what strength it has, the individual aspects of personality, but do not adequately reflect the multiform aspects, the living, moving, and humanistic perspective of personality.

Much has been done to assist or coerce the projective techniques to become psychometric instruments, structured, normed, and quantitative. Projective psychology and projective techniques are still in the process of development of concepts, scoring systems, interpretations, and applications. Quality and quantity of usage continues to be ahead of precise, mathematical verification. If different opinions or contradictions, various interpretations, and inconclusive evidence are created by studies, research, or reports, the better for the scientific study of behavior and the development of special techniques. Such controversial results may increase attention and recognition of problems in personality appraisal and may also enhance momentum to obtain more data and information about theory, validity, reliability, and procedures of projective techniques.

PERSONALITY EVALUATION IN REHABILITATION

The psychological aspects of rehabilitation clients have received increased attention, and appropriate trends in program development have been noted in the rehabilitation literature. Consideration of psychological aspects, personality content and functioning, has been given to psychiatric patients (Richman, 1964), as well as to minority group and economically disadvantaged clients (Scott, DeBellis, and Price, 1969), correctional rehabilitation (Ooley, 1962), the deaf and hearing impaired (Bolton, 1972), the brian damaged (Hirschenfang, Silber and Benton, 1967) and the mentally retarded (Durfee, 1969), the aged (Reiner, 1974), and other physically disabled clients, such as those with hemiplegia (Klocke, 1969), facial disfigurement (Stewart, 1962), cardiovascular impairments (Gray, Reinhardt, and Ward, 1969), and paraplegia (Siller, 1969).

Personnel in rehabilitation agencies and facilities are concerned with structure and function. In regard to such physical disabilities as amputation or quadriplegia, vocational evaluators, physicians, counselors, and instructors are interested in what the disability is, the identification of physical residuals, and resulting dysfunctional and potential functional aspects. In rehabilitation, concepts such as "disability" and "amputation," i.e., upper extremity, lower extremity, unilateral, bilateral, multiple, below knee, above elbow, etc., indicate the emphasis upon the *structural* aspects, the identification of the physical disability. These examples may also serve to illustrate the emphasis upon the *functional* aspects of people with disabilities, because their potential physical functioning is related to the amount of physical loss, strength and mobility of the stump, general health and physical condition of the amputee, as well as the client's psychological reactions and adjustment.

SUMMARY

Projective techniques are recommended as part of the psychodiagnostic battery for personality evaluation. These techniques include brief, general, nonspecific direction, an unstructured task, and provide a global, holistic description of personality rather than focus on the measurement of a particular characteristic. The appropriate use of projective techniques is limited to those who are trained and have supervised experience. These methods are utilized to gain information that is pursued by the clinician and related to the subject's life experiences and other diagnostic procedures. In this manner they may contribute to the total personality picture by providing new information or clarifying and confirming results and impressions from other tests.

Projective methods allow the clinician to observe and record the subject in action, which permits an evaluation of personality organization and functioning. The description of personality, its needs, wishes, attitudes, emotions, and controls, appears to offer information to better prepare and implement appropriate, individualized services in order to enhance the effectiveness of rehabilitation programs.

REFERENCES

Allen, G. W. 1969. The Solitary Singer. New York University Press, New York.

Anderson, H. H., and G. L. Anderson. 1964. An Introduction to Projective Techniques. 8th Ed. Prentice-Hall, Englewood Cliffs, N.J.

Aron, B. 1949. A Manual for Analysis of the Thematic Test: A Method and Technique for Personality Research. Willis E. Berg, Berkeley, Calif.

Beck, S. J. 1964a. Errors in perception and fantasy in schizophrenia. *In* J.

S. Kasanin (ed.), Language and Thought in Schizophrenia. Norton, New York.

Beck, S. J. 1964b. The Rorschach test: A multi-dimensional test of personality. *In* H. H. Anderson and G. L. Anderson, (eds.), An Introduction to Projective Techniques. 8th Ed. Prentice-Hall, Englewood Cliffs, N.J.

Beck, S. J., A. G. Beck, E. E. Levitt, and H. B. Molish. 1961. Rorschach's Test: I. Basic Processes. 3rd Ed. Grune and Stratton, New York.

Bellak, L. 1947. A Guide to the Interpretation of the Thematic Apperception Test. Psychological Corp., New York.

Bellak, L. 1950. The Thematic Apperception Test in clinical use. *In* L. E. Abt and L. Bellak (eds.), Projective Psychology. Knopf, New York.

Bellak, L. 1954. The Thematic Apperception Test and Children's Apperception Test in Clinical Use. Grune and Stratton, New York.

Bolton, B. 1972. Personality studies of deaf adults. Rehab. Res. Pract. Rev. 3:11–17.

Brown, F. 1970. Psychodiagnosis revisited: One version. News Bull. Southwest. Psycho. Assoc. (Austin) 3:2.

Burstein, A. G. 1972. Rorschach. *In* O. K. Buros (ed.), The Seventh Mental Measurements Yearbook. Gryphon Press, Highland Park, N.J.

Cronbach, L. J. 1960. Essentials of Psychological Testing. 2nd Ed. Harper & Row, New York.

Dana, R. H. 1972. Thematic Apperception Test. *In* O. K. Buros, (ed.), The Seventh Mental Measurements Yearbook. Gryphon Press, Highland Park, N.J.

Durfee, R. A. 1969. The misdiagnosis of mental retardation. J. Rehab. 35:22–24.

Exner, J. E., Jr. 1969. The Rorschach System. Grune and Stratton, New York.

Fiedler, L. 1973. Archetype and signature (the relationship of poet and poem). *In* D. J. Burrows, F. R. Lapides, and J. T. Shawcross (eds.), Myths and Motifs in Literature. Free Press, New York.

Freeman, F. S. 1959. Theory and Practice of Psychological Testing. Henry Holt, New York.

Gray, R. M., A. M. Reinhardt, and J. R. Ward. 1969. Psychosocial factors involved in the rehabilitation of persons with cardiovascular diseases. Rehab. Lit. 30:354–359.

Hammer, E. F. 1967. The Clinical Application of Projective Drawings. Charles C Thomas, Springfield, Ill.

Harris, D. B. 1972. The Draw-A-Person. *In* O. K. Buros (ed.), The Seventh Mental Measurements Yearbook. Gryphon, Highland Park, N.J.

Hirschenfang, S., M. Silber, and J. G. Benton. 1967. Psychological appraisal of the brain injured. J. Rehab. 33:23–24.

Holt, R. R. 1964. The Thematic Apperception Test. *In* H. H. Anderson and G. L. Anderson (eds.), An Introduction to Projective Techniques. Prentice-Hall, Englewood Cliffs, N.J.

Klocke, J. 1969. The role of nursing management in the behavioral changes of hemiplegia. J. Rehab. 35:24–27.

Klopfer, B., ed. 1956. Developments in the Rorschach Technique. Volume II: Fields of Application. World Book, New York.

Klopfer, B., M. D. Ainsworth, W. G. Klopfer, and R. R. Holt. 1954. Developments in the Rorschach Technique, Volume I: Technique and Theory. Harcourt, Brace and World, New York.

Klopfer, B., M. M. Meyer, and F. B. Brawer, eds. 1970. Developments in the Rorschach Technique, Volume III: Aspects of Personality Structure. Harcourt, Brace, Jovanovich, New York.

Krutch, J. W. 1972. The tragic fallacy. In W. S. Scott (ed.), Five Approaches of Literary Criticism. Collier-Macmillan, New York.

Levy, S. 1950. Figure drawing as a projective test. In L. E. Abt and L. Bellak (eds.), Projective Psychology. Knopf, New York.

Levy, S. 1967. Projective figure drawing. In E. F. Hammer (ed.), The Clinical Application of Projective Drawings. 2nd Printing. Charles C Thomas, Springfield, Ill.

Lindner, R. M. 1950. The content analysis of the Rorschach protocol. In L. E. Abt and L. Bellak (eds.), Projective Psychology. Knopf, New York.

Machover, K. 1964. Drawing of the human figure: A method of personality investigation. In H. H. Anderson and G. L. Anderson (eds.), An Introduction to Projective Techniques. 8th Ed. Prentice-Hall, Englewood Cliffs, N.J.

Machover, K. 1965. Personality Projection in the Drawing of the Human Figure. 6th Printing. Charles C Thomas, Springfield, Ill.

McArthur, C. C. 1972. Rorschach. In O. K. Buros (ed.), The Seventh Mental Measurements Yearbook. Gryphon Press, Highland Park, N.J.

Murray, H. A. 1943. Thematic Apperception Test Manual. Harvard University Press, Cambridge, Mass.

Ogdon, D. P. 1969. Psychodiagnostics and Personality Assessment: A Handbook. 2nd Printing. Western Psychological Services, Los Angeles.

Ooley, W. R. 1962. It's not hopeless. Rehab. Rec. 3:23–26.

Piotrowski, Z. A. 1965. The Rorschach inkblot method. In B. B. Wolman (ed.), Handbook of Clinical Psychology. McGraw-Hill, New York.

Rabin, A. I. 1964. Validating and experimental studies with the Rorschach method. In H. H. Anderson and G. L. Anderson (eds.), An Introduction to Projective Techniques. 8th Ed. Prentice-Hall, Englewood Cliffs, N.J.

Rappaport, D., M. M. Gill, and R. Schafer. 1968. Diagnostic Psychological Testing. Rev. Ed. International Universities Press, New York.

Reiner, M. L. 1974. Aging—What does it mean? J. Rehab. 40:14–15, 42, 44.

Richman, S. 1964. The vocational rehabilitation of the emotionally handicapped in the community. Rehab. Lit. 25:194–202, 209.

Rosenthal, M. L. 1970. The New Poets: American and British Poetry since World War II. Oxford University Press, New York.

Schafer, R. 1965. The Clinical Application of Psychological Tests. 11th Ed. International Universities Press, New York.

Scott, E., E. DeBellis, and R. L. Price. 1969. Formation of a hardcore project. J. Rehab. 35:30–31.

Scott, W. S. 1972. The psychological approach: Literature and psychological theory. *In* Five Approaches of Literary Criticism. Collier-Macmillan, New York.

Shneidman, E. S. 1965. Projective techniques. *In* B. B. Wolman (ed.), Handbook of Clinical Psychology. McGraw-Hill, New York.

Siller, J. 1969. Psychological situation of the disabled with spinal cord injuries. Rehab. Lit. 30:290–296.

Stewart, M. I. 1962. Surgery only first step. Rehab. Rec. 3:27–30.

Tomkins, S. S. 1947. The Thematic Apperception Test. Grune and Stratton, New York.

Wyatt, F. 1947. The scoring and analysis of the Thematic Apperception Test. J. Psych. 24:319–330.

8 | Vocational Inventories

**LENORE W. HARMON, VIJAY SHARMA,
and ANN B. TROTTER**

The ultimate goal of rehabilitation is to assist the disabled person in learning to lead the most productive, satisfying life of which he is capable. To achieve this goal, the rehabilitation counselor in the State-Federal rehabilitation office or in a private agency works with the client to formulate the steps needed or the most suitable rehabilitation plan to achieve this goal. For most clients, selecting, preparing for, and eventually entering a satisfying occupation is the desired outcome of the rehabilitation process. Because work comprises a major portion of a person's life, through a successful work experience the disabled person is not only able to meet his financial needs and responsibilities, but he is also able to attain the dignity and feeling of self-worth afforded by society to productive persons.

VOCATIONAL INTEREST AND ATTITUDE INVENTORIES

Vocational interest and attitude inventories can be of considerable assistance to the rehabilitation counselor in helping the client to select potential occupations for further exploration via occupational information, job observation, and work evaluation. The ever-increasing complexity of the labor market and the numerous variety of individual jobs, many of which can be adapted for the severely disabled, make occupational selection increasingly difficult for even the most sophisticated counselor and almost impossible for the client who may be relatively naïve about the world of work. The problem of vocational choice is compounded for the client who has been disabled from birth or an early age. Disabled children frequently are over-protected or sheltered by their parents and have little opportunity to observe the work world and to gather data on which to base appropriate career choices. Merely asking the client what he is interested in, his expressed interests, may provide little information to the counselor working with a disabled client who has had limited exposure to the world outside his home, a hospital, or an institution. Hence, vocational inventories provide the counselor and the client with information to enable the client to make a better informed occupational choice. Certainly high interest alone is not sufficient for success in a given career, but a person with both interests and abilities suitable for a given occupation will be more likely to do well and be satisfied in that occupation (Cronbach, 1960). Vocational inventories are one component of career planning, and the rehabilitation counselor must be cognizant of the need to consider information gained from these instruments only in combination with data on client aptitudes, personality characteristics, and physical and mental limitations.

Information on Vocational Options

The first use of vocational inventories with the disabled is thus to provide the client with information to increase the number of vocational options open to him. In this regard, rehabilitation clients generally may be divided into two categories: 1) disabled youth with little or no vocational experience or work exposure, and 2) adults who, through disablement, are no longer able to pursue their former occupations. In dealing with the young client, the counselor can select and use several instruments to delineate job fields of possible interest. Testing can be followed with providing the client occupational information, site visits permitting him to observe workers in action, work sample and evaluation techniques, and, ultimately, the training needed to enter the chosen occupation.

In the past, interest measurement has been geared primarily to clients with professional potential and goals. However, a variety of innovative instruments now exists that can be used to explore interest in the skilled trades and subprofessional areas. Instruments also are available for clients who may not possess the intelligence or reading ability to take the more commonly used instruments, e.g., the Strong Vocational Interest Inventory (SVIB) or the Kuder Preference Test. Vocational inventories that can be used to meet the needs of a broad gamut of disabled clients will be reviewed in subsequent sections of this chapter.

For the disabled youth, inventories also can be used to gain an understanding of the client's level of work orientation and vocational maturity. Inventories assess both attitudes toward oneself as a worker and knowledge of the process of career choice, which may have been profoundly influenced by the experience of being disabled. It seems likely that the prevailing parental attitude toward over-protecting disabled children might lead to both a lack of work orientation and a lack of understanding of the choice process and its elements. If constructive attitudes toward work and career choice processes have not been developed, it is obviously a mistake for the rehabilitation counselor to plunge immediately into a consideration of specific vocational choices. Attention first should be devoted to assisting the client in better understanding himself and the decision-making process.

The rehabilitation counselor also will find vocational inventories useful in assisting the older client who, because of disease or trauma, can no longer pursue his former occupation. For example, a client who has been primarily oriented toward physical activity in occupations such as logging and trucking and becomes a paraplegic will be forced to select a new career and in all probability will have to drastically alter his life style. Kunce (1969) examined the relationship between measured vocational interests and rehabilitation outcome, and he found that although a major interest in physical activities may pose considerable problems for the severely physically disabled in restructuring their lives to include more sedentary occupations, an interest in physical activities may actually be an asset to other clients. Using vocational inventories to understand the older client's work orientation and to help him explore alternative careers is an important component of the rehabilitation process.

Client Participation in the Counseling Process

In addition to opening avenues for occupational exploration, vocational inventories can be used by the rehabilitation counselor to facilitate communication and interaction with his clients. Although many rehabilitation agencies refer clients to psychologists or other resources for psychological testing, the rehabilitation counselor can administer many of the less complex vocational inventories himself. Discussion centered around these instruments and their results frequently can be of value in communicating with the nonverbal client. Instruments such as the Geist Picture Inventory or the United States Employment Service Interest Check List may stimulate client participation in the counseling process, and careful observation by the counselor can better enable him to understand the client's needs and thought processes. Frequently nonexpressive clients may be considered "unmotivated" and therefore determined to be ineligible for rehabilitation services. In many cases the client may simply appear to be "unmotivated" because he has no idea of the actual options available to him. Exploring the variety of career opportunities through the use of vocational inventories may increase client involvement in and motivation for rehabilitation.

In discussing vocational inventories with the client, the counselor must remember that interest per se is not predictive of success in a given occupation and that he must help the client to distinguish between interest and aptitude as well as to recognize the limitations imposed by the client's disability. The rehabilitation counselor must understand what a given instrument acutally measures and clearly convey this to the client.

Preparing the Client for the Testing Process

Finally, vocational inventories can be of use to the rehabilitation counselor in preparing the client for and understanding the overall psychological testing process. Many disabled clients have had limited exposure to psychological evaluation and may be extremely threatened when told, "Go take some tests." In general, vocational inventories are less threatening to the client than aptitude or personality tests, and they may be used to provide the client with an orientation to the testing process. Interpretation of vocational inventories also may be less threatening to the client and can be used to initiate this phase of client understanding.

Summary

Vocational inventories can be used by the rehabilitation counselor to provide the disabled client with information on which to make broader and more appropriate career choices, to facilitate client participation in the counseling and career development process, and to prepare the client for psychological assessment in general. Although many rehabilitation counselors may not actually administer these inventories themselves, understanding the variety of the instruments available, what they measure, and their limitations can result in more informed and appropriate referrals to psychologists and other testing resources and can enable the rehabilitation counselor to use the data reported in psychological evaluations more effectively.

CRITERIA FOR SELECTING VOCATIONAL
INSTRUMENTS FOR REHABILITATION COUNSELING

A psychological test or inventory should never be used without a full inspection of all the testing materials and the accompanying manual. Most test publishers make available a specimen set of these materials at nominal cost so that such an inspection can be made before making a decision to use the instrument. To facilitate test review and selection, the following criteria have been identified and defined.

General Criteria

Some criteria apply to all tests and inventories, not just to instruments to be used with rehabilitation clients. First, it should be stated clearly in the manual what the instrument is designed to measure. If the purposes for developing and using the test are not fully explicated, it is questionable whether the instrument has any specific purposes and impossible to tell whether the inventory will do what the user wants it to do. Only in instances where no other instrument is available should an inventory without an explicitly stated purpose be used. If such an instrument is selected, its use should be considered experimental, and plans should be made to assess its usefulness in the specific situation.

Second, the instrument should possess adequate reliability, preferably of the test-retest type. Internal consistency measures have their uses, but often there is no reason for interest scales to be internally consistent as discussed by Campbell (1971). Interest inventories frequently are used for prediction; thus, it is important that consistency over time be demonstrated. Most measures of interests and values have reliabilities of 0.80 to 0.85 or more over short time periods (Brown, 1970). Lower reliability estimates should alert the user to the fact that the results for clients may contain considerable error. Actually, in the ideal situation the individual report of scores should contain a simplified reference to the standard error of measurement either verbally or graphically.

Third, evidence of validity should be available for the instrument. Validity is related to the stated purpose of the instrument. The author or publisher should be able to present evidence that the instrument accomplishes what it was developed to do. Thus, if an author publishes an instrument designed to measure attitudes toward work, that author should be able to show that the measure is statistically related to other measures and behaviors that are logically related to attitudes toward work. This is a demonstration of construct validity. In addition, evidence of criterion-related validity, either concurrent or predictive, should be presented for most vocational measures because these instruments are used to help make decisions about the future vocational behavior of clients. Thus, if an inventory purports to measure vocational maturity, there should be evidence that people who are vocationally mature score high or that people who eventually make good vocational adjustments score high on the inventory. If an inventory purports to measure interests in specific occupations, data should be presented indicating that people in those occupations score high or that people who eventually enter those occupations score high.

Fourth, it is important that vocational measures used by rehabilitation counselors have norms that are appropriate for their clients. This does not necessarily mean that there should be specific norms for the disabled. Norms, however, should be available for the appropriate age range and educational level of the clients tested. For example, norms based on adolescents generally are not suitable for the older disabled worker. Occasionally, it will be possible to develop local norms that incorporate people of the appropriate age and educational levels for use with rehabilitation clients. Whether these norms should include only rehabilitation clients is debatable. If the inventory being normed is to be used predictively, one might argue that a broader norm group is necessary. If the rehabilitation goal is competitive employment, comparison of the client with workers in general or in a specific occupation may be useful. If the results are to be used to stimulate discussion and exploration, norms based on the specific client population might prove more fruitful. Unfortunately, most vocational measures are so complex that it would be extremely difficult for many agencies to develop local norms.

Special Criteria

Some criteria for vocational measures apply specifically to their use by rehabilitation counselors. First, the readability level of the instrument is especially important because many rehabilitation clients have limited educational skills. These limitations often are a result of the disability and its treatment; thus, the vocational measures used by rehabilitation counselors must allow the client to explore a full range of potentialities without being restricted by the instrument itself. Too frequently clients are given tests that they simply cannot read or understand, and decisions are based on essentially invalid data.

Second, for the same reason, it is important that rehabilitation counselors use vocational measures that are suitable for administration to clients with physical limitations. In general, measures without time limits and/or measures that do not necessitate the use of complex mechanical apparatus are best adapted for rehabilitation clients. Again, it may be necessary to collect norms on certain inventories for people working under specific handicaps. A number of interesting questions arise around these procedures. For instance, would the reading of interest inventory questions to a blind client affect the answers given? Would a more valid set of responses result if a tape recording were used?

A related but separate problem is the third special criterion. Inventories for rehabilitation clients should have validity scales that indicate whether the clients are responding appropriately or merely randomly because of poor abilities or lack of motivation. If possible, the instruments also should have validity scales that indicate consistency of response. These scales are desirable in inventories to be used with any clients but are particularly necessary with rehabilitation clients who may be relatively naïve about the world of work and operating from a somewhat different experiential and motivational framework than the usual client.

To assist rehabilitation counselors and psychologists in selecting and using vocational inventories, the authors prepared detailed descriptive summaries of 22 vocational instruments and brief reviews of several other instruments and batteries. The major instruments are listed under five categories:

General Interest Inventories

1. Strong Vocational Interest Blank
2. Strong-Campbell Interest Inventory (SCII)
3. Kuder Preference Record
4. Kuder Occupational Interest Survey
5. Kuder General Interest Survey
6. Minnesota Vocational Interest Inventory (MVII)
7. Vocational Preference Inventory (VPI)
8. The Self-Directed Search (SDS)
9. Ohio Vocational Interest Survey
10. California Occupational Preference Survey
11. Occupational Interest Inventory (OII)
12. Guilford-Zimmerman Interest Inventory (GZII)
13. Gordon Occupational Checklist
14. Other General Interest Inventories

Pictorial Interest Inventories

1. The Geist Picture Interest Inventory (GPII)
2. Picture Interest Inventory (PII)
3. Vocational Interest and Sophistication Assessment (VISA)
4. Other Pictorial Inventories

Value Inventories

1. Allport-Vernon-Lindzey Study of Values (SV)
2. The Hall Occupational Orientation Inventory (HOOI)
3. Super's Work Values Inventory (WVI)

Measures of Career Maturity

1. Career Maturity Inventory (CMI)
2. Career Development Inventory (CDI)
3. Cognitive Vocational Maturity Tests (CVMT)

Multiple Test Batteries

1. Career Planning Program (CPP)
2. Comparative Guidance and Placement Program (CGP)
3. Vocational Planning Inventory

Reviews of seven instruments that were judged to be potentially most useful in rehabilitation counseling are presented below. The relationship of each of the 22 instruments to the selection criteria will be presented in the last section of this chapter.

Reviews of Selected Vocational Instruments

Strong-Campbell Interest Inventory (SCII) 1974. D. P. Campbell. Stanford Press, Stanford, Calif.

A) Form: T235
B) Purpose: To give persons information about themselves that will help them to make sound decisions about their life plans; to provide information to professionals, such as rehabilitation counselors, who make decisions about others; to help in studying groups of persons.
C) Description: The SCII is a 325-item inventory containing the best 325 items from the 1966 revision of the SVIB for men (Form T399) and the 1969 revision of the SVIB for women (From T398). Most of the items are presented in the "Like-Indifferent-Dislike" format and are arranged in seven sections: Occupations, School Subjects, Activities, Amusements, Types of People, Preference between Two Activities, and Your Characteristics. Three types of scores result: six General Occupational Themes based on Holland's typology (Holland, 1973), 23 Basic Interest Scales, and 124 Occupational Scales. In addition, administrative indices show total responses, percentages of like, indifferent, and dislike responses, and infrequent or unpopular responses.

The average respondent can complete the inventory in one half hour. The reading level is about sixth grade, but most respondents that young do not have stable interest patterns. More typically, interest inventories of this type have been administered to persons more than 17 years of age.

Scoring is too complex to be completed by hand; a scoring service must be used. Profiles that relate the General Occupational Themes to the Basic Interest and Occupational Scales are the usual output, although some scoring services provide interpretive profiles printed individually by computer.

D) Norms: The General Occupational Themes and Basic Interest Scales have been normed on General Reference Samples of 300 men and women. The mean for the group is set at a standard score of 50 and a standard deviation of 10. Because there are sex differences, the profile and interpretive material make it possible to determine how an individual stands on norms for the appropriate sex (and in the case of the Basic Interest Scales, the opposite sex).

The Occupational Scales have been normed on the criterion group of people employed in the occupation who were used to develop the scales. In general, these included people who liked their work and had been employed in their occupation for a minimum of 3 years. Most occupational groups contain 200 or more members. The mean and standard deviation for each group are 50 and 10, respectively. Unlike the other scales, these scales were developed on workers of one sex or the other. Several occupations are represented by two scales developed and normed on males and females separately.

E) Reliability: Two-week and 30-day test-retest correlations are presented for each set of scales. Median correlations, even for the shorter Occupational Theme and Basic Interest Scales, are above 0.86 for the 30-day interval and above 0.90 for the 2-week interval.

F) Validity: The Occupational Theme and Basic Interest Scales have content validity due to the item selection procedure. Only the Occupational Theme Scales are related to a theory (Campbell and Holland, 1972). Each type of scales presented has concurrent validity, i.e., persons in specific occupations score high on appropriate scales. Some discussion of the predictive validity of the Basic Interest Scales is available in the SVIB Handbook (Campbell, 1971). Extensive evidence regarding the predictive validity of previous Occupational Scales is available.

G) Comments: This new revision of the SVIB Handbook has two major advantages. First, measured interests are related to a theory for the first time (Holland, 1973), and second, the problems of having separate forms for each sex are eliminated. The addition of Holland's typology will permit the counselor to discuss broad general themes that may be more appropriate for rehabilitation clients than specific occupations. Caution should be used in discussing occupational scales normed for one sex with a client of the opposite sex (AMEG Commission, 1973; Johansson and Harmon, 1972).

Kuder Occupational Interest Survey 1966. C. F. Kuder. Science Research Associates, Chicago, Ill.

A) Form: DD
B) Purpose: To assess individual preferences, likes, and dislikes for activities and compare them with those of other persons in a wide range of occupations. The goal is to help individuals to narrow the field for further exploration.
C) Description: The Kuder Occupational Interest Survey contains 100 triads of three activities. In each triad the respondent picks the most preferred and the least preferred activity. Responses are recorded on an answer sheet; machine scoring is mandatory. Most people can complete the survey in about 30 minutes. Kuder DD contains 114 occupational scales; 37 were developed using female criterion groups and 77 using male criterion groups. There are 48 college major scales; 19 were developed using female subjects and 29 using male subjects. A verification scale is included to assess respondent carelessness and insincerity. Scores may be reported on all the scales for either sex, on the male scales for men, or on a set of scales including all the female scales and some of the male scales for women.

   The scores are expressed as correlation coefficients that express the relationship between the subject's responses and the responses of a criterion group in the occupation or college major. The various types of scales are listed alphabetically on the profile, but the highest scores for each type (if over 0.30) are ranked at the bottom of the profile. Scores within 0.06 of the highest score are recommended for consideration. Differences of 0.07 or more are considered significant. Comparisons between subjects are not meaningful.
D) Norms: The criterion groups provide the norms in a sense. These groups are fairly well described in the manual as to number, source, average age, educational level, and job satisfaction.
E) Reliability: The reliability of individual profiles over 2 weeks has a median value of 0.90. Over approximately 3 years the median reliability for individual profiles was 0.89. This type of comparison correlates individual profiles rather than scales. No test-retest measures of scale reliabilities are available.
F) Validity: Validity has been assessed in terms of errors of classification of employed subjects. Concurrent validity thus defined is ade-

quate for the 30 scales studies and more impressive than concurrent validity on the Kuder Form D, which utilizes a different scoring system. No evidence of predictive validity is available.

G) Comments: The availability of college major scales of Form DD of the Kuder is an interesting innovation about which much more information is needed. Evidence of predictive validity and the relationship between college major and occupational scales would be helpful. The Survey could be very helpful to rehabilitation counselors in narrowing down the number of occupational fields or academic majors for further consideration by the client. The selection of occupational scales, fortunately, was not limited to fields requiring college training.

Minnesota Vocational Interest Inventory (MVII)   1965–1966. K. E. Clark and D. P. Campbell. Psychological Corp., New York.

A) Form: Males
B) Purpose: The MVII was designed specifically to measure the interests of males 15 years of age and older in nonprofessional areas.
C) Description: The client's interest patterns are compared with those of men in various nonprofessional occupations. One hundred and fifty-eight forced choice triads (in which the respondent chooses the most and least preferred) are used for the Occupational Activity scales. Twenty-nine Occupational scales, such as Baker, Printer, and Sheet Metal Worker, are available. Nine Area scales are provided: Mechanical, Health Service, Sales Office, Office Work, Electronics, Food Service, Carpenter, Clean Hands, and Outdoors. The MVII has one form, with two editions: National Computerized Service (NCS, test-answer sheet with scoring service) and Measurement Research Center (MRC separate acswer sheets, profiles, and hand scoring or scoring service available). Machine scoring is preferable; the possibility of committing some errors with hand scoring does exist. The MVII takes from 45 to 90 minutes to administer. Thus, it is relatively long and may exhaust the rehabilitation client and influence response patterns. A verification scale has been developed for the MVII (Campbell and Trockman, 1963) but has not been incorporated in the inventory.
D) Norms: Norms on two types of scales are provided. Norms for Occupational scales were derived by setting the mean of a criterion group of men in each occupation at 50 with a standard deviation of 10. Area scales (homogeneous scales) were derived through intercorrelation methods (items that had high positive correlations with each

other were included), and norms were developed by scoring a Tradesmen in General group (TIG). The samples on which the scales and norms were derived were mostly selected from the Minneapolis-St. Paul area. The TIG group is not described very specifically.

E) Reliability: Test-retest reliability coefficients for 30-day intervals ranged from the 0.70s to the 0.80s. The coefficients were based upon a sample of 98 industrial institute trainees rather than on high school students or on tradesmen in general.

F) Validity: Concurrent validity for the Occupational Scales was demonstrated by the fact that the scales clearly separated criterion groups and the TIG group. In addition, the results of several studies supported the effectiveness of the MVII in differentiating vocational interests of vocational and technical high school and junior college students (Barnette and McCall, 1964; Bradley, 1958; Johnson and St. John, 1970). The construct validity of the Area Scales was demonstrated through the item content of each scale and the pattern of scores earned on these scales by the criterion groups. Zytowski (1968, 1969) intercorrelated the same or similarly named scales of the MVII, the SVIB, and the Kuder Occupational Interest Survey. Correlations ranged from 0.19 to zero (one negative correlation was obtained: Printer on MVII and Kuder). From these findings, it appears that the MVII scales are not highly related to other interest inventories commonly used in the field.

G) Comments: At present, the MVII seems to be one of the most useful inventories for measuring the nonprofessional interests of adult males. Kauppi and Weiss (1969) demonstrated the instrument's effectiveness with rehabilitation clients. Nonprofessional occupations such as those measured by the MVII frequently are desired and appropriate occupational choices for rehabilitation clients. Unfortunately, the length of the instrument and the relative difficulty of some of the items may limit its use with clients with lowered attention spans or low reading levels. Further research to study the impact of the more difficult items on the scores obtained and on adapting a shortened version of the MVII would be valuable for rehabilitationists. Because scores on the SVIB, which was developed in the same way as the MVII, have been demonstrated to not be generally reliable for students less than 17 years of age, it would be useful to examine the reliability of the MVII for the high school students for which it is recommended.

The TIG groups should be described more completely. Both Occupational Criterion groups and the TIG groups would be more useful to the counselor if they were representative of adults employed in the various occupations (by sex, ethnic groups, and geographic area). In its current form, the use of the MVII with culturally different group members is questionable. The reader is referred Clark (1961) for further information on the MVII.

The Self-Directed Search (SDS) 1970. J. L. Holland. Consulting Psychologist's Press, Palo Alto, Calif.

A) Form: 1970
B) Purpose: The SDS was designed to provide the user with a "vocational counseling experience" in the absence of a counselor. More specifically, an assessment booklet is used to obtain the subject's occupational code as explained in Holland's theory (1973). The code is then used to locate related occupations in a booklet, The Occupations Finder.
C) Description: The SDS has five sections (228 items) in various item formats. The sections are: Occupational Daydreams, Activities, Competencies, Occupations, and Self Estimates. They are used to assess the subject's similarity to each of six personality types: Realistic, Investigative, Artistic, Social, Enterprising, and Conventional. Subjects compile their scores from each section and arrive at a summary code consisting of three of the types in rank order (i.e., Realistic, Enterprising, Aesthetic = REA). The code is compared with the Occupational Daydreams and used to enter The Occupations Finder to locate related occupations. The Occupations Finder also contains Dictionary of Occupational Title codes permitting the user to obtain additional information on specific jobs. The occupations cover jobs held by 95 percent of the United States labor force. They were classified into Holland's codes by a method that was, for the most part, empirical (Holland, 1973). Thus, the final product of completing the SDS is a code type and a list of appropriate occupations for further exploration. Most people complete the SDS in 40 to 60 minutes. Although there are no validity codes as such, extensive suggestions are presented in the manual about what to do when inconsistencies in responding are observed.
D) Norms: Because the product is not a score in the typical sense, there are no norms in the usual sense. Data about the type of people found in many occupations are presented in The Occupations Finder, and this information might be considered normative.
E) Reliability: No test-retest correlations are available. Kuder-Richardson-20 estimates of internal consistency for the subscales range from

0.53 to 0.88. Supposedly, these estimates would have been higher if the estimates had been based on the total scales. Since the total scales produce a code and not a score, total scale reliabilities are not available.

F) Validity: The SDS has impressive construct validity relating it to Holland's (1973) theory. The work of Campbell and Holland (1972) provides evidence of concurrent validity for Holland's theoretical formulation but not for the SDS itself. Evidence is not available on the predictive validity in the scales.

G) Comments: Holland's theoretical formulation provides a powerful basis for relating personal types and work environments; however, more evidence of test-retest reliability and criterion-related validity are needed for this particular instrument. The procedure used in the SDS gives considerable responsibility to the client that may be a step in the right direction, but some counselors may not find it an asset for many rehabilitation clients. The SDS could be of considerable use to the rehabilitation counselor with a large caseload; the use of the instrument could stimulate vocational choice exploration and possibly reduce the time required in face-to-face contact with the client. It should be noted that devising a code type requires good arithmetic skills that some clients may lack. The results seem well suited to a general exploration of careers.

Vocational Interest and Sophistication Assessment (VISA) 1968–1970. J. J. Parnicky, H. Kahn, and A. D. Burdett. Ohio State University, Columbus, Ohio.

A) Form: Male and female
B) Purpose: The VISA is a nonreading, pictorial inventory that was designed to measure selected vocational interests and knowledges of mildly retarded adolescent and adult males and females.
C) Description: The male and female forms contain 85 and 60 pictures, respectively. The male form has seven sophistication pictures to measure knowledge about jobs, three explanation pictures to identify worker-supervisor roles, and 75 interest pictures; the female form has four sophistication, three explanatory, and 53 interest pictures. In addition to the test booklet, separate answer and inquiry sheets are needed to record client responses. The VISA must be administered individually; instructions are presented verbally, and the subject responds verbally to each item. Administration follows the order of sophistication or job area knowledge, explanation of task, and interest inquiry, e.g., "Would you like to do this job?"

Administration requires 20 to 40 minutes depending on the client's cooperation and response patterns. The picture sketches are large and clear in an attempt to avoid undue time pressures and to maintain the client's interest and attention. VISA yields seven scores for males in the following occupational areas: Garage, Laundry, Food Service, Maintenance, Farm and Grounds, Material Handling, and Industry. Only four scores are available for women: Business and Clerical, Housekeeping, Food Service, and Laundry and Sewing. Sophistication level scales are obtained for both sexes. The explanatory pictures serve as a link to the next task of interest measurement only; hence, they are not scorable. Profile sheets have been devised for presenting results and interpretation. A detailed description of scoring procedures is included in the manual.

D) Norms: Norms based on 3,007 educable mentally retarded (EMR) clients enrolled in institutions, schools, or sheltered workshops are provided for both sophistication level and interest patterns. The normative subjects ranged in age from 14 to 35 and in IQ levels from 45 to 84. The sample was drawn mainly from the Northeastern states, and representativeness across socioeconomic and urban-rural dimensions was assured. The relevance and appropriateness of the norms for EMRs in general has not been demonstrated.

E) Reliability: Test-retest reliabilities of the VISA over an interval of 12 to 18 months ranged from 0.46 to 0.97 (Material Handling and Garage) for 1,021 males and from 0.94 to 0.99 (Business-Clerical to Laundry) for 973 females.

F) Validity: Reliability and validity data are not presented in the manual. Other sources, however, provide this information (Parnicky, Kahn, and Burdett, 1968, 1969, 1971; Parnicky and Presnell, 1973). Construct validity has been inferred from factor analysis, which suggested similar factors, " . . . emerging with independent samples and repeated measurements and out of varied data matricies" (Parnicky and Presnell, 1973, p. 7). VISA interest scores have been found to compare closely with clients' verbal responses and supervisor's impressions of clients' major job interests (Parnicky, Kahn, and Burdett, 1971). Predictive validity and the relationship of the instrument to job satisfaction over a period of time have not been explored.

G) Comments: VISA, like its predecessor, The Geist Picture Interest Inventory, is a promising instrument for rehabilitation and guidance counselors working with higher level retardates and other rehabilitation clients. Since the existing norms have some limitations, the development of local norms in the specific facility is recommended. The counselor is cautioned to interpret the results only in terms of the client's needs, previous growth, and experiences.

Super's Work Values Inventory (WVI) 1970. D. E. Super. Houghton Mifflin, New York.

A) Form: 1970
B) Purpose: The Work Values Inventory was designed to measure extrinsic and intrinsic work values of adolescent boys and girls and adult males and females to facilitate sounder occupational choices and to increase the possibility of job satisfaction.
C) Description: The WVI contains 45 value statements, such as, "Create something new" and "Gain prestige in your field." The respondent is directed to answer each item on a five-point scale: 5 = very important, through 3 = moderately important, to 1 = unimportant. Separate answer sheets of the grid form are available in an attractive format; directions are relatively complicated. Value statements are clear and comprehensible for eighth graders, with a few exceptions, e.g., "Add beauty to the world" and "Have a way of life . . . that you like." There is no time limit, but the WVI usually takes from 10 to 20 minutes to complete. Hand scoring stencils and machine scoring services are available. Hand scoring requires 15 to 20 minutes. A weight of "3" is assigned for skipped items; the author failed to give any explanation for this practice. The WVI yields 15 value scales: Altruism, Aesthetic, Creativity, Intellectual Stimulation, Achievement, Independence, Prestige, Management, Economic Returns, Security, Surroundings, Supervisory Relations, Associates, Way of Life, and Variety.
D) Norms: Grade and sex norms for the WVI are very extensive (grades seven through twelve) and carefully designed. The norms are reported in percentile scores, along with means and standard deviations for each scale. At present, adult norms are not available. Because ". . . work values do not seem to change overall with age (and grade) to a marked degree . . ." (Tiedeman, 1972, p. 1480), the grade norms given in the manual also can be used for college students and adults. Super plans to develop occupational norms that may be more applicable for adults. While interpreting the scores, the counselor can emphasize both the relative hierarchy of the client's various values as well as the relationship to sex and grade norms.
E) Reliability: For a 2-week interval, test-retest reliabilities of the various WVI scales range from 0.74 to 0.88.

F) Validity: The WVI was based on very solid construct, content, and concurrent validity studies. Since the initial form of this inventory has been available for over 20 years, comprehensive validity data are provided in the manual. Factor analysis of the items suggested four major value dimensions: Material, Goodness of Life, Self-expression, and Behavior Control. Data on predictive validity are not available.

G) Comments: The WVI is a result of the author's synthesis of several theories and psychometric technology. The results of numerous studies have substantiated the importance of values in curriculum selection, setting goals and aspirations, and job satisfaction (Shah, 1969; Singer and Stefflre, 1954; Super and Kaplan, 1967). Future research may indicate other uses for the WVI in vocational counseling. At present, detailed information on what the counselor should do with the value scores and how to relate them with personal meanings and to the decision of career planning is not given in the manual. Rehabilitation counselors, however, may find Super's (1973) discussion of values along with vocational interests very helpful.

Career Maturity Inventory (CMI)   1973. J. O. Crites. CTB/McGraw-Hill, Monterey, Calif.

A) Form: Form A-1
B) Purpose: The CMI was designed to assess the maturity of attitudes and competencies that are needed to make sound career decisions. It may be used in career counseling to assess client need for counseling and to evaluate career education and counseling programs.
C) Description: The CMI contains two major parts, attitude and competencies. The "Attitude Scale" has 50 true, false questions. The questions were designed to tap five attitudinal dimensions: Involvement in the Choice Process, Orientation toward Work, Independence in Decision Making, Preference for Career Choice Factors, and Conceptions of the Choice Process. The "Competence Test" measures five career choice competencies: Self Appraisal, Occupational Information, Goal Selection, Planning, and Problem Solving. A 20-item multiple choice subtest measures each competency. Items were chosen to express an underlying developmental theory (Crites, 1973a). Admirable attention was given to the effects of grammatical form and item format. The instructions suggest time limits of 20 minutes each for "Attitude Scale" and each subtest of the "Competency Test," a total of 2 hours. Answer sheets may be hand or machine scored. The profile contains raw scores, percentiles,

and a right response scale that is useful in determining a client's specific problems.

D) Norms: The author suggests that local norms, which can be provided when groups of answer sheets are machine scored, are most appropriate. Norms are available for grades six through 13 on the "Attitude Scale" and grade six to 12 on the "Competency Test." No claim for representativeness is made.

E) Reliability: The test-retest reliability of the "Attitude Scale" was 0.71 over a 1-year period for over 1,500 students in grades six through 12. Since items were selected to measure increasing maturity with age, it would be surprising to find a very high test-retest correlation. The only measures of internal consistency available are those for the "Competency Test." Kuder-Richardson-20 correlations ranged from 0.58 to 0.90 with all four of the correlations below 0.75 on part five (Problem Solving) in the lower grades.

F) Validity: Content validity was assured by the great care that was taken in determining the content, form, and scoring of the items. Criterion-related validity is evidenced by the fact that scores on these sets of items are related to grade level, which is itself a measure of maturity. Evidence from studies using more stringent criteria, such as decisiveness and realism of career choice, is not conclusive but suggests that the "Attitude Scale" has criterion-related validity.

G) Comments: The construction of this inventory has been careful and thorough. At this time more evidence of criterion-related validity is needed because the counselor needs to know that a client with a high level of competency as measured by the CMI is, in fact, able to make mature, appropriate decisions. Crites has paid commendable attention to the effects of sex and socioeconomic class on career maturity in his discussion.

AVOCATIONAL INTEREST MEASUREMENT

Increasing consideration is being given to avocational activities in rehabilitation. The constructive and satisfying use of leisure time is important for the satisfaction of individual needs and for the maintenance of a stable and integrated society. Handicapped people are more limited in the avocational activities that they may pursue, yet in many cases they are in more need of avocational activities than the nonhandicapped in order to lead meaningful lives. Employment per se may be limited by the disability; the counselor should be prepared to help the client identify alternatives to work.

Constructive and satisfying use of leisure time does not come easily. Making adequate choices of avocations presents the same problems as making adequate vocational choices. Problems frequently include a lack of knowledge of self, avocational self-concept problems, a lack of knowledge of avocations, a lack of knowledge of community resources, and choice anxiety.

Avocational counseling, sometimes called recreational or leisure time counseling, is beginning to emerge as a distinct body of knowledge and skills. An overall view of philosophy and goals has been prepared by Witt (1973). A model for avocational counseling, paralleling vocational counseling, has been developed by Overs (1970) who developed a system for classifying and coding 800 avocational activities, the Avocational Activities Inventory (1971). Avocational Activities for the Handicapped (Overs, O'Connor, and Demarco, 1974) describes activities in terms of their phenomenological and other psychological dimensions and the social settings in which they occur. Environmental and social-psychological factors are listed for each activity, and impairment tables are provided to show whether a person with a certain type of impairment can do the activity. Energy output tables listing the energy requirements of the activity are useful in determining the suitability of activities for individuals with severe systemic impairments.

At least five avocational interest inventories are currently available (Hartlage, 1968; Hubert, 1969; McKechnie, 1972; D'Agostini, 1972; and Mirenda, 1973). The inventories developed by D'Agostini and Mirenda were based on the Overs' avocational activity classification system. The Hubert inventory was based on Kaplan's leisure typology (1960), with some modifications based on empirical evidence. The McKechnie inventory (1974) was based on an empirically derived cluster system. Hartlage's system (1968) was also derived empirically.

Other avocational choice instruments have been developed by the Research Department, Curative Workshop of Milwaukee: 1) The Avocational Title Card Sort (Overs and Page, 1974), in which the client chooses the activities in which he is interested from over 800 cards, each containing an avocational activity title; 2) the Avocational Picture Card Sort (Overs, Taylor, and Adkins, 1974), in which 163 pictures of avocational activities, classified and coded according to the Avocational Activities Inventory classification, are presented to the client who records on an answer sheet numbers for pictures which represent activities in which he is interested; and 3) a Slide-Projected Picture Sort, which can be used to present the same pictures as those used in the Avocational Picture Card Sort.

Three additional instruments are in early stages of development at the Research Department, Curative Workshop of Milwaukee. An Avocational Magazine Picture Card Sort uses pictures clipped from magazines. Experimental use suggests that, used clinically, it is extremely valuable in eliciting deep-seated feelings and attitudes about avocational activities. The Avocational Plaque Sort is more specialized and consists of samples of craft and collection activities mounted on 6" X 6" plywood plaques. Because this instrument is both concrete and three dimensional, it may be more useful in stimulating choices among certain types of clients, such as the blind, those with low vision, and the mentally retarded. The Milwaukee Avocational Satisfaction Questionnaire, adapted from the Manual for the Minnesota Satisfaction Questionnaire (Weiss et al., 1967), is a 24-item, five-step instrument to measure how well clients like the avocational activities they are pursuing. In addition to being an evaluation tool, it shows promise for use in determining what satisfactions are most important in which activities.

In summary, these varied instruments can be used to assist the handicapped in finding meaningful involvement in avocational activities. As these instruments become more sophisticated, avocational counseling with the handicapped will make a significant contribution to rehabilitation.

INSTRUMENTS VERSUS CRITERIA: RATING CRITERIA

All instruments listed above were rated by the authors on the selection criteria. Ratings by consensus and pertinent information on reading level and validity scales are presented in Table 1.

The purpose of each inventory was rated as plus (+) if it were clearly stated in the test manual. If the manual did not contain this information, the instrument received a minus (−) rating. Test-retest reliability was assessed for each inventory. Ratings were determined as follows: plus (+), test-retest reliability coefficients of 0.69 and above; minus (−), coefficients lower than 0.69; zero (0), reliability information not presented in the test manual.

Construct, concurrent, and predictive validity were assessed for each instrument. Ratings for construct validity were established as follows: plus (+), factor analysis studies available and/or instrument developed on sound theoretical base; minus (−), construct validity evidence available but limited; zero (0), information not available. Concurrent validity ratings were as follows: plus (+), evidence indicates significant relationship to existing, well established instruments, such as the SVIB or Kuder's, or with external criteria; minus (−), evidence available but limited; zero (0), information not available. Predictive validity ratings were as follows: plus (+), adequate evidence of predictive validity; minus (−), evidence available but limited; zero (0), information not available.

Ratings for appropriate adolescent and adult (age 18 and older) norms were defined as follows: plus (+), available; minus (−), available but limited; zero (0), no information. For readability level, the recommended minimum reading level is given if available; zero ratings indicate that this information was not available. The criterion of appropriate validity scales was rated as plus (+) if a validity scale was described in the test manual. On this criterion, a zero (0) rating indicates that validity scales information was not available in the manual.

Initially, the authors also intended to rate each instrument on its appropriateness for various disability groups. It rapidly became apparent, however, that the vast majority of instruments reviewed posed the same limitations for specific disability groups and that a listing of limitations would prove to be extremely redundant. All paper and pencil inventories reviewed necessitate hand and finger dexterity if the client is to take the instrument himself following standardized directions. Persons with motor paralysis or severe dysfunction cannot take these instruments unassisted. With the exception of Bauman's (1973) and Bauman and Hayes' (1951) work with the blind, the effects of reading vocational inventories to clients who cannot physically handle the test materials have received little research attention. Bauman's work is particularly important in view of the fact that few of the inventories reviewed are appropriate in their current forms for blind or partially sighted clients. It is hoped that Bauman's (1973) new instrument will meet this crucial need; see Chapter 14 for further information on this instrument.

The majority of vocational inventories also are inappropriate for the mentally retarded, illiterate persons, and persons with limited reading abilities. The pictorial inventories, especially the Vocational Interest and Sophistication Assessment (Parnicky, Kahn, and Burdett, 1968), will offer promise for these clients if further research substantiates their effectiveness. Finally, the use of vocational inventories for clients from differing cultural and experiential backgrounds has received little research attention. The counselor must exercise caution in administering to these clients instruments designed for and standardized on the dominant white culture.

Table 1. Evaluation of vocational inventories on selection criteria

Instrument	Purpose	Test-retest reliability	Validity			Norms		Readability level	Validity scale
			Construct	Concurrent	Predictive	Adolescent	Adult		
Strong Vocational Interest Blank									
Men	+	+	0	+	+	0	+	9th grade	+
Women									
Strong-Campbell Interest Inventory	+	+	+	+	0	0	+	6th grade	+
Kuder Preference Record (C)	+	+	+	-	0	+	+	9th grade	+
Kuder Occupational Interest Survey (DD)	+	+	+	+	0	-	+	6th grade	+
Kuder General Interest Survey (E)	+	+	+	0	0	+	-	6th grade	+
Minnesota Vocational Interest Inventory	+	+	0	+	0	0	+	9th grade	0
Vocational Preference Inventory	+	+	+	+	0	0	+	0	+
The Self-Directed Search	+	0	+	0	0	-	0	8th grade	0
Ohio Vocational Interest Survey	+	+	-	0	0	+	-	8th grade	+

Test								Grade
California Occupational Preference Survey	+	+	+	-	0	-	-	0	0
Occupational Interest Inventory	+	+	-	-	0	+	+	0	7th grade
Guilford-Zimmerman Interest Inventory	+	0	-	0	0	0	-	0	0
Gordon Occupational Checklist	+	+	-	0	0	-	0	0	8th grade
The Geist Picture Interest Inventory	+	+	-	+	0	-	-	0	NA[1]
Picture Interest Inventory	+	+	+	+	-	+	+	0	NA[1]
Vocational Interest and Sophistication Assessment	+	+	+	-	0	+	+	0	NA[1]
Allport-Vernon-Lindzey Study of Values	-	+	+	-	-	+	+	0	12th grade
The Hall Occupational Orientation Inventory	+	+	+	+	-	-	-	+	0
Super's Work Values Inventory	+	+	+	+	0	+	0	0	8th grade
Career Maturity Inventory	+	-	+	+	0	+	-	0	6th grade
Career Development Inventory	+	-	+	+	0	-	-	0	6th grade
Cognitive Vocational Maturity Tests	+	0	0	+	0	0	0	0	2nd grade

[1] NA=not applicable.

156   Harmon, Sharma, and Trotter

REFERENCES

Association for Measurement Evaluation in Guidance Commission on Sex Bias in Measurement: AMEG Commission report on sex bias in interest measurement. 1973. Meas. Eval. Guidance 6:171–177.

Barnette, W. L., Jr., and J. N. McCall. 1964. Validation of the Minnesota Vocational Interest Inventory for vocational high school boys. J. Appl. Psych. 48:378–382.

Bauman, M. K. 1973. An interest inventory for the visually handicapped. Vis. Handicap. 5:78–83.

Bauman, M. K., and S. P. Hayes. 1951. A Manual for the Psychological Examination of the Adult Blind. Psychological Corp., New York.

Bradley, A. D. 1958. Estimating success in technical and skilled trade courses using multivariate statistical analysis. Doctoral thesis, University of Minnesota, Minneapolis.

Brown, F. G. 1970. Principles of Educational and Psychological Testing. Dryden Press, Hinsdale, Ill.

Campbell, D. P. 1971. Handbook for the Strong Vocational Interest Blank. Stanford University Press, Stanford.

Campbell, D. P. 1966. Strong Vocational Interest Blank Manual, Revised from E. K. Strong, Jr. Stanford University Press, Stanford.

Campbell, D. P. 1974. Strong Vocational Interest Blank Manual for the Strong-Campbell Interest Inventory T325, Merged Form. Stanford University Press, Stanford.

Campbell, D. P. 1969. 1969 Supplement to the SVIB Manual. Stanford University Press, Stanford.

Campbell, D. P., and J. L. Holland. 1972. A merger in vocational interest research: Applying Holland's theory to Strong's data. J. Vocat. Behav. 2:353–376.

Campbell, D. P., and R. W. Trockman. 1963. A verification scale for the Minnesota Vocational Interest Inventory. J. Appl. Psych. 47:276–279.

Clark, K. E. 1961. Vocational Interests of Nonprofessional Men. University of Minnesota Press, Minneapolis.

Clark, K. E., and D. P. Campbell. 1965. Manual: MVII. Psychological Corp., New York.

Crites, J. O. 1973a. Career Maturity Inventory: Administration and Use Manual. CTB/McGraw-Hill, Monterey.

Crites, J. O. 1973b. Career Maturity Inventory: Theory and Research Handbook. CTB/McGraw-Hill, Monterey.

Cronbach, L. J. 1960. Essentials of Psychological Testing. 2nd Ed. Harper and Brothers, New York.

D'Agostini, N. D. 1972. Avocational Interest Index. Sutter Community Hospitals, Sacramento.

Hartlage, L. C. 1968. Avocational Guidance, Inc. Indiana University, Indianapolis.

Holland, J. L. 1973. Making Vocational Choices: A Theory of Careers. Prentice-Hall, Englewood Cliffs, N.J.

Holland, J. L. 1973. The Self-Directed Search. Consulting Psychologists Press, Palo Alto.

Hubert, E. E. 1969. The development of an inventory of leisure interests. Thesis, University of North Carolina. University Microfilm Inc., Ann Arbor.

Johansson, C. B., and L. W. Harmon. 1972. Strong Vocational Interest Blank: One form or two? J. Counsel. Psych. 19:404–410.

Johnson, R. W., and D. E. St. John. 1970. Use of the Minnesota Vocational Interest Inventory in educational planning with community college "career" students. Vocat. Guid. Quart. 19:90–96.

Kaplan, M. 1960. Leisure in America: A Social Inquiry. Wiley, New York.

Kauppi, D. R., and D. J. Weiss. 1969. Comparison of single item and triad verification keys for the MVII. Research report no. 24, work adjustment project, University of Minnesota, 1969. Also, abstract proceedings of the 77th Annual Convention, 4:149. American Psychological Assoc.

Kuder, G. F. 1966, 1970, 1971. Kuder DD Occupational Interest Survey General Manual. Science Research Assoc., Chicago.

Kunce, J. T. 1969. Vocational interest, disability, and rehabilitation. Rehab. Counsel. Bull. 12:204–210.

McKechnie, G. E. Leisure Activities Blank (LAB). Consulting Psychologists Press, Palo Alto. (In press.)

McKechnie, G. E. 1972. A study of environmental life styles. Unpublished doctoral dissertation, University of California at Berkeley.

Mirenda, J. J. 1973. Mirenda Avocational Interest Finder. Marquette University, Milwaukee.

Overs, R. P. 1971. Avocational activities inventory, no. 5A. In Milwaukee Media for Rehabilitation Research Reports Series. Curative Workshop, Milwaukee.

Overs, R. P. 1970. A model for avocational counseling. J. Health Phys. Ed. Recreat. 41:36–38.

Overs, R. P., E. O'Connor, and B. Demarco. 1974. Avocational Activities for the Handicapped. Charles C Thomas, Springfield, Ill.

Overs, R. P., and C. M. Page. 1974. Avocational title card sort. no. 5F. In Milwaukee Media for Rehabilitation Research Reports Series. Curative Workshop, Milwaukee.

Overs, R. P., S. Taylor, and C. Adkins. 1974. Avocational Counseling in Milwaukee. Final report on project H233466, no. 5D. Curative Workshop, Milwaukee.

Parnicky, J. J., H. Kahn, and A. D. Burdett. 1968. Standardization of the Vocational Interest and Sophistication Assessment (VISA): A Reading-Free Test for Retardates. Johnstone Training and Research Center, Bordentown, N.J.

Parnicky, J. J., H. Kahn, and A. D. Burdett. 1969. Standardization of the VISA (Vocational Interest and Sophistication Assessment) Technique. Abstract Proceedings of the 77th Annual Convention. Vol. 4, p. 165–166. American Psychological Assoc.

Parnicky, J. J., H. Kahn, and A. Burdett. 1971. Standardization of the (VISA) Vocational Interest and Sophistication Assessment Technique. Amer. J. Men. Defic. 75:442–448.

Parnicky, J. J., and D. M. Presnell. 1973. Interest inventories and the retarded client. (Unpublished manuscript).

Shah, V. 1969. Work values and job satisfaction. Unpublished doctoral dissertation, Teachers College, Columbia University, New York.

Singer, S. A., and B. Stefflre. 1954. The relationship of job values and desires to vocational aspirations of adolescents. J. Appl. Psych. 38:419–422.

Super, D. E. 1973. The work values inventory. In D. E. Zytowski (ed.), Contemporary Approaches to Interest Measurement, Chapt. 8. University of Minnesota Press, Minneapolis.

Super, D. E., and H. Kaplan. 1967. Work values of school counselors attending NDEA summer guidance institutes. Pers. Guid. J. 46:27–31.

Tiedeman, D. V. 1972. Review of Super's Work Values Inventory. In O. K. Buros (ed.), The Seventh Mental Measurement Yearbook. Gryphon Press, Highland Park, N.J.

Weiss, D. J., R. V. Dawis, G. W. England, and L. H. Lofquist. 1967. Manual for the Minnesota Satisfaction Questionnaire. In Minnesota Studies in Vocational Rehabilitation. Vol. 22. University of Minnesota, Minneapolis.

Witt, P. 1973. Leisure Counseling and Leisure Education Resource Kit. University of Ottawa, Ottawa, Ont.

Zytowski, D. G. 1968. Relationships of equivalent interest scales on three inventories. Pers. Guid. J. 47:44–49.

Zytowski, D. G. 1969. A test of criterion group sampling errors in two comparable interest inventories. Meas. Eval. Guid. 2:37–40.

III
APPLICATIONS
IN REHABILITATION

⑨ Diagnostic Assessment in Rehabilitation

Diagnostic assessment in rehabilitation is different from diagnostic assessment or testing in other contexts. Exactly why this seems to be the case will be elaborated on in the section of this chapter concerning the purposes, procedures, processes, and goals of such assessment.

PURPOSE OF DIAGNOSTIC ASSESSMENT

In working with clients who present themselves or who are presented as candidates for rehabilitation, the basic purpose is to assist in finding and exploring potentially viable habilitation alternatives. So stated, it is obvious that evaluative testing, while it has a critical role in the total effort, does not have an exclusive role.

It might be helpful to elaborate on this. When tests are used for selection purposes, as in personnel selection contexts, they are used to select the more promising candidates and to exclude the less promising (always running the risk of poor acceptances, false positives, and of poor rejections, false negatives). In the rehabilitation context, tests are not used with a purpose of exclusion; rather, they are used, first, to assess the client's particular strengths and weaknesses, and on the basis of such indicators to attempt to work toward a program that "plays to his strengths."

Second, diagnostic assessment in rehabilitation is not simply classificatory. Categories derived from other contexts, however well validated and useful in those contexts, do not inevitably, let alone

161

precisely, have any easily or directly applicable implications for the rehabilitation efforts with a particular client. It may be important to know, from the interview or the history, that this client is a schizophrenic in remission, or that he has an educational history of intellectual retardation, or that he is a stroke victim, but these are rubrics that may specify the problem without definitively prescribing the solution. Attempting to find and to implement a solution is the domain of the total rehabilitative process. Assessment has a role in defining some of the significant variables in that process.

PROCEDURES OF DIAGNOSTIC ASSESSMENT

The exposition of procedures might well begin with some specification of what diagnostic assessment is not. It is not simply "objective testing," however objective and well validated the tests and procedures may be. Good objective tests may be helpful in suggesting promising leads to follow in ability, aptitude, or interest terms. Such suggestive leads are filtered through the subjective impressions and receptivity toward them of the client on whose behalf the efforts are being made. This is but another way of stating the recognition that although the client need not be totally in accord with all such leads, active resistance or objection must be addressed and resolved if optimal cooperation and full participation in the program are to be achieved. This point is made here because it is often the case that, with good objective tests, there is a strong and understandable inclination to view their findings as absolute truths, which may still be a long way from making them workable truths in a fundamental, pragmatic sense.

In a related sense, the assessment is not an "examination" of the client. Examination is a one-way process, and to so view diagnostic assessment in the rehabilitation context would be not only to unduly limit the procedure but also to subject it to possible unnecessary error. The client, faced with an examination situation, will be much influenced not only to put his best foot forward but to present his best aspect. In a recent study conducted by the Chicago Jewish Vocational Service (Gellman, 1974), it was noted that clients in this project "overwhelmingly stated that they would prefer to work even if the job were not steady, was low-paying, had no future, was not interesting or was dirty" (p. 32). By contrast, "Most clients did not impress the counselors as having (such) strong motivation to work. Only 22 per cent were characterized as having very strong work motivations" (p. 34). This citation is relevant here to underline the social desirability aspects of response that may operate to produce bias in the picture presented under conditions where social desirability considerations exert a strong influence on the respondent. An orientation that stresses examination as the basic function maximizes these influences, particularly when failure on such an examination carries with it the threat or the consequence of exclusion from, or forfeiture of, some desirable outcome or state, such as a particular job, the promise of help, some kind of recognition, or some kind of resulting status. Of course, no evaluation procedure, particularly a formalized one such as a test, can be free of such considerations nor can it be entirely without some stress. No professional charged with a diagnostic assessment can, by simple fiat or by good intentions, completely exclude for the client the stress that is part of trying to do one's best in a challenging task situation. His own orientation that he can convey to his client may serve, however, to minimize some of the atypicality or nonrepresentativeness of response that a hard-nosed examination atmosphere promotes. In the rehabilitation context, the interest is not in some peak performance but rather in a level of consistent and sustainable performance. An analogy might serve as an illustration of this consideration. In rehabilitation the interest is usually in such things as whether the client can stand on his feet for an 8-hour day, rather than in whether he can run 100 yards in 10 seconds.

For many of the reasons cited above, assessment is not an "evaluation" in any pass-fail sense. In a context of "playing to the strengths" of the client, evaluation has some selective consequences, but these do not select for or against the client; rather, they select for or against areas of emphasis for exploration and/or development. This is an important distinction. It is the underlying basis upon which a cooperative effort between client and professional can be mounted with the understanding that assessment is a useful avenue for furnishing, in a relatively short time and with relative economy, information concerning promising directions for exploration and development. Even when the client's understanding is less than complete, it can be furthered by the accretion or accumulation of concrete specifics, all informed by the cooperative orientation toward the enterprise promoted by the involved professional or professionals.

Finally, assessment is not even an inventory-taking in terms of achievement as an end product, a compendium of discrete skills or specialized abilities or personality traits favorable or unfavorable to some goal. No simple listing can encompass the dynamic aspects that are crucial to the rehabilitation process, such as that subtle blend of factors that are classified as the client's "motivation," the amounts and kinds of support that can be made available to him and that he can utilize, the shoring up of his viable defenses and the "variables" often critical to his successful rehabilitation that are intuited rather than measured objectively or even assessed unambiguously.

All of the above strictures concerning what diagnostic assessment is *not* must be understood as indicating that it is not any one of these alone. In varying degree, assessment may selectively utilize all of the above described procedures in cooperation with the client and/or his counselor. The point to be made in all of the above is that the overall perspective must be more inclusive than any single component element, each of which may play a useful and helpful contributory role in the process.

The armamentarium of the professional concerned with diagnostic assessment will now be considered in a classificatory context. Many of the chapters in this text detail specific instruments in that armamentarium. For the purposes of this chapter, they will be divided into short-term versus long-term procedures, or brief versus extended evaluation. The short-term procedures are analogous to a snap-shot description, whereas the extended procedures can be considered descriptive of process, of change and development, as sequences of snap-shots.

Short-term Procedures

The Intake Interview and Life History Under the short-term procedures are included the following techniques or activities: first, the intake interview and history taking. One's past may not necessarily be the best or most reliable indicator of the future. In fact, the rehabilitative enterprise may be viewed as a concerted attempt to modify, if not precisely reverse, such rigid determinism. However, everyone has a highly individual life history that conditions the further extrapolation of discernible trends in that life history, as well as conditioning the revision of such trends.

For the purposes of assessment, the impact of life history items individually and in combination are to help understand the client as a particular individual, to generate hypotheses or hunches concerning him that will further the understanding of him as a person. For example, the client's father died when he was 9 years old. The effects of such an item can fluctuate widely depending upon the total context. To conjecture freely but not all-inclusively, it will make a difference if there had been a grandfather in the picture who helped to fill the gap in the family structure. It will make a difference if and when a step-father became part of the picture, and what kind of person he was to the client. The reader can generate quite readily another half dozen factors conditioning the effect that the loss of a father at age 9 may have had.

The important point to be emphasized is that such potentially influential items, while in themselves highly specific, are, in their implications, highly conjectural. One can wander far afield unless conjectures are checked out by supportive additional data, both from the life history as a kind of internal consistency check and from conversation with the client or from related data that might be obtained, for instance, from a sentence completion test.

Taking a good intake interview and history is the indispensible first step in the process of rehabilitation. The questions raised in this first step will in part determine the answers to be sought in the subsequent assessment procedures.

Test Administration and Interpretation   The second large category included in short-term procedures is test administration and interpretation, which in turn includes the preparation for the task, observation and recording of the performance, scoring and interpretation, and finally, elaborating the implications of the findings.

The preparation for the task encompasses not only preliminary notification that testing is in prospect, but also some preliminary discussion of what the purposes of the various tests are and, where possible, what kinds of questions relevant to the client's rehabilitation will be answered by the testing. In school, in industrial selection, the inclusion of testing is often so routine and expected as to require no explanation. This is not a useful assumption to make in the rehabilitation context. At the very least it may be conducive to a passivity, to a more or less willing submission to procedures visited upon the client without fostering either insight or curiosity concerning their relevance, thereby promoting disengagement. At the worst it may present a kind of vaguely sensed threat, a necessary obstacle that the client must encounter if he is to prove himself worthy or deserving of further efforts on his behalf. The specific directions that explain to the client what the task is and how he shall perform it are, therefore, not the first but rather the last step in the procedures of preparing him for the test task.

Observation of the test performance, provided it is an individually administered test rather than a group administered test, involves alertness not only to the scorable aspects of the performance but incidental relevant observations and volunteered information that are not part of the "scorable response." A comment like "Oh wow" can reveal something of the perceived difficulty of the task from the client's point of view.

Idiosyncracies in the content of even "failed" items on particular tests can be informative, often more so than the more readily classifiable correct responses.

The scoring and interpretation of the test responses, particularly with reference to the appropriate norm population, serve to rate the client on the basis of his performance or responses with respect to things such as abilities, interests, personality traits, levels of achievement, etc. Such an objectified rating enables both the client and the counselor to make an assessment of where the client stands or where the client is with respect to a number of variables that are important to the conduct of rehabilitation efforts on his behalf. If he has unusually good finger dexterity it may open up options different from those that may obtain if indeed he has a great deal of difficulty with, and performs poorly on, such an isolated task skill. It should be noted that the scoring and interpretation were characterized as resulting in an objectified "rating." This does not connote the precision of the term "measurement." However, on the one hand, this permits a more realistic appreciation of the assessment procedures themselves while, on the other hand, it gives enough good and reliable information to be adequate to the purposes of the rehabilitation effort.

Thus, the results of any one test, however excellent the test and however skilled the administrator, cannot be the final word. Suitable reservations and/or allowances for error[1] must also be made, as well as changes that may occur over time. Any test interpretation must include this tentative, working hypothesis quality to be maximally useful for rehabilitation purposes.

Elaboration of Test Findings   Third, the process of elaborating the

---

[1] The concept of "error" in psychological measurement is a separate chapter in its history and is a separate two chapters in this volume (Chapters 2 and 3). There is a special sense in which it is considered here, however (Meister, in preparation). In psychological measurement, the traditional tools of assessing validity (and reliability) have been the correlational techniques. In such an orientation, the validity of a test has been considered an attribute of the test, substantiated by studies demonstrating the correlation of the test's scores with the scores on some criterion measure, using a relevant population, i.e., one whose characteristics are "representative" of the population with whom the test will be used in actual testing practice. However, in the single instance ($N = 1$), the considerations of correlation do not apply.

Von Neuman (1951, 1956) suggested that probabilistic considerations might apply for components that cannot be completely error free. In a test situation, replication of testing with different but comparable tests is suggested for the single case. In the diagnostic assessment context of rehabilitation, probabilistic validation considerations are achieved by considering the process of assessment as one of successive approximations, i.e., the replication of findings is achieved by extending those findings over time.

implications of the test "findings" not only shades into but, in a functional sense, may be inseparable from elaborating or evolving a plan to guide exploration of rehabilitation alternatives. This aspect is considered more explicitly in the section on the diagnostic process.

Long-term Procedures

The longer term procedures that play a critical role in the carrying out of rehabilitation efforts include assessment tools such as Work Sample Evaluation, On-site or Vestibule Evaluation, and Work Shop Performance. They are the subject of a detailed consideration in the next chapter of this text. However, because they must be considered an integral aspect of diagnostic assessment in rehabilitation, some of their characteristics bearing on assessment should receive attention here.

Work Sample Evaluation   Although the evaluation of work samples may extend over a period as long as 2 weeks to provide ratings on all of the samples included in such a battery, work samples may be more properly considered as a short-term technique in terms of their findings and the limitations on their findings. A particular task item may take as long as several hours, and it does represent performance over time as contrasted with the generally short time spans of conventional tests. However, these samples do share the limitation of any one-shot, time-limited look at a performance that is without implications for the kind of sustained performance required of actual competitive work that requires between 7 and 8 hours a day, 5 days a week, month in and month out. They can suggest general areas of promises and comparative skill and aptitude, i.e., suggest where the client may begin to seek either a job or job training.

In general work sample evaluations are adequate for making good and pertinent suggestions for such general areas of exploration. But the work sample evaluation as an assessment technique in terms of refinement of performance criteria and precision of norming and most especially in terms of validating studies is in the infancy of its development. It should not be judged by the same standards that are applied to well accepted psychometric instruments.

Finally, from the standpoint of diagnostic assessment, the work samples involve single performances. Thus, they are, psychologically speaking, a short-term technique as they apply to the client and his orientation, even though in programming treatment they may extend over a longer period of time.

On-site or Vestibule Evaluation   The really long-term assessment procedures include not only aspects of evaluation but also of on-site training as well. This is not so much a contamination or confounding of function as it is a reflection of the fact that actual working is an integrated experience for the client that may serve, differentially, assessment and training purposes. This chapter, of course, deals with the assessment aspects. Furthermore, the evaluation conducted in an on-the-job training or vestibule performance is more evaluative than diagnostic; i.e., it is diagnostic for correcting or improving performance in a program to which the client is already committed but not diagnostic in the sense of prescribing rehabilitative procedures.

Work Shop Performance   By comparison, work shop evaluation is a more versatile assessment instrument in the long-term category because it permits a wider range of work assignments, tolerates a wider range of behaviors in an assessment context, and can implement novel and innovative conditions of work. It shall, therefore, serve as the target for this passing commentary on long-term techniques of diagnostic assessment.

In brief, then, an assessment period in a work shop milieu can address the *sustained* aspects of performance as well as critical aspects of job adjustment (not present in the short-term situations), such as regularity of attendance, punctuality, avoidance of the appearance of idleness, adequate productivity of adequate quality, and appropriate relations with supervisors and fellow workers; and it can do so under a *planned* variety of work conditions. These considerations apply with special force to clients with a marginal work history and/or limited experience.

THE DIAGNOSTIC PROCESS

Diagnostic assessment in the rehabilitation context is considered a process not only because it extends over time but also, more dynamically, because it attempts to transcend the limitations of a single event assessment of static entities. Thus it provides the opportunity for detecting change and assessing its extent in various categories of client functioning, i.e., it "looks for" improvement.

As such, diagnostic assessment is not only part of the rehabilitation process but also is functionally continuous with that process, and in practice it is inseparable from it. It is oriented toward treatment and always stresses the implications of its findings for treatment. Thus, the paradigmatic question for diagnostic assessment in rehabilitation is this: With these *liabilities* and these *assets,* what can be worked out for this *particular* client at *this* time or stage in *his* life? Diagnostic assessment attempts to make assessments in the first two italicized categories and then to particularize those findings for a program for a specific, indeed, even an idiosyncratic client. In such a context, diagnostic categories from the medical, psychological, and psychiatric areas may be helpful, but they are hardly definitive in any prescriptive-of-procedures sense. "What can be worked out," therefore, is informed by an understanding of the client as he sees himself and as the professional sees him. It is implemented by dedicated, on occasion, innovative, exploration of suggested alternatives with a sharing of conclusions and with a subsequent workable reconciliation of any discrepancies in conclusions. A viable, effective, mutual participation in the rehabilitation effort demands no less than this.

Counselor as Participant-Observer

In carrying out his task of diagnostic assessment, the rehabilitation professional has a combined role of participant-observer. This concept is borrowed from the late Harry Stack Sullivan and comes from a psychiatric context, but it is very much applicable to the assessment context because it involves the interaction of two persons in a psychologically complex and many faceted situation. Diagnostic assessment is not simply a testing situation in which an examiner or observer, after securing "rapport," thereafter presents tasks and observes the client's performance on those tasks. The potential and actual complexity of this interaction has been pointed out in the article on the dynamic and reality factors in the diagnostic testing interview (Schlesinger, 1973).

The implications of such an orientation pervade the entire assessment process, not only in its procedures but also in its findings. Thus, in his concern for objectivity and criterion referencing, the professional must also be aware of his personal, unique contribution to the total interaction and make it an explicit part of the total "evaluation." How did the client see him and how did he respond on the basis of this "sizing up" or evaluation of his evaluator? With another professional, somewhat different perceptions might have occurred for both parties.

Therefore, rather than attempting to be a neutral "sounding board" against which the client gets "fixed" in a sonar analogue fashion, the professional should recognize and selectively utilize a range of role options depending on his perception of the client's needs, those inferred conditions for the client's optimal functioning.

The professional's own observation of the quality of the interaction between himself and the client should be a legitimate part of the assessment, not merely to "make allowances" for sub-optimal conditions, but, more importantly, to specify a context within which the "testing" took place, thereby placing it in perspective. A very distracted client or one who at the time is only marginally engaged should have his overall performance considered in the light of such conditions as they are perceived by the assessor.

The assessment is meaningful and has its ultimate purpose in its contribution to planning a program of rehabilitation. Ideally, therefore, the implications for programming should not be spelled out unilaterally but should engage both the client and/or the client's counselor (if there is such a professional involved who is separate from the assessment person). The assessment should produce some determination of the possible needs of and services required by the client. But before the initial prescription is arrived at, the potential efficacy of the information generated can be improved by contributions of the client and/or his counselor when they can be made available. Expertise, even of the highest order, while it is a most necessary ingredient in effective planning, is not by itself sufficient. Such a view is not a pronouncement of either modesty or reticence; rather, it is an informed perception of the dynamics of the rehabilitation process.

If there is a single pervasive role for the rehabilitation professional, it is one of fostering an open-minded exploration of the client's potentialities, with an enthusiasm restrained by a basic respect[2] for the client.

Continuing Nature of the Diagnostic Process

Earlier, it was suggested that diagnostic assessment is functionally inseparable from the process of rehabilitation. This is a commentary upon the *continuing* nature of the diagnostic process. To assume that diagnostic assessment is an isolated, discrete, once-and-for-all, circumscribed event is to foreclose prematurely on the role it should fulfill. It might most profitably be viewed as a matter of successive approximations informed by the on-going feedback of results and outcomes. In such a process orientation, the initial diagnostic picture forms the basis for a "first step." This is followed by a "trial" (definite in format but tentative in expectations) of the recommendations or procedures derived from the "diagnosis." The trial is characterized by a feed-back on the results of the procedures being tried. The feed-back in turn is integrated into the

---

[2] The word "respect" is used here in the same sense that "acceptance" was used in a psychotherapy context (Meister and Miller, 1946). There, acceptance was defined as a "man-to-man" regard for the client, characterized (ideally) by the understanding of empathy without the erratic quality of identification or the supportiveness of sympathy, a regard characterized by permissiveness and tolerance rather than by agreement (yet without the condescension implied by "permissiveness" and "tolerance"). In that context, the client's perception and report of his behavior, his behavior as perceived by the counselor, and his need to behave as he does are all accepted, i.e., respected as "where the client is at," the position from which all subsequent change and improvement will occur if they are to occur.

diagnostic and rehabilitative process by indicating changes or revisions in the initial recommendations and procedures. This stage forms the "second round" of diagnosis. This same sequence characterizes "rounds of diagnosis" subsequent to the second. All the successive approximations approach the asymptote that is the goal of rehabilitation.

THE GOAL AND ITS REQUIREMENTS

The goal of rehabilitation is always the achievement of some viable, rewarding, self-actualizing "modus vivendi" for the client, whatever the nature, origin, or classification of his presenting difficulty. Its requirements include good, well informed, knowledgeable observation and good descriptive reportage followed by imaginative, creative generation and exploration of prescriptive alternatives. All of these are then integrated into an implementable program of rehabilitation and, finally, the pursuit of that program to some mutually acceptable outcome.

Viewed globally, its requirements are to understand the client and, meaningfully aided by such understanding, to enlist not merely his cooperation but his active participation in all steps of the rehabilitation process. From such a perspective in rehabilitation assessment, *understanding the client,* with all that that phrase implies is "the name of the game."

REFERENCES

Gellman, W. 1974. Changing Career Patterns for the Vocationally Disadvantaged in a Polyethnic, Multicultural Model Cities Area: Final Report. Jewish Vocational Service, Chicago.

Meister, R. K., and H. E. Miller. 1946. Dynamics of nondirective psychotherapy. J. Clin. Psych. 2:59—67.

Meister, R. K. 1974. Validity considerations in the limiting case of n = 1. (In preparation.)

Schlesinger, H. J. 1973. Interaction of dynamic and reality factors in the diagnostic testing interview. Bull. Menninger Clinic 37:495—518.

von Neumann, J. 1951. The general and logical theory of automata. In L. A. Jeffress (ed.) Cerebral Mechanisms in Behavior: The Hixon Symposium. Wiley, New York.

von Neumann, J. 1956. Probabilistic logics and the synthesis of reliable organisms from unreliable components. In C. E. Shannon and J. McCarthy (eds.), Automata Studies (Annals of Mathematics Studies, No. 34). Princeton University Press, Princeton, N.J.

10 | Vocational Evaluation

WILLIAM GELLMAN and ASHER SOLOFF

Vocational rehabilitation is in a state of rapid transition from an empirical and pragmatic discipline to a theoretical one. A similar movement is occurring in vocational evaluation, though at a much slower rate. The relative dearth of sustained consideration of the theory and principles underlying vocational evaluation practice is striking. The omission of evaluative aspects in developing the theoretical and applied aspects of rehabilitation retards the growth of evaluation at the purely empirical stage. The pragmatic use of methods and techniques results in the accretion of fashionable approaches without appraisal. Evaluators devote their efforts to day-to-day problems at a time when rapid societal changes are transforming the world of work and bringing new types of clients with a variety of problems. Socioeconomic forces are generating an increase in rehabilitation service demands without creating a resource base for meeting service needs. The atheoretical position of vocational evaluation ensures repetition of present practices without increased probability of methodological innovation. There is need for sustained, critical examination of the field of evaluation that will analyze the underlying assumptions and formulate a body of practice principles that will facilitate vocational evaluation's shift from an empirical to an applied discipline.

CURRENT NEED FOR THEORETICAL APPRAISAL

Theory assumes greater importance in a period such as the present in which rehabilitation resources are being stretched to the utmost to meet service demands. A current objective of rehabilitation as defined in the Rehabilitation Act of 1973 is to aid an increasing number of the more

173

severely disabled without a comensurate increase in funding. The ratio of client to service unit is increasing in rehabilitation facilities. At the same time, the possibilities of expanding programs are limited by economic considerations and questions as to the effectiveness of rehabilitation. The result is a continuing drive to improve and to increase service without providing for a proportionate growth in funds to ensure the quality of service.

Concurrently, rehabilitation places an increasing emphasis upon defining and measuring effectiveness of client service and the ability of agencies to reach goals. Agencies and counselors confront the task of establishing priorities for client service and for the use of restricted resources in programming for various categories of clients. Administrators must choose which clients to serve, the extent of service to be given to clients, and the type of program that will maximize the benefits derived by clients. The pressures upon agencies, administrators, and counselors are heightened by conflicting socioeconomic demands and spiraling costs that decrease the benefit-cost ratios of rehabilitation programs.

The demands for increasing and improving client services can be met if rehabilitation were to become more effective. Evaluation can be the key to enhancing the effectiveness of rehabilitation if a body of principles can be formulated that will generate methods for appraising evaluative techniques and improving predictive efficiency. Such principles will be concerned with methods of assessing the rehabilitative potentials of clients, specifying the characteristics of treatment plans, analyzing the nature of vocational adjustment and maladjustment, assessing the properties of pretests, maximizing the predictive validity of appraisals of vocational adjustment, and establishing the premises for analyzing the interrelationship between the client and the work environment. This chapter will outline and examine a theory-based model of vocational evaluation and present the practice principles governing the application of evaluation to rehabilitation clients. The instrumental qualities of evaluation, its orientation toward the goal of facilitating the ability of handicapped persons to become productive, self-sufficient members of society, will be stressed.

GOALS OF VOCATIONAL EVALUATION

The goal of vocational rehabilitation is the enablement of the handicapped client to become more productive until he is able to function adequately in achievement-demanding work settings. The activity may be remunerative or nonremunerative. Vocational evaluation's primary role in the enablement process is to speed the client's vocational development toward this productive goal. Evaluation accomplishes this task by observing the client as a vocational man and by generating a picture of his work personality, thereby permitting determination of his work potential and of the nature of his future interaction with the possible work environments.

The instrumental character of vocational evaluation, with respect to the rehabilitation goal, dictates a future orientation for evaluative observations and conclusions. A second purpose is to preview the client's future work behavior, using a workshop or a work setting as an experimental laboratory, and to predict the nature and extent of the client's vocational development. The prism for observing and analyzing the client's behavior in workshops and work settings is the question of what changes will occur. The future perspective in evaluation directs the evaluator's attention toward questions such as 1) whether a client will be able to work, 2) what type of work he will be able to undertake, 3) what type of adjustment he will make in the work settings in which he will function, and 4) what types of training will actualize his work potential. These areas of examination for forecasting purposes subsume the factors typically considered in evaluation, such as skills, aptitudes, motivation, abilities, and physical capacities. Evaluation's predictive aim integrates both types of data in terms of projected changes in the client's work behavior and the factors influencing the client's vocational development and maturation.

A third aim of evaluation is to specify client behavioral patterns in various types of work or training situations and the level of his adjustment in such situations. This is done by means of predictive equations that are a statement of the client's interaction with a work environment. The differential predictions are hypotheses about client work behavior in typical work settings. The equations are posed in the if-so-then format, i.e., if X occurs, then the client will behave in Y manner. By specifying the situational conditions in the work environment and the relevant inter-personal dimensions, one can examine and forecast the handicapped client's reactions to variations in the social, physical, and productive aspects of the work environment. The hypotheses constituting the skeletal structure of the equation are subject to verification at both the workshop and the competitive employment levels. Quasi-experimental designs may be used to test the validity and predictive power of the equation in workshops and in work settings.

The preparation of a treatment plan for a client is a fourth goal of evaluation. The plan serves as a chart for selecting programs to shape a client's work behavior in conformity to culturally acceptable work roles. A treatment plan for the work adjustment phase presupposes that the evaluator will have obtained the following information: 1) knowledge of the client's work personality, including its developmental possibilities, 2) estimates of the impact upon the work personality of a loss or injury, 3) determinations of the possibilities that the client will compensate for the loss or injury, 4) a projection of the client's future occupational levels, 5) an analysis of his capacity for and ability to profit from vocational training, and 6) a statement of the characteristics of the work environments typical of his projected occupations.

To summarize, the goals of vocational evaluation as an empirical discipline flow from the operational needs of the rehabilitation process, including the achievement of the rehabilitation aim. The goals of vocational evaluation are oriented toward placing the client in productive activity and adjusting him to work. Evaluation's goals necessitate a future perspective in assessing a client's vocational problems and potentials and in preparing a treatment plan. The conclusions derived from the evaluative process are embodied in differential equations that predict client behavior under varying conditions in differing types of work settings. The validity of the evaluative equations is measured by client responses to treatment and by the client's on-the-job adjustment. Formal testing of equations during treatment provides a basis for modifying the equations to improve forecasts of the client's future work adjustment.

THEORETICAL ASSUMPTIONS

Vocational evaluation is an applied discipline using practice principles derived from vocational psychology and vocational rehabilitation. The application of these principles presupposes the use of theoretical variables that can serve as the structural base for carrying out the primary evaluative functions of assessing work potentials and capacities, and formulating a treatment plan for facilitating the client's work adjustment. The theoretical assumptions link the theory of vocational evaluation as derived from vocational psychology with the principles guiding the practice of evaluation in rehabilitation settings.

This section discusses the assumptions that are basic to evaluation in a rehabilitation setting. Theoretically, the evaluative process can be viewed as a method for acquiring information about the goal-oriented, productive behavior of handicapped persons in the work sector. Empirically, vocational evaluation defines the data to be observed and assessed, and it specifies the variables facilitating vocational maturation and adjustment. The techniques used reflect both the assumptions underlying vocational evaluation and its objectives of analyzing the work environment, of assessing the behavioral configuration of capacities, potentials, and attitudes, and of appraising the interaction of the client and the work environment.

Constructs of the Theoretical Variables

The following constructs are suggested as theoretical variables governing the application of vocational evaluation to rehabilitation.

The Work Sector In an industrial society the work sector is differentiated from other specialized societal areas such as home, school, or recreation. The work sector is the subcultural field including productive activities, work, and concomitants or derivatives of work. The work sector is characterized by goal-directed, achievement-oriented behavior using developmentally acquired behavior patterns and skills to attain economic objectives. The term "productive" includes remunerative and nonremunerative activities that society, the client, and the vocational rehabilitation agency see as contributing to the economic well-being of the community.

The Work Personality The work personality is the characteristic pattern of work activity displayed in a work situation or in an achievement-demanding setting. The work personality incorporates work attitudes, behavioral work patterns, value systems, incentives, and abilities—the behavioral configuration regarded as necessary to function effectively in a work setting. It is a personality constellation adapted to allow the person to operate in the job seeking and job choice areas and to enact appropriate work roles in a selected work setting.

Development Aspects The work personality is developmental, that is, acquired during growth. The formation and shaping of the work personality begins in early childhood and continues through the sequence of activities that pattern the growth of infants and young people. In an industrial society, the family furnishes motivation and achievement-oriented values; school and after-school activities provide the prerequisites for industrial know-how and practice in meeting extrafamilial social norms. Summer and part-time jobs provide an introduction to the world of competitive employment. The process of orientation is completed during the first stage of full-time work when the work personality matures.

Work Roles Each culture uses selected types of work personalities as ego models for training, selecting, and rewarding people who are or will become productive. Such socially selected work personalities become typed as the work roles that are deemed appropriate and suitable for the productive system. The work roles are incorporated into various types of work settings and work activities. Each occupational and work situation category has a limited number of work roles that are deemed suitable.

The emphasis of the work society upon appropriate behavioral patterns in work situations reinforces developmental pressures to meet norms and standards. During the developmental period, the work personality prepares for vocational maturity by enacting preparatory work roles that will be consonant with the occupational level and type of work that the person will undertake when he enters the work world. The testing of the work personality tends to take place in those portions of the occupational structure and work areas that are accessible to maturing youth. As the work personality develops, it integrates stimulus and response cues into its work role repertoires, which facilitate adaptation to the social expectations and productive demands of coworkers and supervisors.

Job Adjustment   The level of adjustment in a work environment is a function of the degree of compatibility between the work role potentials of the disabled client (work personality) and the work role demands of the work environment.

Work Environment   The work environment conjoins, first, the work activity system with its demands for competencies and skills; second, the physical setting with its relevant physical demands and capacities; and third, the social function with its web of relationships to coworkers and supervisors. The work roles, as enacted by the employees in the work situation, embody the characteristics and behavior deemed minimally adequate or suitable for the particular work environment.

Continuity of Work Personality   The primary task of vocational evaluation, the projection from present to future work behavior, assumes the continuity of the work personality. In the absence of major changes in the psychological substructure or in the work environment, the work personality observed in a workshop or in a work assessment program will resemble that work personality exhibited in industrial work settings. The developmental trends that created and adapted the work personality for a given band of work positions persist into maturity and continue to maintain and to shape work behavior and attitudes. Because work personalities are modifiable, evaluation should be viewed as a continuing analysis of intraindividual and extraindividual change-agents that may alter developmental trends in a client's work personality.

WORK ENVIRONMENT AND WORK PERSONALITY

The most direct way of theorizing about the relationships between work environments and work personality is by categorizing both constructs in the same dimensions. In order to assess a client's potential for performance in a given setting it is necessary to ask how each of the attributes of his work personality, and how the pattern of attributes that uniquely characterize him, relates to the demand characteristics of that environment. Conversely, it is necessary to relate demand characteristics to potential worker attributes (including work personality attributes) in order to select persons most likely to perform well in particular environments. When the same dimensions are employed for both constructs, measurements that suggest or buttress or question evaluation decisions are possible.

Needs and Press Congruent Measurement

A general procedure for categorizing personality and context dimensions in the same terms and for measuring degrees of correspondence and difference was developed by Stern, Stein, and Bloom (1956) and continued by Stern (1970). Basing their work on the psychological theories of Henry Murray, Stern and his associates constructed and tested instruments for the simultaneous measurements of "needs" and "press." Needs were the dimension of personality, press the dimensions of environmental pressures. Stern (1970) devised and used scales for measuring press in several types of settings, thus offering a general approach to building measurement procedures to index environmental demands and congruent dimensions of personality.

The closest approximation in rehabilitation research to Stern's model is that offered by the Work Adjustment Project at the University of Minnesota (Lofquist and Dawis, 1969). Based on a theory of work adjustment (Chapter 13), this group has provided congruent scales for measuring work needs and work environments. They have also provided outcome scales using the same dimensions as used in the need and environment scales. These instruments are imbedded in a system for choosing optimal work environments for people with specified work needs and for choosing modal need patterns for success in specific work settings. The Minnesota group has generated Occupational Reinforcer Patterns to fit need patterns. They have not yet, so far as we know, studied the relations between actual work settings and worker needs.

Their Job Description Questionnaire (Borgen et al., 1968) provides a set of 21 categories for describing and analyzing work environments. These categories are equivalent to the 21 need categories that appear in the Minnesota Importance Questionnaire (Gay et al., 1971). While 21 categories provide a good opportunity to study demand patterns that fit need patterns, there are too many categories for a useful analytical characterization of major types of work environments to build on in a theory of vocational evaluation.

An alternative set of "person" categories to which a reasonable set of environmental categories could be matched were derived from A Scale of Employability for Handicapped Persons (Gellman, Stern, and Soloff, 1963). A factor analysis of the Workshop Scale (the scale in which work behavior was directly described) yielded the following independent categories: 1) attitudinal conformity to work life, 2) speed of production, 3) maintenance of quality, 4) acceptance of work demands, and 5) interpersonal security.

A classification for work environments congruent with this list of client qualities would be one in which each dimension varied from high to low in the degree to which a work setting demanded. It can be assumed that all work settings require a minimum degree of capacity in each dimension, but settings will vary in the pattern of demands required for success.

It is important to recognize both the qualitative and the quantitative distinctions among work environments. Patterns of work demands are frequently qualitatively distinct and may best be responded to by groups of people whose patterns of needs and competencies are equivalently distinct. Each pattern is, however, a consequence of quantitative differences in the demand levels of one or more dimensions. This relationship between qualitative and quantitative differences is necessary when one defines both environment and person along the same dimensions.

The vocational evaluator must be concerned with two classifications of work environment, the first corresponding to the types of work situations that may be available for clients after rehabilitation. The second is a classification of rehabilitative work environments. The evaluator must be prepared to structure workshop environments so as to contribute to changes deemed desirable for clients and to provide settings in which a client's readiness to change can be assessed.

Establishing work environments for rehabilitative and evaluative purposes demands a great deal of flexibility. The evaluator or rehabilitator must not only relate work demands to client needs; he must also distinguish, as much as he is able, the work environments of different clients in the same workshop. The latter task is difficult to do with any degree of planning, but it may appear more possible if one realizes that variations in supervisory practice represent variations in work demands. To some degree all clients (and all workers in competitive settings) are subject to different environments. Beginning with that recognition, a taxonomy needs to be developed that can aid in specifying the characteristics of the environment needed to bring about the desired change in a client with specific characteristics.

It is not always easy to construct meaningful congruent scales to measure work personality and work environments. There are demand characteristics of work environments that can be stated as personality characteristics in only the most superficial way. Scales based on relatively superficial personality statements are more useful for theory testing with many clients than for evaluating (specifying the problems and suggesting solutions for) individual clients. Also, there are aspects of environment, such as degree of centralization and amount of job differentiation, that might have consequences for which congruent work personality items can be written but for which there are not likely to be direct translations into personality terms. The construct of work role, described in an earlier section, helps to bridge the conceptual gap.

The term "work role," like the term "role" generally, places the person in the environment. Any person's work role represents the integration of all the influences that bear upon him in performing the functions of his position. It reflects not only work personality and environment, which are measurable momentary states, but also the more general processes of vocational development, personal development, and institutional development, which serve as "ground" for the current situation. It also reflects the forces that control the integration of work personality and work environment about which less is known than either personality or environment.

Work Role Deficiency Measurement

An alternative to congruent scaling and the characterization of work problems by the "degree of fit" between measured work personality and work environments is the characterization of work problems according to work role deficiencies. Such a classification is presented in Table 1, which is adapted from a previous statement by Gellman (1973), relating the problems on a theoretical basis to vocational development and the goals around which the work personality is organized. Columns 2, 3, and 4 have separate but intertwined implications for treatment. A goal for evaluation is to distinguish the problem so as to select an environmental procedure that will optimize the chances of overcoming it. At this point in the understanding of work programs, it is an open question whether all types of work role problems can be successfully handled in the same setting.

The measurement problems inherent in this schema are more complicated than those that are derived from theories that can be

Table 1. Classification of the vocationally disadvantaged[1]

(1) Type of vocational deficiency	(2) Its work role problem	(3) Level of vocational development	(4) Goal orientation of work personality
Vocationally arrested	Unable to function on a protracted basis because of inner goal conflict	Limited but able to progress	Subculture and dominant work culture
Vocationally maladjusted	Unable to function because of goal conflict with work culture	Complete	Subculture
Vocationally displaced	Unable to function because of loss of occupational skill	Complete	Dominant work culture
Vocationally nonadjusted	Unable to function because of lack of vocational development	Limited	Work personality partially formed from dominant work culture

[1] Adapted from Gellman (1973).

reflected by congruent scales. Both congruent and noncongruent scales are needed, and a procedure for integrating them in the manner suggested by the chart is called for.

SOME EMPIRICAL WORK

Much of the measurement work and a number of the innovations introduced at the Chicago Jewish Vocational Service (CJVS) involving vocational evaluation have derived from and were fed back into the approach to evaluation described in this chapter. The content of A Scale of Employability for Handicapped Persons (Gellman, Stern, and Soloff, 1963) was based on several of the theoretical constructs suggested previously. The results of the factorial study provided some dimensions of work personality that can serve as the basis for evaluating clients. Other results made it clear that work personality dimensions unrelated to other constructs, such as potential work settings, provide weak predictions of employment success, even if the levels of prediction are statistically significant.

Subsequent studies using employability scales adapted from the original Scale demonstrated that work personality can change in therapeutic work settings among mentally retarded adolescents (Shulman, 1967), disturbed adolescents (Chicago Jewish Vocational Service, 1969), and older workers (Soloff and Bolton, 1969). Unfortunately, no effort was made in any of these studies to characterize or to measure work environments. The factors promoting change were identified only through informed speculation by service staff and were not systematically related to the degree of change in aspects or dimensions of work personality.

Chicago Jewish Vocational Service Observation Manual

The interrelatedness for evaluation purposes of the many theoretical and empirical constructs mentioned in this chapter has been underscored by two projects conducted by the CJVS Research Utilization Laboratory (Chicago Jewish Vocational Service, 1974). The purpose of the CJVS-RUL was to devise, test, and disseminate innovations based on knowledge derived from research to be used by direct service personnel in vocational rehabilitation settings. The first innovation was an Observation Manual designed to help floor supervisors in rehabilitation and sheltered workshops evaluate work problems and work potentials for clients (Soloff, Goldston, and Pollack, 1972). The Manual and the guide that accompanies it describe behavior that is likely to be associated with successful post-program work performance. The 12 activities to which attention is drawn in the Manual include several that have to do with client-supervisor relationships, several that occur in client-peer relationships, and several that describe the client's personal efforts. The floor supervisor is helped to recognize and to interpret client behavior in the 12 areas. He is provided with a set of simple scales by which to measure client behavior in each area, and he is encouraged to relate the evaluations he makes to planning for subsequent client services.

The choice of areas was entirely empirical, the intent being to illustrate how one might develop a systematic evaluation procedure by observing work in a workshop. Theory-building was going on from the perspective of a practitioner, nevertheless. A systematic framework that could be applied to observing and interpreting client behavior was provided. Attention was drawn to specific areas of behavior that set the major terms in which all clients had to be analyzed and evaluated. Measurement was simultaneously taking place because definitions for use in differentiating kinds of behavior were provided, and degrees of performance in each area were required.

It was from reports on experiences in using the Observation Manual that the need for systematic consideration of interrelations among evaluation goals, rehabilitation process, and the theoretical assumptions about clients and work environments became clear. Most striking was the way in which the use of a common evaluative language by practitioners of different disciplines (counselors, floor supervisors, and psychologists, for example), clients, and employers led to unanticipated changes in client behavior, shorter evaluation and work adjustment programs, and more satisfactory job placements. A change in the client's work environment, originally intended to sharpen the evaluative skills of floor supervisors, led to unexpected changes in client work personalities, changes in the predictive equations needed by staff for planning adjustment procedures and for sharpening the descriptions, and choices of future optimal work environments.

Structured Role-playing Techniques

The second relevant CJVS-RUL project was one in which structured role-playing techniques were designed to contribute to work adjustment programming (Pollack, 1972). Workshop personnel were trained to set up role-play situations dealing with behavior problems at work for use with workshop clients. As was true with the Observation Manual experience, results with structured role-playing demonstrated the interdependence of the elements of the rehabilitation system, even with respect to the measurement of each element. Clients and staff became conscious of new elements that had to be systematically considered in evaluating performance (which is embryonic theory building), and staff were placed in the position to realize that the definition and degree of existence of a client characteristic was in part a function of how staff defined and anticipated it.

The efforts at the CJVS to improve evaluation by enriching the interaction of theory and measurements have been only partial. Nevertheless, some of those efforts, especially those carried out by the RUL, have demonstrated that it is possible to bring about more effective and more efficient programs as a result of building theory and anchoring that theory in new forms of measurement.

SUMMARY

Necessary improvement in vocational evaluation can best be achieved through strengthening its theory and the principles for applying theoretical assumptions and propositions. The major goal of vocational evaluation is instrumental: to provide data for speeding clients' vocational development toward the objective of vocational rehabilitation. Companion goals are: 1) to preview each client's future work behavior and predict the nature and extent of his vocational development, 2) to specify each client's behavioral patterns in various types of work or training situations and the level of his adjustment in such situations, and 3) to prepare a treatment plan for each client that takes advantage of data in at least six areas of knowledge.

The theoretical assumptions with which the evaluator works constitute the structural base for carrying out the evaluation and for formulating the treatment plan. These assumptions must include definitions of and propositions relating the following constructs: 1) the work sector, 2) work personality, 3) personal and vocational development, 4) work role, 5) job adjustment, 6) work environment, and 7) continuity of the work personality.

The practice of vocational evaluation must take into account the principal aspects of rehabilitation practice, including its goals, its long-term and sequential nature, its insulation from the world of work, its need to make decisions with insufficient data, and its recognition of the masking effects of disability.

Vocational evaluation must take place within a context of simultaneous concern for work personality and work environment. At the same time, there must be concern for the measurement of all variables in a manner that allows concern for the relationships among them. Some of the recent work at the Chicago Jewish Vocational Service, particularly work done by the Research Utilization Laboratory, highlights some of these needs.

REFERENCES

Borgen, F. H., D. Weiss, H. Tinsley, R. Davis, and L. Lofquist. 1968. The Measurement of Occupational Reinforcer Patterns. Minnesota Studies in Vocational Rehabilitation, No. 25.

Chicago Jewish Vocational Service. 1969. The integration of vocational services with existing treatment programs for emotionally disturbed adolescents in residential, group, and foster home placement. (Final Report to U.S. Children's Bureau, Grant No. D-80.) Chicago.

Chicago Jewish Vocational Service. 1974. Innovation in vocational rehabilitation programs through research utilization. (Final Report for SRS Grant No. RD-22-P-55182.) Chicago.

Gay, E. G., D. Weiss, D. Hendel, R. Davis, and L. Lofquist. 1971. Manual for the Minnesota Importance Questionnaire. Minnesota Studies in Vocational Rehabilitation, No. 28.

Gellman, W. 1965. The workshop as a clinical rehabilitation tool. Rehab. Lit. 26:34–38.

Gellman, W. 1968. The principles of vocational evaluation. Rehab. Lit. 29:98–102.

Gellman, W. 1973. Fundamentals of rehabilitation. In J. F. Garrett and E. S. Levine (eds.), Rehabilitation Practices with the Physically Disabled. Columbia University Press, New York.

Gellman, W., D. Stern, and A. Soloff. 1963. A scale of employability for handicapped persons (Final Report for SRS Project No. 108.) Chicago Jewish Vocational Service, Chicago.

Lofquist, L., and R. Dawis. 1969. Adjustment to Work: A Psychological View of Man's Problems in a Work-oriented Society. Appleton-Century-Crofts, New York.

Pollack, R. 1972. Basic Guidelines for Role-playing in Rehabilitation Settings. Chicago Jewish Vocational Service, Chicago.

Shulman, L. 1967. The Vocational Development of Mentally Handicapped Adolescents: An Experimental and Longitudinal Study. Chicago Jewish Vocational Service, Chicago.

Soloff, A., and B. Bolton. 1969. The validity of the CJVS scale of employability for older clients in a vocational adjustment workshop. Ed. Psych. Meas. 29:993–998.

Soloff, A., L. Goldston, and R. Pollack. 1972. Observation and Client Evaluation in Workshops: A Guide and Manual. Chicago Jewish Vocational Service, Chicago.

Stern, G. G. 1970. People in Context: Measuring Person-Environment Congruence in Education and Industry. Wiley, New York.

Stern, G., M. I. Stein, and B. S. Bloom. 1956. Methods in Personality Assessment. Free Press, Glencoe, Ill.

11 The USES Testing Program

ROBERT C. DROEGE and HENDRIK D. MUGAAS

Occupational tests serve an important function in the activities of about 2,000 local offices of state employment services. The tests are used in vocational counseling and in the selection of persons for specific jobs. The development and validation of these tests is a continuing activity of the cooperative federal-state employment service test research program.

TEST DEVELOPMENT AND VALIDATION

Organization and Funding

Leadership for the cooperative test research program is provided by a small staff of research psychologists in the national office of the United States Employment Service (USES), U.S. Department of Labor. They set the priorities, prepare test specifications for new tests needed, develop designs for test research, do data analysis, and prepare test research reports, test manuals, and guides for test development and validation. Test research field centers in Detroit, Raleigh, and Salt Lake City, staffed with state employment service personnel, act as extensions of the USES national office. Personnel in these centers train state employment service test development technicians, coordinate their activities, and consolidate data collected for test research studies. At present, 42 state employment services participate in the test research program. They employ test development technicians who carry out data collection for test development and validation projects in accordance with experimental designs developed by the national office.

187

Underlying Concepts

The programs of development and use of occupational tests in the employment service are based on the principle of individual differences, not only in degree of occupational skills already acquired, but also in potential for acquiring skills and on the fact that these differences can be measured. The concepts listed below guide the conduct of the test development program.

Occupational Orientation   The tests developed must be occupationally oriented if they are to be useful in vocational counseling and selection in the employment service.

Independent Measures   In the long run, it is more efficient to develop an independent measure of each of the most important factors in the range of occupational performance than to develop a global measure for each specific occupation. This is particularly relevant when the users of the assessment measures are concerned with measuring a client's qualifications for many different occupations.

Dictionary of Occupational Titles   The tests developed should be oriented as much as possible to the USES *Dictionary of Occupational Titles* used by placement interviewers and counselors in the employment service.

Variety of Uses   The tests must be applicable for use with a wide variety of clients. This is necessary because the employment service serves both young and old applicants, the well educated and the educationally deficient, inexperienced applicants for entry jobs and experienced and trained applicants, applicants for the skilled trades and applicants for semiskilled and laborer jobs.

Simplicity   The tests must be simple to administer and to score, and the results must be readily interpretable; these are important requirements because of the varying qualifications of the personnel who use the tests in the employment service.

Types of USES Tests and Their Applications

A variety of USES tests have been developed for use by vocational counselors and employment interviewers; they are as follows.

Aptitude Tests   Aptitude tests measure occupational potentialities. They are useful in the following situations: first, in the selection of persons for referral to occupational training or to job openings for which neither training nor previous experience is required. The purpose of the tests is to aid in selecting persons with the capacity to acquire the skills involved in a specific job. Second, they are useful in employment counseling for choice of vocational goals and planning for required training. The purpose of the tests is to help compare a client's aptitudes with the requirements of many areas of work so that a realistic vocational plan can be developed.

Clerical Skills Tests Clerical skills tests measure the variety of clerical jobs skills a client has acquired through job experience or training.

Literacy Skills Tests Literacy skills tests measure the basic skills in reading and arithmetic that are important in occupational training and on the job. They are used to determine whether the client meets the literacy requirements of the occupation(s) or occupational training being considered. They also provide information that can be used to group persons with similar levels of skills for literacy training.

Interest Inventories Interest inventories provide information on occupational interest.

Pretesting Orientation Techniques Pretesting orientation techniques help prepare a client to take tests and help to alleviate anxieties about test taking.

GENERAL APTITUDE TEST BATTERY

Description

The General Aptitude Test Battery (GATB) consists of 12 tests measuring nine aptitudes; the aptitudes are as follows.

1. *Intelligence—General Learning Ability (G)* The ability to "catch on" or to understand instructions and underlying principles; the ability to reason and to make judgments (measured by Part 3—Three-dimensional Space, Part 4—Vocabulary, and Part 6—Arithmetic Reason).

2. *Verbal Aptitude (V)* The ability to understand meaning of words and the ideas associated with them, and the ability to use them effectively; the ability to comprehend language, and to understand relationships between words, and to understand meanings of whole sentences and paragraphs; the ability to present information or ideas clearly (measured by Part 4—Vocabulary).

3. *Numerical Aptitude (N)* The ability to perform arithmetic operations quickly and accurately (measured by Part 2—Computation, and Part 6—Arithmetic Reason).

4. *Spatial Aptitude (S)* The ability to comprehend forms in space and to understand relationships of plane and solid objects; frequently described as the ability to "visualize" objects of two or three dimensions, or to think visually of geometric forms (measured by Part 3—Three-dimensional Space).

5. *Form Perception (P)* The ability to perceive pertinent details in objects or in pictorial or graphic material; the ability to make visual comparisons and discriminations and to see slight differences in shapes and shadings of figures and widths and lengths of lines (measured by Part 5—Tool Matching, and Part 7—Form Matching).

6. *Clerical Perception (Q)* The ability to perceive pertinent detail in verbal or tabular material; the ability to observe differences in copy, to proofread words and numbers, and to avoid perceptual errors in arithmetic computation (measured by Part 1—Name Comparison).

7. *Motor Coordination (K)* The ability to coordinate eyes and hands or fingers rapidly and accurately in making precise movements with speed; the ability to make a movement response accurately and swiftly (measured by Part 8—Mark Making).

8. *Finger Dexterity (F)* The ability to move the fingers and to manipulate small objects with the fingers rapidly and accurately (measured by Part 11—Assemble, and Part 12—Disassemble).

9. *Manual Dexterity (M)* The ability to move the hands easily and skillfully; the ability to work with the hands in placing and turning motions (measured by Part 9—Place, and Part 10—Turn).

Finger dexterity and manual dexterity are measured with the use of apparatus tests, while the other aptitudes are measured by paper-and-pencil tests.

GATB Manual: Description

The Manual for the USES General Aptitude Test Battery (U.S. Department of Labor, 1970a) consists of separately bound sections; they are as follows.

Section I—Administration and Scoring, B-1002 Section I contains procedures for administration and scoring of the 12 tests comprising the GATB and the tables used in converting raw test scores to aptitude scores.

Section II—Occupational Aptitude Pattern Structure Section II contains the GATB Occupational Aptitude Pattern structure used for counseling purposes. Occupational Aptitude Patterns (OAPs) for 62 occupational groups are shown for adults and for ninth and tenth graders. These OAPs are combinations of GATB aptitudes and cutting scores, indicating aptitude requirements for groups of occupations.

Section III—Development Section III contains technical information on the development of the GATB, procedures for GATB occupational validation research, techniques used in developing Specific Aptitude Test Batteries (SATBs), and the GATB Occupational Aptitude Pattern (OAP) structure. It also has information on the effects of age, minority group status, cultural exposure, disabilities, sex, and training on aptitude scores; and guidelines for using GATB test results.

Section IV–Norms: Specific Occupations   Section IV contains the GATB minimum aptitude requirements for specific occupations and includes alphabetical and industrial indexes to the occupations covered.

Development

The original edition of the General Aptitude Test Battery was published in 1947 (Dvorak, 1947). Historically, the GATB evolved from the work of the Occupational Research Program in the U.S. Employment Service (Shartle et al., 1944) and the previous work of the Minnesota Employment Stabilization Research Institute (Paterson and Darley, 1936).

The basic assumption underlying the GATB is that the few basic aptitudes underlying the large variety of tests once used by the employment service can be identified through factor analysis and that a large variety of occupations can be clustered into groups according to similarities in the aptitudes required. This makes it feasible to test most of a client's important vocational aptitudes in one sitting and to interpret his scores in terms of a wide range of occupations.

The nine GATB aptitudes were identified by factor analytic studies of more than 50 tests that the employment service had been using over a period of years, and 12 tests were chosen to provide for an adequate measure of all nine aptitudes (Staff, Division of Occupational Analysis, 1945). Two criteria were applied in choosing the tests: factorial validity and empirical validity against an external criterion. Sometimes the test with the highest factorial validity was disregarded in favor of a test that had acceptable factorial validity but also had repeatedly demonstrated its practical validity against criteria of success for a number of jobs.

To provide a common scale for the nine GATB aptitudes, a general working population sample of workers in a wide variety of occupations was tested with the tests chosen to measure these aptitudes. The data from this sample were used to develop tables for converting raw test scores to standardized scores with a mean of 100 and a standard deviation of 20 for each aptitude of the GATB (Mapou, 1955).

Since its publication in 1947, the GATB has been researched in a continuing program of development and occupational validation of Specific Aptitude Test Batteries (combinations of two, three, or four aptitudes with associated cutting scores for specific occupations) and Occupational Aptitude Patterns (combinations of three aptitudes with associated cutting scores for groups of occupations). This research is

described in the Manual for the USES General Aptitude Test Battery—
Section III: Development.

Adminstration and Scoring

USES General Aptitude Test Battery Administration of the GATB
requires about 2.25 hours. All of the paper-and-pencil tests, except Part 8,
are arranged in two booklets for which answer sheets are provided. Part 8
is on a separate sheet, and no answer sheet is required. Scoring stencils are
used for hand scoring.

Raw scores are converted to aptitude scores by use of conversion
tables. When more than one test is used to provide a measure of a given
aptitude, the converted scores for each test are summed to obtain the
aptitude score.

Occupational Aptitude Patterns Occupational Aptitude Patterns
(OAPs) are combinations of three GATB aptitudes with associated cutting
scores. OAPs indicate the aptitude requirements for groups of occupations.
There are 62 OAPs, and they cover more than 1,200 occupations. The
OAP-aptitude score matching process, described in detail in the Manual for
the USES General Aptitude Test Battery—Section I: Administration and
Scoring, is as follows: a client's GATB aptitude scores are compared with
the aptitude cutting scores for the OAPs and a letter grade of H, M, or L is
assigned for each OAP. Letter grades are assigned as follows.

1. If a client's obtained scores meet or exceed all of the cutting scores, a
letter grade H is assigned.
2. If a client's scores plus one standard error of measurement (SE_m) meet
or exceed all of the cutting scores, a letter grade of M is assigned. (The
standard error of measurement of an aptitude is an index of the accuracy
or reliability of individual scores on the aptitude. The SE_m is expressed in
the same units as the aptitude score itself. The SE_ms vary for the nine
aptitudes and differ for the GATB and NATB.)
3. If a client's scores plus one standard error of measurement (SE_m) do
not meet all of the cutting scores, a letter grade of L is assigned.

A nationwide scoring service is available when NCS or Intran answer
sheets are used. The service includes converting raw scores to aptitude
scores, matching aptitude scores with OAPs, and printing a Test Record
Card with the results.

Specific Aptitude Test Batteries Specific Aptitude Test Batteries
(SATBs) are combinations of two, three, or four aptitudes with associated
cutting scores. SATBs reflect aptitude requirements for specific occupations against which a client's aptitude scores can be matched. There are

more than 400 SATBs, and the SATB-aptitude score matching process is the same as that for OAPs.

Interpretation

A client's performance on the GATB is interpreted in terms of his scores (H, M, or L) on OAPs and SATBs. The interpretation of the letter grades is as follows.

H: A client's scores equal or exceed those of workers judged to be satisfactory in the occupations. If he is also qualified on the basis of factors other than aptitudes, there is a good probability that he will do well on the job.

M: A client's scores are close to those of workers judged to be satisfactory in the occupations. The chances of his doing well on the job are somewhat lower than those of persons in the H category.

L: A client's scores are similar to or below those of workers found to be unsatisfactory in the occupations. The chances of his being satisfactory on the job are low, and he should be considered for other jobs that utilize his stronger aptitudes.

The OAPs and the occupations covered by each are shown in the Manual for the USES General Aptitude Test Battery—Section II: Occupational Aptitude Pattern Structure. The SATBs are shown in Section IV: Norms: Specific Occupations.

Applications to the Deaf

The deaf population presents unique problems in aptitude measurement. Test administration procedures must be modified to accommodate hearing loss. Measurement of general learning ability requires special attention because of deaf persons' difficulty with verbal tests used in many intelligence tests. Both of these problems have been overcome to an extent through modification of the GATB for use with the deaf.

The research described below, originally reported by Botterbusch and Droege (1972), provides a basis for obtaining measures of occupational aptitude for deaf individuals through a modified GATB.

Procedure Test data from 1958 through 1969 were collected by four state employment service agencies (Connecticut, Louisiana, Michigan, and New Mexico). At the time of testing, all subjects were students in various schools for the deaf. Instruments used were the General Aptitude Test Battery and the USES Nonreading Measure of General Learning Ability (Nonreading G), a weighted composite of scores on the first three parts of the Cattell Culture Fair Test (Part 1—Figure Series, Part 2—Figure

Classification, and Part 3—Matrices) and Part 7—Form Matching of the GATB (U.S. Department of Labor, 1963).

The GATB was administered to all state samples; the Nonreading G was administered only in Louisiana and New Mexico. The instruments were administered by teams composed of state employment service personnel and school instructors.

Results In all samples the mean scores obtained on Aptitudes G (General Learning Ability), V (Verbal Aptitude), and N (Numerical Aptitude) were lower than the mean scores obtained on Aptitude S (Spatial Aptitude), P (Form Perception), Q (Clerical Perception), K (Motor Coordination), F (Finger Dexterity), and M (Manual Dexterity). As would be expected, the mean score on Aptitude V was the lowest mean aptitude score in each sample. The standard deviations of Aptitude V ranged from 6.0 to 8.3, indicating that most subjects scored within a relatively narrow range. The weighted mean scores on Aptitudes G, V, and N were approximately one standard deviation below the GATB mean of 100, the general working population sample. On the other aptitudes the deaf students scored near or above average. Consistently high mean scores were obtained for Aptitude P, a nonverbal measure of perceptual speed. Scores averaged almost 10 points higher on Aptitude P than on Aptitude Q, a perceptual speed measure involving verbal content.

The deaf students obtained scores considerably lower than the general working population mean on GATB Aptitudes G, V, and N, which are measured by tests with verbal content. On aptitudes not measured by tests with verbal content, the students obtained mean scores as high as or higher than the general working population mean. In addition, the deaf subjects obtained much higher mean scores on the Nonreading G than on GATB Aptitude G. Thus, the deaf students consistently obtained higher scores on nonreading and nonverbal tests than on reading and verbal tests.

Discussion Three arguments can be given for the inappropriateness of using the entire GATB with a deaf population. First, because of their handicap, deaf people comprise a special population that is not comparable to the general working population, for which the GATB was originally developed and normed. Second, many parts of the test require verbal and reading skills, in which the deaf tend to be deficient. Third, standardized GATB administration procedures cannot be followed on any of the 12 parts. For these reasons it could be concluded that the results obtained in this study are questionable because of the characteristics both of the subjects tested and the instrument itself.

The results of the study, however, indicate that these arguments are not entirely valid. The students scored near or above the population mean on all GATB aptitudes except G, V, and N. This is a strong indication that modifications in administration procedures to meet the needs of the deaf were successful. It also indicates that the students' handicap did not limit their performance on the entire GATB. What is needed, however, is a measure of Aptitude G that is more appropriate for use with the deaf. Such a measure has been developed. The Nonreading G developed by the U.S. Employment Service measures general learning ability with the use of nonverbal test materials.

Caution must be used in interpreting these results in terms of the OAP structure. Because a person passes a specific set of OAP norms with Nonreading G does not necessarily indicate that he has the literacy skills needed for a specific job; it implies only that he has the potential. The literacy level required for a specific job or job training should be determined, and reading achievement tests should be given to determine if this level is met by the deaf person. Operational use of the GATB for measuring Aptitudes S, P, Q, K, F, and M and the Nonreading G appears justified when test administrators and counselors are aware of the unique situation of the deaf. When used with proper caution, these instruments will provide an adequate assessment of the deaf person's aptitudes.

Applications to the Mentally Retarded

One of the contributions of the GATB is that it provides for measurement of a variety of aptitudes important for occupational success, not just "intelligence." If such differential aptitude measurement is important generally in the vocational counseling of clients with normal intelligence, it is critically important in counseling intellectually retarded clients. Several GATB studies have been conducted to determine the extent to which retarded persons perform well on tests of aptitudes other than intelligence.

Local Office Applicants This study was described in detail in articles by Murray (1956a, 1956b). In 1955 GATB data were collected on 249 persons with Aptitide G scores of 75 and under from local offices in New York City, Erie, Pennsylvania, and Philadelphia, Pennsylvania. Analysis of the data from these 249 persons showed that 71, or 28.5 percent, had scores of 110 or better on one or more of the other aptitudes; 131, or 52.6 percent, had scores of 100 or better on one or more of the other aptitudes; and 187, or 72.1 percent, had scores of 90 or better on one or more of the other aptitudes.

Table 1 shows the number and percentage of persons with G scores of 75 and under who achieved scores of 100 or higher on other aptitudes. It will be noted that no one with a G score of 75 or less had a score of 100 or better on Verbal Aptitude, but on each of the other aptitudes some

Table 1. Proportion of persons who had G aptitude scores of 75 or below and scores of 100 or higher on other aptitudes

Aptitude	Cases with scores of 100 or higher	
	Number	Percent
Verbal	0	0
Numerical	2	1.5
Spatial	6	5
Form perception	34	27
Clerical perception	23	18
Motor coordination	70	54
Finger dexterity	42	33
Manual dexterity	56	44

achieved higher than average scores. A large number achieved above average scores in Motor Coordination, Finger Dexterity, and Manual Dexterity. As the scores indicate, not all of those in the group possess average abilities, but a great many do. Moreover, while it cannot properly be said that a person compensates for low intelligence with higher aptitudes in other areas, above average aptitudes frequently do appear concurrently with low intelligence.

Rochester, New York, Students In 1965 the New York State Employment Service completed a study in which the GATB was administered to a total of 112 males and 46 females classified as "slow learners" and to 46 males and 47 females classified as "educable mental retardates" in order to explore their occupational potential. The classification slow learner was determined by an IQ in the approximate range of 76 to 89 and/or evidence of a low level of academic functioning. The mentally retarded group consisted of persons who, in general, has IQs of 75 and below. All were students enrolled at four high schools in Rochester, New York, and were tested in their terminal year in special programs designed to prepare them to enter occupations. Two groups of "normal" high school seniors (a total of 336 males and 348 females) were used for comparison purposes. For the retarded and slow learner groups, more than the usual number of testing personnel were present at the time of testing to facilitate handling of the practice exercises and to maintain the motivation and pace needed for optimum performance.

Significant differences were found among the mean scores of the three groups on all aptitudes, with retardates scoring the lowest and "normals" the highest. On all subtests of the GATB, the normals attempted more items than the slow learners, who in turn attempted more items than the mentally retarded.

There has been some question regarding the reliability of the GATB when used with persons of low ability. A test that is very difficult for lower ranges of ability might result in inordinate guessing or in the failure to differentiate among persons at these lower levels. However, analyses of the data indicated that for most subtests of the GATB guessing was not a factor for the items attempted by the mentally retarded and slow learner groups, and that the items attempted were at a level of difficulty that permitted differentiation among examinees.

Less than half of the mentally retarded group (39 percent of males and 45 percent of females) qualified for one or more Occupational Aptitude Patterns (OAPs), but more encouraging results were obtained concerning the occupational potential of slow learners. In this group, 76 percent of the males and 63 percent of the females qualified for one or more OAPs.

Minnesota Studies A series of studies involving the GATB was conducted on mentally retarded persons from two sources, sheltered workshops throughout Minnesota and clients of the Minnesota Division of Vocational Rehabilitation (Lofquist, Dawis, and Weiss, 1970). The general conclusion reached was that the GATB is an appropriate tool for multifactor assessment of abilities for the mentally retarded. The authors state:

> The findings concerning the GATB strongly support the feasibility of a multidimensional (multifactor) approach to the assessment of "vocational potential" (work potential) in mentally retarded individuals. This approach contrasts sharply with, on the one hand, the IQ approach (wherein the IQ is the basic determiner of the range of work possibilities to be considered for the individual) and, on the other hand, the work sample approach (wherein vocational rehabilitation counseling is based on work try-out experience). In the latter approaches, the range of work possibilities that can be considered are limited—by invalidity of the IQ in its lower ranges as a predictor of job success, and by time and space constraints on the number of work samples that any constraints on the number of work samples that any one individual can attempt to try out (p. 94).

One purpose of the studies was to investigate the need for modification of GATB tests and testing procedures to accommodate the needs of the retarded. The authors' conclusion in this regard is as follows:

> Rather than revise the content of the GATB tests, it was thought that modifying test administration procedures would enable the

meaningful use of these tests with mentally retarded persons. Consequently a series of studies was conducted to investigate the effects of the following test administration modifications: (a) eliminating the separate answer sheet; (b) increasing the number of practice problems; (c) individual (vs. group) administration of the GATB tests; (d) administering the tests under untimed conditions; (e) eliminating items that correlate significantly with verbal ability; (f) simplifying test instructions and directions; and (g) simplifying practice problems. *None of these modifications was found consistently to exert any significant influence on the test performance of the mentally retarded subjects.* One might conclude that the GATB as presently administered can yield useful work-personality information about mentally retarded individuals in the higher IQ ranges (the "borderline" category). Individuals in the "mild" or lower categories would be better served by a new ability test battery which would have to be constructed in such a way as to calibrate with the GATB (italics added for emphasis) (p. 99).

NONREADING APTITUDE TEST BATTERY

Description

The Nonreading Aptitude Test Battery was designed for use with educationally deficient persons who do not have sufficient literacy skills to take the GATB. It measures the same aptitudes as the GATB. The nine aptitudes and the tests used to measure these aptitudes are:

1. Intelligence (G) Measured by Test A: Picture-Word Matching; Test B: Oral Vocabulary; Test D: Design Completion; and Test F: Three-dimensional Space.
2. Verbal Aptitude (V) Measured by Test A: Picture-Word Matching, and Test B: Oral Vocabulary.
3. Numerical Aptitude (N) Measured by Test B: Oral Vocabulary; Test C: Coin Matching; and Test D: Design Completion.
4. Spatial Aptitude (S) Measured by Test F: Three-dimensional Space.
5. Form Perception (P) Measured by Test E: Tool Matching, and Test G: Form Matching.
6. Clerical Perception (Q) Measured by Test I: Name Comparison.
7. Motor Coordination (K) Measured by GATB Part 8: Mark Making.
8. Finger Dexterity (F) Measured by GATB Part 11: Assemble, and GATB Part 12: Disassemble.
9. Manual Dexterity (M) Measured by GATB Part 9: Place, and GATB Part 10: Turn.

Following is a brief description of tests that make up the Nonreading Aptitude Test Battery.

Picture-Word Matching (Test A)   Test A consists of 42 items in which the examinee must determine which of five pictures associates best with a stimulus word read by the examiner. These items are arranged in order of increasing difficulty for persons of low education levels. It measures Aptitudes G and V.

Oral Vocabulary (Test B)   Test B contains 45 items that must be read to the examinee. The examinee must decide whether the two words are the same, opposite, or different. These items are in order of increasing difficulty for persons of low education levels. It measures Aptitudes G, V, and N.

Coin Matching (Test C)   Test C consists of 63 items in which the examinee must indicate whether two groups of coins have the same value. It measures Aptitude N.

Design Completion (Test D)   Test D contains 29 matrix type items that are in order of increasing difficulty for persons of low education levels. It measures Aptitudes G and N.

Tool Matching (Test E)   Test E consists of a series of 48 exercises containing a stimulus drawing and four black-and-white drawings of simple shop tools. The examinee indicates which of the four black-and-white drawings is the same as the stimulus drawing. Variations exist only in the distribution of black and white in each drawing. It measures Aptitude P.

Three-dimensional Space (Test F)   Test F consists of a series of 40 exercises containing a stimulus figure and four drawings of three-dimensional objects. The stimulus figure is pictured as a flat piece of metal which is to be either bent, or rolled, or both. Lines indiate where the stimulus figure is to be bent. The examinee indicates which one of the four drawings of three-dimensional objects can be made from the stimulus figure. It measures Aptitudes G and S.

Form Matching (Test G)   Test G consists of two groups of variously shaped line drawings. The examinee indicates which figure in the second group is exactly the same size and shape as each figure in the first or stimulus group. It measures Aptitude P.

Coin Series (Test H)   Test H contains three subtests: Part I has 72 items and Parts II and III have 46 items each. The examinee must mentally manipulate the coins according to the assigned system. It measures Aptitude N.

Name Comparison (Test I)   Test I consists of two columns of names. The examinee inspects each pair of names, one in each column, and indicates whether the names are the same or different. Contains 150 items. It measures Aptitude Q.

Mark Making, Place, Turn, Assemble, and Disassemble These are the same as GATB Parts 8 to 12.

NATB Manual: Description

The Manual for the USES Nonreading Aptitude Test Battery (U.S. Department of Labor, 1970b, 1971) is composed of the separately bound sections described below.

Section 1—Administration, Scoring, and Interpretation Section 1 contains procedures for administration and scoring of the 14 tests comprising the NATB, tables used in converting raw test scores into aptitude scores, and interpretation of aptitude scores using the Occupational Aptitude Pattern structure of the GATB and Specific Aptitude Test Batteries (SATBs).

Section 2—Development Section 2 contains technical information on the development of the NATB.

Development

The Occupational Aptitude Patterns (OAPs) to be used are those developed for the GATB. Information on OAPs is obtained by reference to the Manual for the USES General Aptitude Test Battery, Section II: Occupational Aptitude Pattern Structure.

The GATB was used as the model for the development of the NATB because the GATB measures the most important vocationally significant aptitudes, and also because the GATB has been validated extensively against occupational criteria. The tests making up the NATB were selected on the basis of multiple correlations with GATB aptitude scores and standardized on the basis of data from disadvantaged groups. A detailed account of the development and standardization of the NATB is presented in the Manual for the USES Nonreading Aptitude Test Battery, Section 2: Development, and in an article by Droege et al. (1970).

At its present stage of development, the validity of the Nonreading Aptitude Test Battery can only be inferred. It has not been validated against hard criteria of job and training success with disadvantaged persons. It derives what validity it has on the basis of its relationship to the GATB, which has been validated extensively against job criteria.

Additional development work is underway to improve the NATB. The goals are to decrease testing time and to develop better measures of Verbal Aptitude, Numerical Aptitude, and Clerical Perception.

Administration and Scoring

The paper-and-pencil tests, A through I, of the NATB are printed in eight booklets. There are no separate answer sheets, and the examinee marks his answers in the booklets. Form A is the only form available. Administration time is about 3.5 hours, and no more than six examinees may be tested at one time. Directions for administration and scoring the NATB are contained in the Manual for the USES Nonreading Aptitude Test Battery, Section 1: Administration, Scoring, and Interpretation. A machine-scoring service is available that provides for scoring the test booklets, converting raw scores to aptitude scores, matching aptitude scores with Occupational Aptitude Patterns, and printing test record cards and Permascore labels. This service is available from two sources, the National Computer Services, Inc., and the Intran Corporation, both of Minneapolis, Minnesota.

Interpretation

A client's performance on the NATB is interpreted in terms of his scores (H, M, or L) on Occupational Aptitude Patterns (OAPs), which are the same as those used for the GATB.

Applications to the Educationally Deficient

Recent research on 342 educationally deficient blacks, Indians, Mexican-Americans, and whites tested with both GATB and NATB shows that the NATB is more appropriate than the GATB for those with a deficiency in basic literacy skills. However, the counselor must be cautious and conservative in interpretation of NATB scores because of the indirect basis for the validity of the NATB and the possibility that disadvantaged clients may lack adequate motivation in the testing situation.

In interpreting results on the nonreading tests administered to disadvantaged clients, the counselor must keep in mind that his client may not have the literacy skills to enter an occupation for which he has demonstrated aptitude. For example, his client's aptitude scores may meet the norms for Machinist (N-80, S-80, and M-80), but his literacy skills may be lower than those required for entering an apprenticeship for Machinist. A separate determination must be made of the extent to which training in literacy skills is needed before the client is ready to enter the occupation or occupational training for which he has aptitude qualifications. This is done by comparing his achievement level, as measured by the Basic Occupational Literacy Test, with the literacy skills requirements for the occupations and training courses being considered.

Applications to the Mentally Retarded

Some research has been completed on application of the NATB to the retarded. In one study (Carbuhn and Wells, 1973), 102 retarded persons were tested at Fairview Hospital and Training Center, Salem, Oregon, and the test scores were correlated with measures of on-the-job-training success. In the discussion of the findings, the authors state:

> Many types of standardized tests are inappropriate for use with the mentally retarded since they require some skill in reading or verbal ability, but the occupations for which the retarded can be competively employed seem to require dexterity, memory, and perhaps what Jensen calls the "ability to learn from looking and doing." The NATB appears to fulfill most of these test requirements quite satisfactorily. An added advantage is group administration (6 to 10 persons) by a less highly trained examiner, with a saving in the examiner's time and effort.

At another point in the discussion the authors make reference to their previous research on applicability of the NATB to the retarded:

> The NATB is not appropriate for use with all levels of mental retardates, since comprehension of instrutions requires a minimum level of intellectual ability (IQ about 40) according to the authors' initial research. In that study, the battery could be appropriately administered to retarded persons whose intellectual level would be classified as moderate and mild retardation (IQ 40–69) as well as those with borderline levels of intellectual ability (IQ 70 and above).

The authors' final comment is as follows:

> Although the research reported here involved institutionalized retardates, the application of the results should be generalizable to students in special education classes or to slow learners in regular public school classes. School and rehabilitation counselors and other guidance personnel should find the NATB an additional source of measurement data for differential assessment of vocational aptitude.

Data from two separate studies on effects of training on NATB test scores for the retarded (U.S. Department of Labor, 1968, 1972b) indicate that occupational training has some effect on test scores. However, the results are not conclusive, and additional research would be useful.

RELATED TECHNIQUES

Basic Occupational Literacy Test

The Basic Occupational Literacy Test (BOLT) (U.S. Department of Labor, 1972a) is a test of basic reading and arithmetic skills for use with educationally disadvantaged adults. Reading skills are assessed by a Reading Vocabulary subtest and a Reading Comprehension subtest. Arithmetic skills are assessed by an Arithmetic Computation subtest and an Arithmetic Reasoning subtest.

BOLT Reading Vocabulary, Reading Comprehension, and Arithmetic Computation test forms are available at four levels of difficulty: Advanced, High Intermediate, Basic Intermediate, and Fundamental. BOLT Arithmetic Reasoning test forms are available at three levels of difficulty: Advanced, Intermediate, and Fundamental. Alternate forms A, B, and C are available for each subtest at each level of difficulty, except the advanced level for which alternate forms A and B are available. The content of BOLT items is generally suitable for adults; content pertaining to school, toys, and other children's activities is not used. In general, reading content is similar to that found in newspapers, popular magazines, or nontechnical instruction manuals.

BOLT Wide Range Scale

This instrument is used as an indicator of appropriate levels of BOLT subtests to administer and as a device to determine whether the GATB or NATB would be more appropriate for a given client. The Wide Range Scale may be administered individually by the counselor or group administered in the testing unit. The Scale takes about 15 minutes to administer and is scored separately for Vocabulary and Arithmetic.

Pretesting Orientation Techniques

Many disadvantaged persons are unfamiliar with tests, do not understand the purpose of testing, and fear group testing situations. As a result, some do not show up for scheduled testing and others tend to score lower than they should because of fear or inadequate motivation.

Pretesting orientation techniques are needed to minimize these problems, and a variety of techniques are required. Techniques to minimize differences in 1) familiarity with test content, 2) ability to understand test directions, and 3) knowledge of the nature and purpose of occupational testing are three examples.

These techniques may be used separately or in combination, depending upon the needs of the applicant. For example, an applicant may be given the "Pretesting Orientation on the Purpose of Testing," then the "Pretesting Orientation Exercises," and finally, for study at home, the booklets "Doing Your Best on Aptitude Tests" and "Doing Your Best on Reading and Arithmetic Tests." Information about these techniques and their availability may be obtained from the Manpower Administration, U.S. Department of Labor, Washington, D.C. 20213. Another possibility is developing techniques adapted to the local setting.

Interest Check List

The Interest Check List is an interviewing aid used to obtain information on the range of vocational interests of a client. It is particularly useful with persons who have no definite work interests or who have limited knowledge of the variety of jobs and occupational fields. The check list enumerates 173 items that have been taken without alteration in wording or sequence and keyed to the Worker Trait Arrangement (WTA) and Occupational Group Arrangement (OGA) of the third edition of the *Dictionary of Occupational Titles* (U.S. Department of Labor, 1965). The numbers in parentheses underneath each group of items in the check list refer to WTA and OGA classifications that should be explored with the client when responses indicate an interest in the activities described. The Interest Check List should be administered in accordance with the separately published Instructions for Administering and Using the Interest Check List.

No score is obtained from the Interest Check List. It is not a test, but rather an interviewing aid. It is an exploratory device from which the counselor and the client can investigate together the range of vocational interests of the client. Details of interpretation are contained in the Instructions for Administering and Using the Interest Check List.

RELEASE OF USES TESTS TO OTHER ORGANIZATIONS

USES tests are developed primarily for use in the public employment service system. They form an important component in comprehensive employment services provided to both applicants and employers. Although designed primarily to meet the needs of employment service interviewers and counselors for assessment of applicants, these tests are also often useful to counselors in other organizations, rehabilitation agencies, prisons, etc. Some of these tests are on public sale, and others are on restricted sale, which means that orders from the suppliers must be routed through the state employment service for approval.

Because of the usefulness of USES tests to other nonprofit organizations, the employment service has developed a procedure for release of USES tests to other agencies, when warranted, for operational use or for research. As an alternative, cooperative arrangements are sometimes made whereby a rehabilitation agency's clients may be referred to the employment service local office for testing. Organizations interested in exploring these possibilities should contact their state employment service.

REFERENCES

Botterbusch, K. F., and R. C. Droege. 1972. GATB aptitude testing of the deaf: Problems and possibilities. J. Employ. Counsel. 9:14–19.

Carbuhn, W. M., and I. C. Wells. 1973. Use of nonreading aptitude tests (NATB) for selecting mental retardates for competitive employment. Meas. Eval. Guid. 5:460–467.

Droege, R. C., W. Showler, S. Bemis, and J. Hawk. 1970. Development of a nonreading edition of the General Aptitude Test Battery. Meas. Eval. Guid. 3:45–53.

Dvorak, B. J. 1947. The new USES General Aptitude Test Battery. Occupations 26:42–44.

Lofquist, L. H., V. R. Dawis, and D. J. Weiss. 1970. Assessing the work personalities of mentally retarded adults. Final report on DHEW Research Grant No. RD-2568-P. Department of Psychology, University of Minnesota, Minneapolis.

Mapou, A. 1955. Development of general working population norms for the USES General Aptitude Test Battery. J. Appl. Psych. 39:130–133.

Murray, E. 1956a. Developing potential skills of the retarded. Employ. Sec. Rev. 23:35–36.

Murray, E. 1956b. The vocational potential of the retarded. Voca. Guid. Quart. 4:87–89.

Paterson, D. G., and J. G. Darley. 1936. Men, Women, and Jobs. University of Minnesota Press, Minneapolis.

Shartle, C. L., B. J. Dvorak, and C. A. Heinz. 1944. Ten years of occupational research, 1934–1944. Occupations 7:387–446.

Staff, Division of Occupational Analysis, War Manpower Commission. 1945. Factor analysis of occupational aptitude tests. Ed. Psych. Meas. 5:147–155.

U.S. Department of Labor. 1963. Technical Report on Development of an Interim Nonreading Measure of Aptitude G of the GATB. Manpower Administration, Washington, D.C.

U.S. Department of Labor. 1965. Dictionary of Occupational Titles. 3rd Ed. U.S. Government Printing Office, Washington, D.C.

U.S. Department of Labor. 1968. Technical Report on Effects of Training on Aptitude of Educable Mentally Retarded High School Students. Manpower Administration, Washington, D.C.

U.S. Department of Labor. 1970a. Manual for the USES General Aptitude Test Battery, Sections I, II, III, and IV. U.S. Government Printing Office, Washington, D.C.

U.S. Department of Labor. 1970b. Manual for the USES Nonreading Aptitude Test Battery, Section 2: Development. U.S. Government Printing Office, Washington, D.C.

U.S. Department of Labor. 1971. Manual for the USES Nonreading Aptitude Test Battery, Section 1: Administration, Scoring, and Interpretation. U.S. Government Printing Office, Washington, D.C.

U.S. Department of Labor. 1972a. Manual for the Basic Occupational Literacy Test, Sections 1 and 2. U.S. Government Printing Office, Washington, D.C.

U.S. Department of Labor. 1972b. Technical Report on Effects of Training on Aptitudes of the Trainable Mentally Retarded. Manpower Administration, Washington, D.C.

U.S. Department of Labor. 1973. Manual for the GATB-NATB Screening Device. U.S. Government Printing Office, Washington, D.C.

12 | Measurement of Client Outcomes in Rehabilitation

RICHARD T. WALLS and M. S. TSENG

In order to maintain a proper perspective while dealing with the issues of measuring client outcomes in rehabilitation, the rehabilitation system will be viewed in this chapter as an input-intervention-output paradigm (Figure 1). A paradigm is a model or pattern that portrays the temporal, spacial, causal, or logical relationships of events by use of boxes, connecting lines, and positions on vertical and horizontal dimensions. Conceptualizing an input-intervention-output paradigm of rehabilitation permits systematic, orderly, and useful approaches to the identification and assessment of issues involved in the measurement of client outcomes.

INPUT-INTERVENTION-OUTPUT PARADIGM

As can be seen in Figure 1, this paradigm of the rehabilitation system assumes three basic stages, input, intervention, and output, that complete a looping cycle. Each stage is described below.

Preparation of this manuscript was supported in part by the Social and Rehabilitation Services (HEW) through the West Virginia Regional Rehabilitation Research and Training Center. Appreciation is expressed to John Stuart, David Hassick, James DiFebo, and William Pierce for their assistance.

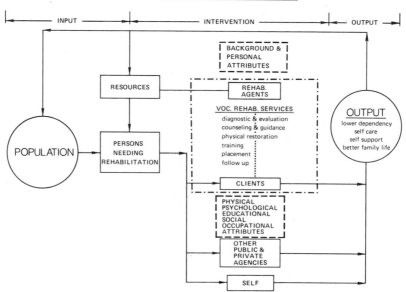

VOCATIONAL   REHABILITATION   SYSTEM

Figure 1. An input, intervention, output system.

Input

The input end includes the components of 1) a general population, 2) a sub-population consisting of people who need rehabilitation, and 3) another sub-population of those who serve as rehabilitation resources.

Intervention

The second stage, "intervention," represents the phase during which rehabilitation takes place. The disabled person may complete this stage 1) entirely on his own resources, 2) through the assistance of public and private agencies other than those of vocational rehabilitation, or 3) via the services of vocational rehabilitation agencies. The primary role of the vocational rehabilitation agencies is portrayed in Figure 1 by the largest box (formed by broken lines) in which diagnostic and evaluation, counseling and guidance, physical restoration, training, placement, and follow-up services serve as vehicles for intensive client-rehabilitation agent interactions. The client brings into this box with him his physical, psychological, educational, social, and occupational strengths and weaknesses. The rehabilitation agent who is to help the client also brings his background and personal attributes into the picture. Interactions between the client and the rehabilitation agent through various services allow pooling of the client's own resources and the environmental resources to facilitate his rehabilitation.

Output

The client then moves on to the output stage where, ideally, his dependency is lower, self care improved, self support attained or retained, and family life strengthened (taken from the SRS program objectives, 1968). The client then re-enters the general population. From a strictly client-centered perspective, this input-intervention-output paradigm may be viewed as an intake-process-outcome model where rehabilitation intake, process, and outcome constitute rehabilitation input, intervention, and output, respectively.

Figure 2 illustrates how the client goes through the rehabilitation process (or intervention) stage with the assistance of the state vocational rehabilitation agency within the paradigm. This flow chart (Leary and Tseng, 1974) makes use of the rehabilitation statuses (00 to 30) that are currently in use by vocational rehabilitation agencies across the nation. Every two-digit number in the chart represents a rehabilitation status that identifies a particular phase in the rehabilitation system.

The first status at which the client enters the intervention (or process) stage is 00 (referral). A client obtains referral status once the agency records his name, address, disability, age, sex, date of referral, source of referral, and social security number. When the client indicates that he would like to work with vocational rehabilitation and signs the application he moves to status 02 (applicant). It is sometimes necessary to determine eligibility for services. The client goes to status 06 when extended evaluation up to 18 months is needed. The 04 status has recently been deleted. If the client is not eligible for rehabilitation services, or if eligibility cannot be determined, the case is closed at status 08. The client then goes back, through the exit point 08, to the general population in the input stage of the paradigm.

The client moves to status 10 if he is eligible for rehabilitation services, and a rehabilitation plan is prepared. He goes on to status 12 when the rehabilitation plan is approved. For some reason, a case may have to be closed from statuses 10 or 12. If so, the client leaves the intervention stage, as far as the vocational rehabilitation agency is concerned at this point, through status 30. The client moves on to status 14 when receiving counseling and guidance, to status 16 while receiving physical restoration service, or to status 18 when he is being educated or trained. After all necessary services have been provided, the client is ready for employment. He is in status 20 if he does not return to or obtain employment immediately. He goes to status 22 if he obtains new employ-

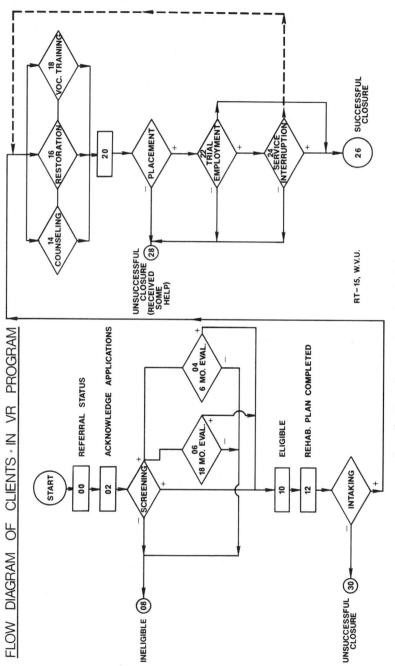

FLOW DIAGRAM OF CLIENTS IN VR PROGRAM

Figure 2. Flow diagram of vocational rehabilitation.

ment or returns to former employment. At times, the client's services can be interrupted. If so, he moves to status 24 and remains there during the period of service interruption.

When the client has been provided with the services that were planned for him and has reached the point in his rehabilitation process where he cannot be additionally assisted by the agency, his case is closed. If the client is not employed and the case is closed, he moves to the output stage of the paradigm through status 28. On the other hand, when the client is productively employed and the case is closed, he moves out of the system through status 26 and enters the output stage of the paradigm.

It is clear from the above description that clients who enter this vocational rehabilitation system are to move out of it after intervention through four exits, or outcome statuses. They are statuses 08, 30, 28, and 26. While status 08 signifies those referred cases *rejected* for services, statuses 30, 28, and 26 provide exits for those referred cases *accepted* for services.

Of the cases accepted for services, those who have received some assistance and are closed unemployed are routed to status 30, which signifies unsuccessful closure; those who have received all necessary services and are closed unemployed are branched to status 28, which indicates another unsuccessful closure; and those who have received all necessary services and are employed reach the desired exit point status 26, which represents a successful closure. The various categories of employment induced within the status 26 rehabilitation and their associated interpretation difficulties are discussed in a separate publication.[1]

Obviously, rehabilitation intervention (or process) should have positive impact not only on client employability but also on a host of other aspects of the client's functioning, including his occupational, physical, economic, educational, social, and psychological well being. Any specific attributes in these different dimensions that are operationally defined to yield valid and reliable measures can be used as criteria of success for assessing the effectiveness of rehabilitation intervention (or process).

REVIEW OF OUTCOME VARIABLES

The broad mission of the Rehabilitation Services Administration (RSA) has been stated as, "In conjunction with other public and voluntary

[1] Walls, R. T., and M. S. Tseng. Measurement of Client Outcomes in Rehabilitation. *In* J. B. Moriarty (ed.), Resource for Evaluating VR Programs. West Virginia Rehabilitation Research and Training Center, Morgantown, West Virginia.

agencies, to stimulate, develop, and implement programs which provide services for the disabled in maximizing their potential for a full and, to the extent possible, a productive life" (RSA Long-Range Plan, 1973). A full and productive life is of course subject to varying interpretation.

Productivity in terms of raw numbers of rehabilitants is obviously an agency program goal. They propose to increase this gross number of rehabilitations to 400,000 in 1975 and to 680,000 in 1979. This pure quantity measure of outcome refers to the total number of "Status 26 Closures."

Vocational Rehabilitation has traditionally operated within this "numbers" framework and has been widely accused of "creaming off the top," or taking the easier cases. There is a natural inclination for state and local programs to spread limited resources to help the most people and to appear favorably in statistics required by the Agency.

Although RSA admonitions for increasing quality as well as quantity have become a tradition with little substance, there is increasing evidence of genuine concern for developing outcome criteria to more adequately represent client accomplishment. This increased concern emerges as vocational rehabilitation begins to reach more deeply into areas of the severely disabled.

The primary concern for improving outcome in terms of earning levels and employment stability is apparent in the sub goals listed by RSA. Services should " ... lead to full or partial participation in the labor force ... to the extent individually possible, [to] become productive in the economy." However, other outcomes are also enumerated, such as reduction of the institutionalized population and their dependency on society (RSA Long-Range Plan, 1973).

Additional evidence of active agency pursuit of alternatives and supplements to absolute number of successful case closures comes from the considerable research projects, programs, and centers supported by the Social and Rehabilitation Services. RSA also recognizes the need for viable outcome alternatives to the 26 closure status system and encourages research in general, as well as suggesting directions for specifically needed research.

General criticisms and resentment of the closure system and the "numbers game" have been growing steadily in rehabilitation for more than two decades. Viaille (1968) contended that the agency closure reporting system encourages: 1) number of closures rather than quality of services, 2) noncomplex cases requiring least counselor time, 3) premature case closure to meet quotas, 4) seasonal demand and uneven case flow, 5) distortion and questionable practices in reporting because of special cases, etc., and 6) no recognition for effort expended in cases closed nonrehabilitated. Similar objections have been noted by other authors (Hawryluk, 1972; Muthard and Miller, 1966; Silver, 1969; Westerheide and Lenhart, 1974).

Present and past attempts to develop weighted closure systems have been seriously damaged by the inadequate closure classifications used as outcome measures. Prerequisite to weighted closure is establishment of clear, unequivocal, operational, outcome variables. Such research makes the prominent error of assuming homogeneous groups exist with regard to both outcome and prediction variables. The typical effort attempts to relate various client factors to the gross agency status outcomes through correlational (correlational, regression, factor analysis) techniques.

It is thus justifiably imperative that high priority be given to development of accurate and more objectively descriptive outcome criteria for rehabilitation. To date, however, an alternative accountability scheme, acceptable to all concerned, has not emerged. The gross concept of the "26 closed rehabilitated" remains. Even such a macro criterion is preferable to no criterion at all.

With such difficulties noted, the following work is presented to provide a context for further discussion and for model explication. The great majority of research has utilized closed-rehabilitated versus not rehabilitated as the criterion. However, a few investigators have attempted creative departures to other outcome variables.

Studies with a "Closed-Rehabilitated" Criterion

The present discussion is not intended as a descriptive or integrative literature review. Several good reviews of success prediction and client characteristics associated with outcome are extant (Grigg, Holtmann, and Martin, 1970; IRI Prime Study Group, 1974; Hammond, Wright, and Butler, 1968; Sankovsky, 1968). Rather, the intent here is to summarize briefly the criterion variables used in such studies. As noted, the vast majority have utilized 26 status (closed-rehabilitated) as the success criterion.

Some potential prediction variables are continuous in nature and may be considered at least ordinal. That is, the order of two data bits may be specified by treating one as greater than the other. Variables such as age at disablement and years of education approach the equal-appearing interval or even a true interval scale with a true zero point. Such scales are considered additive and are appropriate for use in analysis of variance, product-moment correlation, and similar statistical models discussed subsequently. Some variables are clearly noncontinuous; examples are marital status and sex. Of course, a continuous variable such as age may be split into below and above age 30 or some such partition, to create discrete categories. A success versus nonsuccess criterion is also obviously noncontinuous or discrete. Although reader sophistication in statistical concepts is by no means required, the noted distinction between noncontinuous (nominal or discrete) and ostensibly continuous variables is helpful to keep in mind as the discussion continues.

Demographic variables have been the most available data across large numbers of clients. Furthermore, demographic characteristics are in large part relatively objective and thus have been used in a number of research efforts. In one study or another (depending on the local sample or population studied, the scale or split utilized, and the statistical technique employed) all of the following have been found related to successful closure-rehabilitated. The list as reported here is in no way instructive to the reader who wishes to know which level or end of a scale is predictive of success in rehabilitation; it simply indicates that a lot of demography has been found related to the present closure status system. Some variables identified have been: major disability, age, age at disability onset, marital status, number of dependents, education, race, referral source, SSDI status, public assistance, source of income, mobility, socioeconomic status, employment history, home ownership, sociocultural disadvantagement (Aiduk and Longmeyer, 1972; DeMann, 1963; Heilbrun and Jordan, 1968; Miller and Allen, 1966; Tosi and Vesotsky, 1970; Westerheide and Lenhart, 1974).

Less readily available is information of a social and psychological nature. Several studies have attempted to use such factors in predicting successful rehabilitation closure. The MMPI, Army General Classification Test, Rorschach, Kuder Personal Preference Record, and Wechsler Adult Intelligence Scale have been used as predictors with little success (Ayer, Thoreson, and Butler, 1966; Drasgow and Dreher, 1965; Gilbert and Lester, 1970; Goss, 1968; Gressett, 1969; Neff, 1955; Pearlman and Hylbert, 1969). Social Vocabulary Index, the Interaction Scale, the Edwards Personal Preference Schedule (Clayton, 1970; Goss, Morosko, and Sheldon, 1968; MacGuffie, 1970; MacGuffie et al., 1969) have also yielded marginal success. It appears that more acceptable psychological adjustment and health as well as mental agility may be associated with successful closure and placement. However, such general and weak relationships from psychological tests probably contribute minimally to increased understanding or prediction.

A few investigators have also attempted to study social or psychosocial constructs related to client outcome (Barry and Malinovsky, 1963; Lane and Barry, 1970; Salomone, 1972; Westerheide and Lenhart, 1974;

Wright, 1968). For example, social and religious participation, family relationships, motivation, vocational goals, personal characteristics, and employer attitudes toward physical impairment have been discussed as possible predictors. The operational definitions of motivation, for example, are often too broad or variable to facilitate measurement, interpretation, or communication. In short, ego strength and similar psychosocial attitude constructs in the absence of defining and vocationally relevant behaviors appear to hold little promise of reliable aid in prediction of rehabilitation outcome as it presently exists.

Bolton (1972) suggests that although prediction of outcome studies have been popular, the single greatest need in such research is standardization of research procedures and uniformity of reporting format. Bolton states, "Prediction studies in rehabilitation are generally not comparable due to mixed disability samples and differences in referral criteria, criterion definitions and measurements, predictor variables (even biographical data is not comparable because every agency collects slightly different information or records it differently) and methods of data analysis" (p. 17).

Case difficulty ratings have also been based primarily upon the 08, 26, 28, 30 closure criteria. Miller (1965) stated:

> ... it seems reasonable to assume that *fewer* difficult and complex cases result in ... closures (successful). In fact, an operational definition of case difficulty and complexity could be the number of cases—of all like these—which achieved rehabilitation status. Thus, the question of building a set of complexity weights, or "norming" case difficulty, becomes one of figuring out what variables within cases make a difference in terms of later success. We can then build sub-populations of "cases-like-this" to see what percentage of each sub-population is achieving ... closure (successful) status. On the basis of these percentages, we can then "norm" the cases for complexity (p. 31).

Both Miller and Barillas (1967) and Wallis and Bozarth (1971) utilized this general approach. The former system considered major disability, referral source, age, and years of education—with closure status as the outcome. Wallis and Bozarth (1971) used major disability, age, years of education, and type of previous rehabilitation contact—also with a successful closure criterion.

Sermon (1972) developed a case difficulty index from the percent rehabilitated nationally for any given disability category. This plan uses national statistics to establish the difficulty associated with each disability while disregarding other qualifying demographic, psychological, or social characteristics. Obviously, the criterion is the agency rehabilitation, successful versus unsuccessful closure. Several states (e.g., Florida) are experimenting with or incorporating the difficulty index into their data procedures. Florida uses a Composite Difficulty Index that includes: 1) time, 2) cost, 3) number of services provided, and 4) Sermon's index (Zawada, 1973). Zawada reports this composite index to be valuable for program evaluation studies in Florida.

In a study relating case service expenditures to the number of successful closures per counselor, Lawlis and Bozarth (1971) attempted to differentiate quantity from quality. They proposed that increased quantity or number of successful 26 closures is associated with more funds spent on a larger number of clients. In the latter circumstance more complex cases are assumed to require greater appropriations. Possible sources of inaccuracy in such assumptions have been noted (Westerheide and Lenhart, 1974).

Studies with "Other" Criterion Variables

Several departures from the 26 closed-rehabilitated criterion have been attempted. Silver (1969) obtained counselor estimates of difficulty of rehabilitating various disabilities in terms of counselor time and effort. Paired comparison and semantic differential techniques were used in an attempt to rank order gross disability categories according to the time and effort judged by counselors to be necessary to gain successful closure. Although Silver obtained fairly consistent ordering from cerebral palsy (most difficult) through hernia and dental repair, such measures contribute little to objective case outcome study. In fact, the judgements are made in reference to standard closure criteria. Similarly, a difficulty index taking account of total time from client acceptance to closure has the same terminal reference. Goff (1969) computed difficulty in terms of months from acceptance to closure, but of course counts the agency closure status as the end point in the process.

In addition to their previously noted criterion, Miller and Barillas (1967) unsuccessfully attempted to relate their index to a measure of client satisfaction. Kunce et al. (1969) reported a significant relationship between treatment time and job level, but none between treatment time and job placement or salary. Utilizing variables from the RSA-300 having a common sense contribution to gainful employment, Kunce and Miller (1972) sought relationships to three outcome criteria. The 12 predictor variables were: age, selective service, race, number of dependents, years of education, earnings at acceptance, welfare status, SSDI status, number of disabilities, marital status, and previous rehabilitation client. The three criterion variables were closure status, work status at closure, and earnings at closure. Those authors report a number of significant chi square, correlation, and stepwise regression findings in relation to these three outcome metrics (Westerheide and Lenhart, 1974).

Eber (1966) derived two criterion measures from closure and follow-up information. "Vocational Adequacy at Closure" involved differential weights for 1) work status at closure, 2) DOT job code at closure, 3) weekly earnings at closure, and 4) closure code. His "Vocational Adequacy at Follow-up" similarly involved 1) employment at follow-up, 2) work status improvement from closure, 3) job satisfaction, and 4) counselor estimate of success. An 11-step composite work adjustment criterion was used in a follow-up study of former VA clients by Stein, Bradley, and Buegal (1970). These 11 brief descriptions of work adjustment provided indication of current job status, job time, and number of jobs since discharge (Bolton, 1974a). However, as with other novel outcome criteria, these have been used by few researchers or agencies except those developers.

The Regional Rehabilitation Research Institute (RRRI) at Oklahoma University constructed items designed to measure client satisfaction with speed of service, medical service, training service, employment, participation in planning, counselor effort in placement, agency policies, physical facilities, and personal treatment in the Consumer's Measurement of Vocational Rehabilitation (Hills and Ledgerwood, 1972). While such follow-up attempts are laudable, their percent of questionnaire return has been low (13 and 27 percent). Furthermore, the unreliability of such judgmental items as, "The quality of training I received" and "My counselor's ability to help me" may preclude the usefulness of these responses.

In addition to closure status, Ayer, Thoreson, and Butler (1966) used DOT occupational level and an upward mobility rating as outcomes. McPhee and Magleby (1960) used substantial, unsubstantial, and minimal employment. One criterion variable for Neff, Novick, and Stern (1968) was percent of time worked during a 1-year follow-up period. Tseng (1972) found a number of personal and skill characteristics related to successful versus unsuccessful completion of vocational training. Rehabilitation success was in terms of ambulation and self care skills for Ben-Yishay et al. (1970). Several employment related criteria (level, persistance, tenure, stability, looking for work, employer/employee satisfaction) have been examined in relation to various handicaps (Barry, Dunteman, and Webb, 1968; Kilburn and Sanderson, 1966; Miller, Kunce, and Getsinger, 1972; Schletzer et al., 1959; Weiner, 1964). For sheltered workshop clients Nadler (1957) used a composite criterion of: 1) number of jobs a client could perform, 2) his productivity, 3) his steadiness of work, 4) attendance and punctuality, 5) independence, and 6) work quality. Cunningham, Botwinik, and Weickert (1969), Lorei (1967), Lowe (1967), and Taylor (1963) considered remaining out of the hospital and in the community a success criterion for mental patients, while Burstein et al. (1967) considered discharge and employment outcome for a similar sample. Noble (1973) suggests the current U.S. minimum wage as the success closure criterion.

Many authors and professionals presently are suggesting that a measure of client improvement or change from beginning to end of the rehabilitation process is the most profitable outcome consideration. The agency closure criterion or economic indicators are surely inadequate for reflecting accomplishments of an unpaid family worker or homemakers. However, the very economic and vocational changes that are most readily measured are increase in weekly earnings, reduction in welfare grants, and job level. Valid physical and psychological improvements are more difficult, but probably not impossible to measure reliably. Several suggestions for incorporating such change factors (i.e., social, community, and personal living competencies) in outcome metrics have been broached (Cook, 1967; Kelman and Willner, 1962; Krantz, 1971). The States Advisory Committee for Service Outcome Measurement Project (RSA/EV-3-73) listed criteria for administratively feasible change outcomes as 1) being measured for all clients, 2) requiring no changes in service delivery systems, 3) requiring no sophisticated data processing equipment, 4) being easily interpreted, 5) requiring little training, and 6) not requiring more than 10 minutes of counselor time per case. While researchers should attend to such administrative requests for parsimony, the development of suitable rehabilitation outcomes should be the overriding consideration at this point.

A Rehabilitation Gain Scale was constructed by Reagles, Wright, and Butler (1970, the University of Wisconsin Regional Rehabilitation Research Institute) as part of the Wood County Project for rehabilitation of persons with environmental or nonmedical disabilities. The Rehabilitation Gain Scale requires the client to respond to items reflecting vocational success and personal-social adjustment. While client self reports of source of income or weekly earnings, for example, may be accurate, serious methodological problems exist in self estimates of items such as physical condition, chance of getting a job, and emotional adjustment. The scale yields a pre-score, a post-score, and a composite pre-minus post-change score. Bolton (1974b) notes that the averaging of separate dimensions such as vocational success and personal adjustment into a single composite probably limits the interpretation and meaning of the gain score.

The Rehabilitation Gain Scale was expanded by Human Service Systems, Inc., into the Human Service Scale, a self reported degree of change instrument for clients served through various human services. From an initial pool of 300 items, 80 were selected following item analysis and counselor ratings. These 80 items are designed to reflect Maslow's (1954) hierarchy of five basic needs, physiological, safety and security, love and belongingness, esteem, and self-actualization. For example, the question, "How often are you bothered by muscle twitches, trembling, or shakes?" presumably relates to the client's physiological needs. Although the internal consistencies of these separate HSS scales are largely acceptable, they do not appear to support the hierarchical ordering suggested above by Maslow's theory (Bolton, 1974a). The Virginia Department of Vocational Rehabilitation modified the Wisconsin RRRI scale of rehabilitation gain by deleting extravocational items and adding 10 self perception items (Hawryluk, 1974). In general, referral clients closed in status 26 did not differ significantly in composite gain one year later from those still in process or closed not rehabilitated. Other states and research centers (e.g., California, West Virginia, and Michigan) have developed questionnaires that combine objective and subjective information about client outcome that may be used in the pre-post client gain paradigm.

The Rehabilitation Service Outcome Measure was developed by the Oklahoma Service Outcome Measurement Project to examine client gain in six aspects of rehabilitation change: 1) difficulty, e.g., employment prognosis, 2) educational status, e.g., months of on-the-job training, 3) economic and vocational status, e.g., weekly earnings, 4) physical functioning, e.g., mobility, 5) adjustment to disability, e.g., client's confidence in himself as a worker, and 6) social competency, e.g., decision making ability. The Rehabilitation Services Outcome Measure is recorded by the counselor, but the same criticisms apply with regard to unreliability of judgmental items. Although a few counselors participating in a reliability study might produce acceptably reliable ratings from expanded case folders, the possibility exists of gross distortion and errors in judgement in items such as client's confidence or decision making ability (Westerheide and Lenhart, 1973). The Arkansas Division of Rehabilitation Service has been experimenting with an adapted form of the Oklahoma service outcome measure (Thurman, 1973). This adaption has eliminated some of the unreliable items from the Oklahoma Service Measurement Outcome Project, Form A (e.g., Physical Functioning Compensatory Skills with an intercounselor reliability of 0.31). However, Arkansas retained some unreliable items from the Oklahoma Form A (e.g., Work Tolerance, General Health Status other than Disability, Employment Prognosis, Mobility and Vocational Level, with intercounselor reliabilities of 0.55, 0.47, 0.56, 0.57, and 0.42, respectively) (Thurman, 1973; Westerheide and Lenhart, 1973).

Thus, some authors have tried to make a case for use of professional judgement or client judgement in evaluation of rehabilitation gain or outcome. The fact that such judgmental data have been used in attempts to demonstrate improvements in psychological and social functioning in the fields of social work and psychotherapy is not convincing. This whole tack of judgmental evaluation is fraught with difficulties of definition, validity, and reliabilities. Sufficient at this point is the caution that interjudge reliability of "about 0.60," as well as weak definitions and validity of areas such as "personal meanings and experiencing" are inadequate separately (Rogers, 1961; Tomlinson and Hart, 1962). Taken together they are lethal to any such attempted measurement. Similar comment may be directed to the estimated client movement scale developed by Hunt and Kogan (1952).

Hetzler (1963) came nearer to the recording of objective information in his social case work movement survey. He counted the presence in the home of items such as bed space, telephone, and alarm clock before and after services. While the validity of some of Hetzler's items may be questioned, cross rater reliability in such tabulation would be high. The issues of reliability and validity of outcome measures are paramount and integral to assessment of the effect of client, counselor, and administrative success.

TOWARD A SYSTEM OF
REHABILITATION OUTCOME ANALYSIS AND EVALUATION

Program evaluation, weighted closure, case difficulty, and gain scale have become popular "catch" terms in vocational rehabilitation. As previously noted there have been several attempts to operationalize case difficulty or to develop weighted closure systems based on the 26 closure concept (e.g., Miller and Barillas, 1967; Sermon, 1972; Wallis and Bozarth, 1971). Such attempts have been handicapped by that inadequate closure status system. The 1974 IRI Prime Study Document on *Measurement of Outcomes* notes that the 26 closure as a measurement concept fails to consider any success short of ideal. Weighting systems have used case difficulty in the manner of this ideal as a primary determinant of quality. Thus, in most weighted closure procedures a severely retarded client is more difficult and hence more desirable to rehabilitate, from the counselor's standpoint, than a slightly disabled client. Moreover, recent legislation stresses this factor. While one may be more difficult, if both genuine rehabilitations that would not have occurred by spontaneous remission or by some other mechanism, is one of these clients more important to rehabilitate than the other? The heterogeneous 26 category does not provide sufficient outcome information about these two clients so that case difficulty may be viewed in context. Moreover, the IRI group states that analysis debunk the idea of "rehabilitating" X thousands of persons; they ask instead for data that measure impact in specific terms of earnings, job level, and reduction of public assistance.

The IRI Prime Study Group (1974) suggests taking first things first. Conclusive and comprehensive outcome variables and measures are prerequisite to, not dependent upon, effective program evaluation, effective counselor evaluation, and effective client service delivery evaluation. The IRI group essentially endorsed areas proposed by the Oklahoma Service Outcome Measurement Project: Physical, Educational, Vocational, Economic, and Psychosocial. The IRI plan was revised slightly as follows: Psychosocial Functioning, Physical Functioning, Economic Independence, and Vocational Functioning and Potential.

Some of these presently may be measured reliably and validly within a revised VR outcome context. Psychosocial has been omitted for reasons noted previously. It is indeed possible that objective and reliable psychosocial indices may be developed. The current state of such indices does not warrant inclusion at this time. However, researchers and practitioners should be encouraged to continue to seek and to develop accurately reliable measures of psychosocial functioning and gain.

The authors have developed a procedure for quantifying VR outcomes by assigning numbers to closure categories in four areas: physical capacity and mobility increase, public assistance decrease, earning increase, and vocational placement at closure. In order to improve the efficiency of the rehabilitation service process, it is necessary to identify the input and intervention variables that determine successful outcomes in the various areas of client functioning. Illustrations of four statistical models (chi square, analysis of variance, correlation, and multiple regression) that may be used to accomplish this purpose are available in a separate publication.[2]

REFERENCES

Aiduk, R., and D. Longmeyer, 1972. Prediction of client success with vocational rehabilitation in a state mental hospital. Rehab. Counsel. Bull. 15:3–10.

---

[2] See footnote 1 on p. 211.

Ayer, M. J., R. W. Thoreson, and A. J. Butler, 1966. Predicting rehabilitation success with the MMPI and demographic data. Pers. Guid. J. 40:634–637.

Barry, J. R., G. H. Dunteman, and M. W. Webb, 1968. Personality and motivation in rehabilitation. J. Counsel. Psych. 15:237–244.

Barry, J. R., and M. R. Malinovsky, 1963. Client Motivation for Rehabilitation: A Review. University of Florida Regional Rehabilitation Research Institute, Gainesville.

Ben-Yishay, Y., L. Gertsman, L. Diller, and A. Hans, 1970. Prediction of rehabilitation outcomes from psychometric parameters in left hemiplegics. J. Consult. Clin. Psych. 34:436–441.

Bolton, B. 1972. The prediction of rehabilitation outcomes. J. Appl. Rehab. Counsel. 3:16–24.

Bolton, B. 1974a. Introduction to Rehabilitation Research. Charles C Thomas, Springfield, Ill.

Bolton, B. 1974b. A factor analysis of personal adjustment and vocational measures of client change. Rehab. Counsel. Bull. 18:99–104.

Burstein, A., A. Soloff, H. Gillespie, and M. Haase, 1967. Prediction of hospital discharge of mental patients by psychomotor performance: Partial replication of Brooks and Weaver. Percept. Motor Skills 24:127–134.

Clayton, W. H. 1970. Correlates of client-counselor interaction and rehabilitation outcome. Dissertation Abstracts International 31 (4-a):1572-A.

Cook, T. E. 1967. Psychosocial barriers to rehabilitation in Appalachia. Rehab. Counsel. Bull. 11:98–105.

Cunningham, M. K., J. D. Botwinik, and A. A. Weickert, 1969. Community placement of released mental patients: A five-year study. Social Work 14:54–61.

DeMann, M. M. 1963. A predictive study of rehabilitation counseling outcomes. J. Counsel. Psych. 10:340–343.

Drasgow, J., and R. Dreher. 1965. Predicting client readiness for training and placement in vocational rehabilitation. Rehab. Counsel. Bull. 9:94–98.

Eber, H. W. 1966. Multivariate analyses of a vocational rehabilitation system. Multivar. Behav. Res. Mono. No. 66-1.

Gilbert, D. H., and J. T. Lester. 1970. The relationship of certain personality and demographic variables to success in vocational rehabilitation. Unpublished manuscript, Orthopedic Hospital, Los Angeles.

Goff, C. 1969. An objective index for measuring the vocational rehabilitation counselor's case-load difficulty. Unpublished doctoral dissertation, University of Oklahoma, Norman.

Goss, A. 1968. Predicting work success for psychiatric patients with Kuder Preference Record. Ed. Psych. Meas. 28:571–576.

Goss, A., T. Morosko, and R. Sheldon. 1968. Use of the Edwards Personal Preference Schedule with alcoholics in a vocational rehabilitation program. J. Psych. 68:287–289.

Gressett, J. 1969. Prediction of job success following heart attack. Rehab. Counsel. Bull. 13:10–14.

Grigg, C. M., A. G. Holtmann, and P. Y. Martin. 1970. Vocational Rehabilitation for the Disadvantaged. D. C. Health, Lexington, Mass.

Hammond, C. D., G. N. Wright, and A. J. Butler. 1968. Caseload feasibility in an expanded vocational rehabilitation program. Wisconsin Studies in Vocational Rehabilitation, Monograph VI. University of Wisconsin, Regional Rehabilitation Research Institute, Madison.

Hawryluk, A. 1972. Rehabilitation gain: A better indicator needed. J. Rehab. 38:22–25.

Hawryluk, A. 1974. Rehabilitation gain: A new criterion for an old concept. Rehab. Lit. 35:322–328.

Heilbrun, A. B., and B. T. Jordan. 1968. Vocational rehabilitation of the socially disadvantaged: Demographic and intellectual correlates of outcome. Pers. Guid. J. 47:213–217.

Hetzler, S. 1963. A scale for measuring case severity and case movement in public assistance. Social Casework 44:445–451.

Hills, W. G., and D. E. Ledgerwood. Consumer's measurement of vocational rehabilitation in New Mexico (and in North Dakota). Unpublished manuscripts, Regional Rehabilitation Research Institute, University of Oklahoma, Norman.

Hunt, J. M. and L. F. Kogan. 1952. Measuring Results in Social Casework. Family Service Association of America, New York.

IRI Prime Study Group. 1974. Measurement of Outcomes. Research and Training Center Press, Institute, W. Va.

Kelman, H. R., and A. Willner. 1962. Problems in measurement and evaluation of rehabilitation. Arch. Phys. Med. Rehab. 43:172–181.

Kilburn, K. L., and R. E. Sanderson. 1966. Predicting success in a vocational rehabilitation program with the Raven Colored Progressive Matrics. Ed. Psych. Meas. 26:1031–1034.

Krantz, G. 1971. Critical vocational behaviors. J. Rehab. 37:14–16.

Kunce, J. T., R. J. Mahoney, R. R. Campbell, and J. Finley. 1969. Rehabilitation in the concrete jungle. Research series no. 3. University of Missouri–Columbia, Regional Rehabilitation Research Institute.

Kunce, J. T., and D. E. Miller. 1972. Simplified prediction: A follow-up study. J. Counsel. Psych. 19:505–508.

Lane, J. M., and J. R. Barry. 1970. Recent research on client motivation. Rehab. Res. Pract. Rev. 1:5–25.

Lawlis, G. F., and J. D. Bozarth. 1971. Considerations for the development of weighting systems for the evaluation of counselor effectiveness. Rehab. Counsel. Bull. 14:133–140.

Leary, P. A., and M. S. Tseng. 1974. The vocational rehabilitation process–explained. J. Rehab. 40:9, 34.

Lorei, T. 1967. Prediction of community stay and employment for released psychiatric patients. J. Consult. Psych. 31:349–357.

Lowe, C. M. 1967. Prediction of posthospital work adjustment by the use of psychological tests. J. Counsel. Psych. 14:248–252.

MacGuffie, R. A. 1970. Relationship between the Social Vocabulary Index and the Interaction Scale and rehabilitation success. J. Counsel. Psych. 17:289–290.

MacGuffie, R. A., F. V. Janzen, C. O. Samuelson, and W. N. McPhee.

1969. Self-concept and ideal-self in assessing the rehabilitation applicant. J. Counsel. Psych. 16:157–161.

Maslow, A. H. 1954. Motivation and Personality. Harper & Row, New York.

McPhee, W. M., and F. L. Magleby. 1960. Success and failure in vocational rehabilitation. Pers. Guid. J. 38:497–499.

Miller, D. E., J. T. Kunce, and S. H. Getsinger. 1972. Prediction of job success for clients with hearing loss. Rehab. Counsel. Bull. 16:21–28.

Miller, L. A. 1965. An empirical set of complexity weights for "12" closures in state agencies. Cited by Muthard, J. E., ed. 1965. Training guides in case load management for vocational rehabilitation staff, final report, Committee on Caseload Management, Rehabilitation Services Series No. 66-22, U.S. Department of Health, Education, and Welfare, Vocational Rehabilitation Administration, Washington, D.C. p. 31.

Miller, L. A., and G. Allen. 1966. The prediction of future outcome among OASI referrals using NMZ Scores. Pers. Guid. J. 45:349–352.

Miller, L. A., and M. G. Barillas. 1967. Using weighted 26-closures as a more adequate measure of counselor and agency effort in rehabilitation. Rehab. Counsel. Bull. 11:117–121.

Muthard, J. E., and L. A. Miller. 1966. The criteria problem in rehabilitation counseling. College of Education, State of Iowa, Iowa City.

Nadler, E. 1957. Prediction of sheltered shop work performance of individuals with severe physical disability. Pers. Guid. J. 36:95–98.

Neff, W. S. 1955. The use of the Rorschach in distinguishing vocationally rehabilitable groups. J. Counsel. Psych. 2:207–211.

Neff, W. S., B. Novick, and B. Stern. 1968. A follow-up counseling program, final report. Jewish Occupational Council, New York.

Noble, J. H. 1973. Actuarial system for weighting case closures. Rehab. Rec. 14:34–37.

Pearlman, L. G., and K. W. Hylbert. 1969. Identifying potential dropouts at a rehabilitation center. Rehab. Counsel. Bull. 13:217–225.

Reagles, K. W., G. N. Wright, and A. J. Butler. 1970. A scale of rehabilitation gain for clients of an expanded vocational rehabilitation program. Wisconsin Studies in Vocational Rehabilitation, Monograph XIII, Series 2. The University of Wisconsin, Regional Rehabilitation Research Institute, Madison.

Rogers, C. R. 1961. The process equation of psychotherapy. Amer. J. Psychother. 15:27–45.

RSA Long-range Plan. 1973. Rehabilitation Services Administration, Washington, D.C.

Salomone, P. R. 1972. Client motivation and rehabilitation counseling outcome. Rehab. Counsel. Bull. 15:11–20.

Sankovsky, R. 1968. Predicting successful and unsuccessful rehabilitation outcome: A review of literature. Grant No. RT-14. University of Pittsburgh, Pittsburgh. December.

Schletzer, V. M., R. V. Dawis, G. W. England, and L. H. Lofquist. 1959. Factors related to employment success. Minnesota Studies in Vocational Rehabilitation, Bulletin 27. University of Minnesota, Minneapolis.

Sermon, D. T. 1972. The Difficulty Index: An Expanded Measure of Counselor Performance. Minnesota Division of Vocational Rehabilitation, St. Paul.

Silver, D. L. 1969. A look at evaluation of vocational rehabilitation counselor performances. J. Rehab. 35:13–14.

SRS Program Objectives. 1968. Rehabilitation Services Administration, Washington, D.C.

Stein, C. I., A. D. Bradley, and B. Buegel. 1970. A test of basic assumptions underlying vocational counseling utilizing a differential criterion method. J. Counsel. Psych. 17:93–97.

Taylor, F. 1963. The general aptitude test battery as predictor of vocational readjustment by psychiatric patients. J. Clin. Psych. 19:130.

Thurman, D. G. 1973. Outcome measures progress report. Division of Rehabilitative Service, State of Arkansas, Little Rock, Ark.

Tomlinson, T. M., and J. T. Hart, Jr. 1962. A validation study of the process scale. J. Consult. Psych. 26:74–78.

Tosi, D. V., and L. R. Vesotsky. 1970. Successful rehabilitation as a function of client status. Psych. Repts. 27:37–38.

Tseng, M. S. 1972. Predicting vocational rehabilitation dropouts from psychometric attributes and work behaviors. Rehab. Counsel. Bull. 15:154–159.

Viaille, H. 1968. Operations research program in the Oklahoma Vocational Rehabilitation Agency. VRA Grant No. RD-946. Oklahoma Vocational Rehabilitation Agency, Oklahoma City.

Wallis, J. H., and J. D. Bozarth. 1971. The development and evaluation of weighted DVR case closures. Rehab. Res. Pract. Rev. 2:55–60.

Weiner, H. 1964. Characteristics associated with rehabilitation success. Pers. Guid. J. 42:687–694.

Westerheide, W. J., and L. Lenhart. 1973. Development and reliability of a pretest-posttest rehabilitation services outcome measure. Rehab. Res. Pract. Rev. 4:15–23.

Westerheide, W. J., and L. Lenhart. 1974. Case Difficulty and Client Change: A Review of the Literature. Department of Institutions, Social and Rehabilitative Services, Oklahoma City.

Wright, G. N., ed. 1968. Clinical versus Statistical Prediction in Wisconsin Studies in Vocational Rehabilitation. Series I, Monograph VII. University of Wisconsin, Madison.

Zawada, A. R. 1973. Florida Difficulty Index in achieving rehabilitation. Unpublished manuscript, Division of Vocational Rehabilitation, Tallahassee, Florida.

13 | The Minnesota Theory of Work Adjustment

The Minnesota Theory of Work Adjustment began as a simple problem in evaluation. In 1957, Lloyd H. Lofquist and George W. England received a two-year grant from the Office of Vocational Rehabilitation to study the effectiveness of various job placement procedures used with physically handicapped clients. A control group design was contemplated, with the several "treatments" representing the different job placement procedures being evaluated. The investigators, however, quickly became aware of a pivotal problem: What outcome measures should be used? The standard solution was, of course, to review the literature.

The literature review turned out to be a surprise and a disappointment. In the first place, evaluation (outcome) studies appeared to be infrequently reported. An annotated bibliography of evaluation studies on physically handicapped filled no more than 12 pages of a research monograph (Dawis et al., 1958) comprising 61 studies published between 1931 and 1958, half of these appearing in the last 5 years of the period. Easily the most discernible weakness of these studies was the choice and measurement of the evaluation or outcome criteria. It was obvious to the investigators that the problem of outcome measurement (then better known as the "criterion problem") needed immediate attention. Happily, their Federal sponsors saw the wider implications of such outcome research for the field of vocational rehabilitation and agreed to support programmatic research on the criterion problem. Thus, in 1959, did the Work Adjustment Project originate.

THE WORK ADJUSTMENT PROJECT

The concept of "work adjustment" was chosen by the investigators to provide a focus for their research efforts, to integrate the various evaluation criteria found in the research literature, and to designate the general area of research encompassing evaluation criteria. A second review of the literature, which this time spanned not only vocational rehabilitation but also the different fields of applied psychology (counseling, industrial, personnel, occupational, and vocational) as well as related subfields of economics and sociology, resulted in the formulation of a comprehensive definition of work adjustment to provide a research framework for the project.

This definition of work adjustment (discussed in the next section) proved to be a useful framework within which to plan and to conduct research. Studies were undertaken to develop measures of work adjustment variables, both predictor and criterion. Research was undertaken to obtain and to validate work histories of employees, to assess the attitudes of employees and the impact of these attitudes as employment barriers, to develop criterion measures of employment satisfaction and satisfactoriness. Increasingly, however, the prediction and explanation of work adjustment became the major concern of the project.

The history of the Work Adjustment Project is typical of many research programs. The Project's research progressed through three stages: 1) an exploratory stage, in which the investigators staked out the field, identified the guideposts, and tentatively explored the area; 2) a descriptive stage, in which the investigators systematically went over the "ground," developing a "map" (theory) to describe the "area"; and 3) finally, a testing stage, in which the "map" was systematically evaluated (and later on revised and retested). By 1964, the Work Adjustment Project had produced its "map," the Theory of Work Adjustment.

DEFINITION OF WORK ADJUSTMENT

The term work adjustment has many meanings. It can refer to the *process,* as well as to the *outcome* of the process. Work adjustment can be viewed *internally,* from the viewpoint of the client undergoing or experiencing work adjustment, as well as *externally,* from the viewpoint of the professional person or agency providing the work adjustment service, or of the employing organization, or of society. It can occur over the *short term* or over the *long term.* Work adjustment can be reckoned by a simple criterion (e.g., obtaining employment) or by more *complex* criteria. It would behoove any investigator of this topic, therefore, as a first order of business, to specify one's meaning of the term work adjustment.

Work adjustment has a specific usage in the rehabilitation literature. It refers to the treatment-training process at the beginning of rehabilitation (or habilitation, for some clients) designed to develop basic work competencies and work attitudes necessary for competitive and renumerative employment. The basic nature of this training process can be seen in the inclusion of topics such as grooming, job interviewing, and the development of habits of punctuality and reliability. Work adjustment in this sense is a therapeutic process carried on in rehabilitation workshops and work adjustment facilities. It is of relatively short duration, reckoned in weeks rather than years. It has a focused objective: to bring the disabled or disadvantaged client to the level of (for some, becoming once again) a potentially functioning worker in a work-oriented society.

A reading of *A Definition of Work Adjustment* (Scott et al., 1960) will indicate that the conventional rehabilitation usage of the term was not what was intended by Lofquist and his fellow Work Adjustment Project investigators. These investigators used the term work adjustment initially to designate the general area encompassing 1) evaluation or outcome criteria, such as job satisfaction and employee morale, job tenure and labor turnover, productivity and efficiency, mobility and work history patterns, and the like, and 2) factors affecting, and predictive of, such outcomes.

While the definition of work adjustment given in the 1960 monograph provided useful starting points and helpful principles, in time a more elaborated and integrated theoretical statement about work adjustment was felt to be needed. Accordingly, such a statement was developed, and was published in 1964 as *A Theory of Work Adjustment* (Dawis, England, and Lofquist, 1964). A revision of this statement later followed (Dawis, Lofquist and Weiss, 1968). A more complete statement has been published in book form (Lofquist and Dawis, 1969).

BASIC CONCEPTS OF THE THEORY

Speaking at a simple level, a theory is an account of what is happening or what has happened. The Theory of Work Adjustment, then, is an account of what is happening or what has taken place in work adjustment. As an account, the theory is, itself, quite simple.

Tenure, Satisfaction, and Satisfactoriness

When a person goes to work, one of the first objective observations that can be made is that he/she continues on the job for a certain length of time. Tenure, length of time on a job, is a basic concept of the Theory of Work Adjustment. Tenure implies a minimal level of work adjustment. If an employee were to drop below this level, then it is presumed that he/she would leave the job.

Leaving the job may be voluntary or involuntary. If leaving were voluntary, one might infer "personal" reasons; one might infer enough dissatisfaction or not enough satisfaction. If leaving the job were involuntary, one might infer "performance" reasons; the employee may not have been satisfactory enough. Satisfaction and satisfactoriness are basic concepts of the Theory of Work Adjustment. Satisfaction and satisfactoriness are, therefore, viewed as being involved in tenure. Tenure is seen in the theory as depending primarily on satisfaction and satisfactoriness.

Of course, a number of other factors besides satisfaction and satisfactoriness can affect tenure. Tenure may be affected by labor market conditions, by collective bargaining agreements, by laws and other public regulations governing tenure, by social tradition or social practice of long standing, by other personal factors (such as family considerations), and many other factors. Two reasons are advanced for not including these other factors. First, the authors were limiting themselves to the construction of a *psychological* theory, hence nonpsychological concepts would be inappropriate. Second, the authors believed that these other factors could, in large measure, be accounted for by the psychological variables they chose. In truth, one of the "tests" of a theory is the extent to which it can account for and assimilate other explanations.

Tenure, satisfaction, and satisfactoriness, then, are the basic outcomes, or *dependent variables,* of work adjustment. To the extent that work adjustment has taken place, tenure, satisfaction, and satisfactoriness would be manifested to some commensurate extent. That is, they are *indicators* of work adjustment. These indicators point to the basic factors involved in work adjustment. Satisfaction suggests factors on the *individual* side, while satisfactoriness suggests factors on the *work* side (viewing work adjustment as what happens when a person goes to work). At this point, the Theory of Work Adjustment becomes even more explicitly psychological; it turns to psychological concepts for an account of the event that is called work adjustment.

Reinforcement Taking the individual side first: behavior may be explained (largely though not exclusively) by the principle of reinforcement. According to this principle, behavior is shaped and maintained by the consequences of the behavior. Some of these consequences are called reinforcers because they appear to reinforce or strengthen behavior. As a person grows up, he/she is exposed to diverse environmental conditions, many of which are experienced as reinforcing. Such experiences develop in the person certain preferences for reinforcers, many of which have relevance for the work setting. Some people, for example, may prefer (are reinforced by) working alone, while others may prefer working with other people. Some people may prefer situations where they make all the decisions, while others may prefer not to have to make the decisions. These preferences for reinforcers, when classified and categorized into a smaller number of classes, are what might be called *psychological* (as opposed to physiological) *needs* in that people tend to seek them out as consequences of behaving. Meeting the person's psychological needs, in turn, is crucial to job satisfaction. Needs and reinforcers, then, are basic concepts of the Theory of Work Adjustment.

Response Capabilities Taking the work side next: modern work has been organized into more or less standard sets of tasks (required behaviors) called jobs (or more precisely, positions). People are hired for a job presumably because they are capable of doing the job; in more technical terms, they have the behavior, or response, capabilities for the job. Response capabilities do not, of course, appear overnight. They are produced by the long process of learning and the shorter processes of training and are contingent on genetic inheritance. As a person grows up he/she develops a large number of response capabilities (also called *skills*), many of which can be used to meet work requirements. Persons differ in their skills: Some are "good with their hands," others are quick with words or with numbers, still others are socially sensitive or are "good listeners." There are, of course, many more skills than these examples show. The many skills and response capabilities, when categorized into a smaller number of classes, are what might be called *abilities.* A person utilizes abilities to meet the behavior requirements (to perform the required tasks) of the job. Having the appropriate abilities, therefore, is crucial to satisfactoriness. Abilities and ability requirements, then, are basic concepts of the Theory of Work Adjustment.

To summarize, needs and reinforcers are seen as the important factors in the determination (hence, the prediction) of satisfaction. Abilities and ability requirements are identified as the important factors in the determination and prediction of satisfactoriness. Needs and abilities are characteristics of the person. Reinforcers and ability requirements are characteristics of work, that is, of the work environment. What is left is to conceptualize the "encounter" between the individual and work, the interaction between the individual person and the work environment.

Correspondence between Individual and Environment

The most basic concept of the Theory of Work Adjustment is the correspondence between individual and environment.

> Correspondence between an individual and his environment implies conditions that can be described as: a harmonious relationship between individual and environment, suitability of the individual to the environment and of the environment for the individual. Consonance or agreement between individual and environment, and a reciprocal and complementary relationship between the individual and his environment. Correspondence, then, is a relationship in which the individual and the environment are correspondsive, i.e., mutually responsive. The individual brings into this relationship his requirements of the enviornment; the environment likewise has its requirements of the individual. In order to survive, i.e., exist, in an environment, the individual must achieve some degree of correspondence.
>
> It is a basic assumption of the Theory of Work Adjustment that *each individual seeks to achieve and maintain correspondence with his environment.* (Italics in original) Achieving and maintaining correspondence with the environment are basic motives of human behavior (Dawis, Lofquist and Weiss, 1968, p. 3).

Correspondence, then, is a concept that designates the status or condition of the relationship between a person and one's environment, in the case of work adjustment, one's work environment. This status or condition can be studied over the short term or over the long term. Short-term correspondence may include hour-to-hour, day-to-day or even week-to-week interaction between individual and environment; long-term correspondence may refer to the total period of a person's tenure on one job or the total period of his/her working years. Because the study of long-term correspondence was the more urgently needed at the time for purposes of vocational rehabilitation and vocational counseling, the Theory of Work Adjustment was addressed initially to this aspect.

Needs and reinforcers, and abilities and requirements have been singled out as the crucial elements in the determination of satisfaction and satisfactoriness, respectively. By incorporating these elements into the concept of individual-environment correspondence (or, alternatively, by using the concept of individual-environment correspondence to integrate these elements) the Theory of Work Adjustment authors were able to construct the predictors of satisfaction and satisfactoriness. In this formulation, *need-reinforcer* correspondence becomes the predictor of satisfaction, while *ability-requirement* correspondence becomes the predictor for satisfactoriness. Need-reinforcer correspondence and ability-requirement correspondence are therefore the independent (input) variables in a system in which satisfaction and satisfactoriness are the dependent (output) variables.

However, this formulation leaves two separate systems in tandem: one system governing satisfaction and another governing satisfactoriness. Analytically, the systems can exist independently and can be considered separately; nonetheless, some integration is desirable in the interests of a unified or integrated theory. To accomplish this integration, the authors of *A Theory of Work Adjustment* chose to utilize the notion of a "moderator" variable (Saunders, 1956; Ghiselli, 1960). A moderator variable correlates with the *relationship* between independent and dependent variables. For example, if it is found that for younger people practice correlates with (is more strongly related to) subsequent performance while this is not so for older people (that is, for older people practice is not as strongly related to subsequent performance, and the older the group the weaker the relationship), then age is correlated with the relationship between practice and subsequent performance. Thus, age *moderates* the relationship between practice and subsequent performance.

In the Theory of Work Adjustment, satisfaction moderates the relationship between ability-requirement correspondence and satisfactoriness, and satisfactoriness moderates the relationship between need-reinforcer correspondence and satisfaction. In other words, the prediction of satisfactoriness from ability-requirement correspondence is affected by satisfaction: the more satisfied the better the prediction, and the less satisfied the poorer the prediction. Likewise, the prediction of satisfaction from need-reinforcer correspondence is seen as being affected by satisfactoriness: the more satisfactory the better the prediction, and the less satisfactory the poorer the prediction. Satisfaction helps determine satisfactoriness, and satisfactoriness helps determine satisfaction. The determination of satisfactoriness by ability-requirement correspondence is contingent (conditional) upon satisfaction, and similarly, the determination of satisfaction by need-reinforcer correspondence is contingent upon satisfactoriness.

This use of the correspondence concept in the sense of long-term correspondence is premised on one very important assumption: that the relevant characteristics of a person and of the work environment are relatively stable. By stability is meant not only constancy or fixity (within error limits) but also regularity or predictability (in the case of a changing or fluctuating characteristic). Ample evidence in the literature (Anastasi, 1958; Tyler, 1965) supports the assumption that abilities and, to a lesser extent, needs, are relatively stable in the adult years. The stability of a person's characteristics (abilities, needs) enables the conceptualization of this stable characterization of the individual as a unique person as one's *personality,* in the case of work-related abilities and needs, as one's *work personality.* By definition, the work personality is stable. It is important, then, to remember that the Theory of Work Adjustment is premised on a stable work personality.

PROPOSITIONS OF THE THEORY

The following propositions, designed by the authors (Dawis, Lofquist, and Weiss, 1968) to "serve as a basis for research," state the Theory of Work Adjustment more formally:

> *Proposition I.* An individual's work adjustment at any point in time is indicated by his concurrent levels of satisfactoriness and satisfaction.
>
> *Proposition II.* Satisfactoriness is a function of the correspondence between an individual's abilities and the ability requirements of the work environment, provided that the individual's needs correspond with the reinforcer system of the work environment.
>
> > *Corollary IIa.* Knowledge of an individual's abilities and of his satisfactoriness permits the determination of the effective ability requirements of the work environment.
> >
> > *Corollary IIb.* Knowledge of the ability requirements of the work environment and of an individual's satisfactoriness permits the inference of an individual's abilities.
>
> *Proposition III.* Satisfaction is a function of the correspondence between the reinforcer system of the work environment and the individual's needs, provided that the individual's abilities correspond with the ability requirements of the work environment.
>
> > *Corollary IIIa.* Knowledge of an individual's needs and of his satisfaction permits the determination of the effective reinforcer system of the work environment for the individual.
> >
> > *Corollary IIIb.* Knowledge of the reinforcer system of the work environment and of an individual's satisfaction permits the inference of an individual's needs.
>
> *Proposition IV.* Satisfaction moderates the functional relationship between satisfactoriness and ability-requirement correspondence.
>
> *Proposition V.* Satisfactoriness moderates the functional relationship between satisfaction and need-reinforcer correspondence.
>
> *Proposition VI.* The probability of an individual being forced out of the work environment is inversely related to his satisfactoriness.
>
> *Proposition VII.* The probability of an individual voluntarily leaving the work environment is inversely related to his satisfaction.
>
> Combining Propositions VI and VII, we have:
>
> *Proposition VIII.* Tenure is a joint function of satisfactoriness and satisfaction.
>
> Given Propositions II, III, and VIII, this corollary follows:

Corollary VIIIa. Tenure is a function of ability-requirement and need-reinforcer correspondence.

Proposition IX. Work personality-work environment correspondence increases as a function of tenure (pp. 9–11).

In summary, the Theory of Work Adjustment consists of nine propositions, which may be grouped into the following four:

1. One proposition about work adjustment indicators
2. Two propositions about individual-environment correspondence and its relationship to the indicators
3. Two propositions about the indicators as moderator variables
4. Four propositions about tenure.

The last proposition, that individual-environment correspondence increases as a function of tenure, may be considered to be the "work adjustment principle." It provides the foundation for the mechanisms and processes of work adjustment (adjustment to work) to be discussed in a later section.

INSTRUMENTATION OF THE THEORY

A formal test of a theory requires that the theory's concepts be operationalized, i.e., stated in terms precisely and specifically describing the operations by which observations are to be made in order to confirm or to disconfirm the theory or any part of it. This requirement is usually fulfilled through the use of instruments in data collection. For the Theory of Work Adjustment six instruments would be needed to make the requisite observations, measures of the following six concepts: 1) satisfactoriness, 2) satisfaction, 3) abilities, 4) needs, 5) ability requirements, and 6) reinforcer systems. Measures of satisfactoriness and satisfaction would be the outcome or criterion measures. (Tenure is an outcome variable, too, but this can be observed without the need of instrumentation.) Measures of abilities and needs would be required to describe the person while measures of ability requirements and reinforcer systems would be needed to describe the work environment. To enable the measurement of correspondence, one approach would be to develop parallel measures of people and work environments; that is, measures of abilities and ability requirements should utilize the same set of ability dimensions, and likewise, measures of needs and reinforcers should utilize the same set of reinforcement dimensions. This approach was followed in the Work Adjustment Project.

At this point, it is worth noting that the Theory of Work Adjustment does not specify the elements, i.e., the dimensions, of any of the six concepts. For such specification, the Work Adjustment Project investigators had recourse to the psychological literature. For example, the literature on job satisfaction and on work attitudes, needs, values, and interests was reviewed for dimensions to include as likely candidates in the measurement of satisfactions, needs, and reinforcer systems. The literature on abilities and work performance was reviewed for possible directions in the measurement of satisfactoriness, abilities, and ability requirements. This review was summarized and reported in Scott et al. (1960).

Three parallel instruments were developed for the measurement of satisfactions, needs, and reinforcer systems. These were the Minnesota Satisfaction Questionnaire (MSQ), the Minnesota Importance Questionnaire (MIQ), and the Minnesota Job Description Questionnaire (MJDQ), respectively. These three instruments were designed to measure satisfaction with, importance of, and presence of the same 20 reinforcers (or reinforcer dimensions), respectively. These are listed below, followed by a representative statement describing the reinforcer:

1. Ability Utilization—I could do something that makes use of my abilities
2. Achievement—The job could give me a feeling of accomplishment
3. Activity—I could be busy all the time
4. Advancement—The job would provide an opportunity for advancement
5. Authority—I could tell people what to do
6. Company Policies and Practices—The company would administer its policies fairly
7. Compensation—My pay would compare well with that of other workers
8. Coworkers—My coworkers would be easy to make friends with
9. Creativity—I could try out some of my own ideas
10. Independence—I could work alone on the job
11. Moral Values—I could do the work without feeling that it is morally wrong
12. Recognition—I could get recognition for the work I do
13. Responsibility—I could make decisions on my own
14. Security—The job would provide for steady employment
15. Social Service—I could do things for other people
16. Social Status—I could be "somebody" in the community
17. Supervision-Human Relations—My boss would back up the employees (with top management)
18. Supervision-Technical—My boss would train the employees well
19. Variety—I could do something different every day

20. Working Conditions—The job would have good working conditions

These 20 reinforcers or reinforcer dimensions were derived from two sources: The Industrial Relations Center's Employee Attitude Questionnaire (Fox, Albers, and Hellweg, 1954) and Schaffer's influential study (Schaffer, 1953) which, in turn, was derived from Murray (1938).

The MSQ (Weiss et al., 1967) is a Likert-rating-type self-report questionnaire that asks the respondent to rate his/her satisfaction with different job aspects (i.e., reinforcers) on 5-point rating scales. Two forms are available: a 100-item, 21-scale Long Form, and a 20-item, 3-scale Short Form. The MSQ Long Form is scored on satisfaction with each of the 20 reinforcers listed above, plus a General Satisfaction score. Median internal consistency reliabilities for these scores range from 0.78 for Responsibility, to 0.93 for Advancement and Recognition, with more than four-fifths of the reliability coefficients being above 0.80. Median stability coefficients range from 0.83 for a one-week test-retest interval, to 0.70 for a one-year interval. Validity evidences are based primarily on the confirmation of expected group differences. Normative data are available on 25 occupational groups in professional-technical-managerial, clerical-sales, service, and bench work and other blue collar fields.

The MSQ Short Form is scored on three scales: Intrinsic Satisfaction, Extrinsic Satisfaction, and General Satisfaction. Median reliabilities are 0.86 for Intrinsic Satisfaction, 0.80 for Extrinsic Satisfaction, and 0.90 for General Satisfaction. No stability coefficients are reported. Validity evidences are also primarily based on group-difference studies. Normative data are available for seven occupational groups spanning the occupational hierarchy.

The MIQ (Gay et al., 1971) is a 210-item paired comparison instrument that is scored on the same 20 reinforcer dimensions listed above. In this case, however, the scores reflect a person's needs (i.e., preferences for reinforcers) expressed in terms of the importance of specific reinforcers to a person "in (his/her) *ideal* job, the kind of job (he/she) would most like to have." Scores are given as "adjusted scale values" (scale values adjusted to a person's subjective point of indifference, the point separating the important from the not important). Scores range from -4.00 to +4.00.

Median internal consistency reliabilities for the MIQ scales vary from 0.77 to 0.81. Median scale stability coefficients range from 0.89 for immediate retest, to 0.53 for a 10-month interval. Stability coefficients for MIQ profiles are much higher, the medians ranging from 0.95 for immediate retest, to 0.87 for the 10-month interval. A validity score indicates random responding or logical inconsistency (intransitivity of choices).

Validity is supported by a variety of studies, including group differences and correlational studies. Percentage norms are available for DVR clients, vocational-technical school women, college students, employed persons, and a total group of more than 5,000 people. While these norms are useful in the interpretation of scores, the MIQ is best interpreted in conjunction with Occupational Reinforcer Patterns (ORPs), to be discussed next.

The MJDQ (Borgen et al., 1968a) is the instrument developed to describe reinforcers in the work environment. The MJDQ is a rating (more correctly, ranking) instrument in which reinforcers are presented in groups of five for the respondent to rank order. From these responses, the equivalent of paired comparison data can be reconstituted and used to develop normative profiles of reinforcers present in particular work environments. These profiles are similar in form to the MIQ profile, from the set of 20 reinforcer dimensions used, to the numerical scale used to plot scale values. These profiles, known as ORPs, have been developed from supervisor ratings for 148 occupations (Borgen et al., 1968b; Rosen et al., 1972).

Because the MIQ (a measure of individual persons) and the ORPs (measures of work environments) are parallel measures (have the same reinforcer dimensions, are scaled on the same numerical scale), it becomes possible to derive an *index of correspondence,* such as a summated difference score or a measure of profile similarity. Derivation of such an index of correspondence allows for the empirical test of the Theory of Work Adjustment proposition concerning the prediction of satisfaction. Studies involving such an empirical test will be discussed in the next section.

In an analogous manner, an empirical test of the Theory of Work Adjustment proposition concerning the prediction of satisfactoriness is made possible by the availability of instruments and measures describing a person's abilities and the ability requirements of work environments, as well as the development of a measure of satisfactoriness by the Work Adjustment Project (Gibson et al., 1970). Several different measures of abilities were available for consideration, but the most superior by far was the U.S. Training and Employment Service's General Aptitude Test Battery (GATB). Not only was the GATB psychometrically the most technically superior ability instrument available, but also ability-requirement descriptions of work environments in the same ability-dimension terms were available for hundreds of occupations—a feature that could not be claimed for any other comparable ability instrument (see Chapter 11). The GATB, then, and its associated ability-requirement descriptions of work environments, the Occupational Aptitude Patterns (OAPs), were adopted for Work Adjustment Project tests of the Theory of Work Adjustment proposition.

The GATB (U.S. Department of Labor, 1970) is a multiaptitude test battery consisting of 12 separate tests: eight paper-and-pencil and four performance tests. GATB scores are given in standard score form, with a mean of 100 and a standard deviation of 20, standardized in a norm group of 4,000 workers representing the U.S. labor force. Three-month stability coefficients are in the 0.80s for G, V, N, and S, and in the 0.70s for the remaining aptitudes. Validities against training and on-the-job criteria range from the 0.20s to the 0.90s, with the modal values in the 0.60s. These validities are for batteries of three aptitudes whose configuration of cutting scores are known as Occupational Aptitude Patterns (OAPs).

Because OAPs describe the set of cutting scores for three aptitudes that best predict training success or job success, they are good estimates of the ability requirements of jobs. They can thus be used to describe work environments in the same terms (ability dimensions) as ability test descriptions of the individual person. Meeting the ability requirements specified by an OAP can then be taken as ability-requirement correspondence between the individual person and the specific work environment. OAPs are currently available for some 1,200 occupations representing 62 out of a possible 84 OAP combinations (U.S. Department of Labor, 1970).

For the description of satisfactoriness, the Work Adjustment Project departed from its parallel-measures approach and developed a rating scale, the Minnesota Satisfactoriness Scales (MSS; Gibson et al., 1970), based on 28 items commonly used in supervisory ratings. Factor analysis of these items led to the construction of four scales: Performance, Conformance, Dependability, and Personal Adjustment. Because of relatively high inter-correlations among these scales (0.50s to 0.80s), a General Satisfactoriness Scale based on all 28 items was added. Internal consistency reliabilities for these scales ranged from 0.69 to 0.95, with a median of 0.87. Two-year stability coefficients ranged from 0.40 to 0.68, with a median of 0.50. Validity evidences included correlation with tenure, lack of correlation with satisfaction, and observation of expected group differences. Percentile norms are available for the following occupational groups: A) professional, technical, and managerial, B) clerical and sales (separately for male and female), C) service, D) machine trades and bench work, and E) workers-in-general.

To recapitulate, formal tests of the Theory of Work Adjustment propositions require that its basic concepts be operationalized. The following instruments are available for such tests, as well as for other applications of the theory:

MSQ— to measure satisfaction
MSS— to measure satisfactoriness
MIQ— to measure needs
GATB— to measure abilities
ORPs— to measure reinforcers
OAPs— to measure ability requirements

EVIDENCE FOR THE PROPOSITIONS

With instruments such as those described in the preceding section, it was possible for the Work Adjustment Project to conduct research bearing on the propositions of the Theory of Work Adjustment. The following findings from this research constitute evidence supporting the theory's propositions.

Satisfaction and Satisfactoriness Scores

Satisfaction and satisfactoriness scores were found to be relatively independent, i.e., uncorrelated. Mean cross-correlations between MSQ and MSS scale scores ranged from 0.04 for a group of 165 salesmen to 0.15 for a group of 186 clerks, in a study of six occupational groups involving 1,177 people (Weiss et al., 1966). For the total group the cross-correlations ranged from -0.13 (Extrinsic Satisfaction versus General Satisfactoriness) to 0.07 (Extrinsic Satisfaction and Conformance). These findings support the implication in Proposition I of the theory, that the two indicators of work adjustment are relatively independent.

Prediction of Satisfactoriness Scores

Satisfactoriness scores could be predicted from the ability scores of workers in a given occupation. Because ability requirements are presumably the same for all people working in the same occupation, ability scores will correlate perfectly (+1.00) with ability-requirement correspondence scores for these people. Therefore, the correlation of ability scores with satisfactoriness scores will be equivalent to the correlation of ability-requirement correspondence scores with satisfactoriness scores. Such correlations have been reported in Work Adjustment Project research, using the MSS and the GATB, to range from 0.33 (for 97 janitors and maintenance men) to 0.48 (for 133 machinists and assemblers) in one study (Lofquist and Dawis, 1969). Similar correlations in personnel psychology research have ranged up to 0.50 or higher (Ghiselli, 1966). Such findings support Proposition II of the theory.

Prediction of Satisfaction Scores

Likewise, satisfaction scores could be predicted from the need scores of workers in a given occupation. Such correlations between satisfaction scores and need scores would be equivalent to correlations between satisfaction scores and need-reinforcer correspondence scores because the reinforcer system is presumably the same for every one in the same occupation. (To the extent that this presumption is incorrect, the correlation would be diminished.) Correlations between MIQ scores and MSQ scores for 16 different occupational groups have been reported in Work Adjustment Project research to range from 0.01 to 0.48 on cross validation (Lofquist and Dawis, 1969). Other unpublished data using need-reinforcer (MIQ-ORP) correspondence scores in a study of seven occupational groups yielded correlations ranging from 0.13 to 0.40. These findings support Proposition II of the theory.

Satisfaction and Prediction of Satisfactoriness

The prediction of satisfactoriness (MSS) scores from ability (GATB) scores for one occupational group was found to be best for the "high satisfaction" (measured on the MSQ) groups and poorest for the "low satisfaction" groups (Lofquist and Dawis, 1969). The correlations for males were 0.69 (for the high satisfaction group) versus 0.34 (for the low satisfaction group); for females, 0.63 (for the high satisfaction group) versus 0.42 (for the low satisfaction group). These findings support Proposition IV of the theory concerning satisfaction as a moderator variable in the prediction of satisfactoriness from ability-requirement correspondence. No data bearing on Propositions V and VI are currently available from Work Adjustment Project research.

Satisfaction and Termination

Concerning the relationship of satisfaction to termination in Proposition VII, a relevant study is reported by Taylor and Weiss (1972). A group of 475 discount store employees were administered the MSQ. One year later, 20 percent of them were found to have terminated. These "leavers" were found to have significantly lower scores than the "stayers" on 9 of the 20 MSQ scales taken at the beginning of the study. This finding, that tenure can be predicted from job satisfaction data, supports Schuh's (1967) review of the literature, which shows that job satisfaction data are among the best predictors of tenure. Thus, there appears to be strong support for Proposition VII of the theory.

Tenure

That tenure depends on the combination of satisfaction and satisfactoriness (Proposition VIII) is shown in Anderson's study reported in Gibson et al. (1970). Anderson (1969), in a doctoral dissertation, cross-classified 1,508 workers into satisfied-unsatisfied versus high-low satisfactoriness groups and followed them up 2 years later. For the satisfied group she found significantly fewer of the high satisfactoriness group terminating, compared with the low satisfactoriness group. This contrast was not observed for the unsatisfied group. Thus, it was the combination of satisfaction and satisfactoriness that provided the best predictor of tenure, thereby supporting Proposition VIII of the theory.

Personality and Work Environment

No data have been available as yet that bear on Proposition IX of the theory. However, this proposition—that individual-environment correspondence increases with tenure—has provided the basis for an extension of the Theory of Work Adjustment, from the *outcome* side of work adjustment to the *process* side of work adjustment. This is discussed in the next section.

EXTENSIONS OF THE THEORY

Proposition IX, that "Work personality—work environment correspondence increases as a function of tenure," has provided the impetus for logical extensions of the Theory of Work Adjustment into the area of the process of work adjustment (Lofquist and Dawis, 1969, pp. 67–69). The implications of Proposition IX are best understood in the case of discorrespondence as a person's initial condition on the job. If adjustment were to take place, and tenure were subsequently to be observed, some accommodation between individual and work environment presumably would have to occur. Otherwise, the person would have left the work environment or the work environment would have forced him/her out. If correspondence were the person's initial condition, Proposition IX would not be operative because the person would already be "adjusted," i.e., satisfied and satisfactory.

Assuming that perfect correspondence between individual and work environment is the ideal situation and is rarely if at all observed "in nature," different people would differ in the amount of discorrespondence (deviation from perfect correspondence) that they would tolerate before becoming annoyed or bothered enough by the situation to want to do something about it. These differing "tolerances" could be used to define a new personality dimension that could be labeled *flexibility*. The more discorrespondence one can tolerate, the more flexible he/she is, and vice versa. (It should be noted that the same observations might be made of the work environment as of the individual, i.e., with respect to the discorrespondence that the work environment will tolerate before wanting to do something about it.)

When discorrespondence has exceeded the point at which it is minimally tolerable to the person, he/she will presumably attempt to decrease discorrespondence (increase correspondence). Logically, there are two ways by which a decrease in discorrespondence (or increase in correspondence) may be accomplished: One may act on the work environment (manipulate it, shape it, modify it, dominate it), or one may react to environmental demands (accommodate to the environment, modify the expression of one's personality to conform to environmental requirements). In the former approach the initiative is the person's, while in the latter the initative is not. In the former, the person is active while in the latter he/she is reactive. Activity and reactivity are thus two modes of adjustment, and individual differences in utilization of these adjustment modes may be used to define two more new personality dimensions: *activeness* and *reactiveness*. It is recognized that most if not all people use both modes at one time or other in their work careers, and that utilization of one or the other depends in part on situational factors. However, it is reasonable to assume that, in the course of one's response and reinforcement history, a person develops a more or less stable preference for one mode of adjustment. The rate with which a person adjusts (i.e., reduces discorrespondence to more tolerable levels) defines still another new personality dimension.

Thus, from a consideration of the implications of Proposition IX, four new personality dimensions are identified and defined: 1) flexibility, 2) activeness, 3) reactiveness, and 4) rate of adjustment. Because these dimensions are conceptually involved in the *process* of adjustment, are best observed over time, and describe the person in action, they may be categorized as personality *style* dimensions, in contrast to abilities and needs, which are conventionally categorized as dimensions of personality *structure*.

The process of adjustment may now be described in its totality. A person always strives for a tolerable level of correspondence as he/she sees it. If initially this is the case, the person is fortunate. If not, he/she attempts to decrease discorrespondence by either active or reactive adjustment (or, more probably, by some combination of both). This goes on until tolerable correspondence is achieved once again. Different persons differ in the speed with which this adjustment is achieved. Finally, circumstances may arise such that regardless of what the individual does, discorrespondence continues to increase. Soon a point is reached that is absolutely intolerable for the individual, and he/she leaves the work environment. The amount of discorrespondence that a person will tolerate before leaving the work environment may be used to define his/her *absolute* flexibility. Absolute flexibility may or may not correlate with flexibility as previously defined (i.e., the amount of discorrespondence tolerated before the person does anything about it).

Similar adjustment mechanisms may be used to describe the *work environment's* adjustment: The amount of discorrespondence tolerated by the work environment before doing something about the situation or discharging an employee from the organization; active and reactive modes of adjustment; rate of adjustment. Thus, work adjustment, i.e., the achieving and maintaining of individual-environment correspondence, is an *interactive* process.

IMPLICATIONS FOR VOCATIONAL REHABILITATION

The Theory of Work Adjustment, as with any viable theory, may be used as an heuristic device in the exploration and organization of a field of study or a field of application. In this final section, the Theory of Work Adjustment will be utilized in the consideration of the field of vocational rehabilitation.

Rehabilitation might be viewed, at a simple level, as essentially a problem solving field. The problems to be solved in rehabilitation originate from disability as the primary, though not the exclusive, cause. The term vocational rehabilitation further delimits the types of problems considered to those related to the work career and employment. The Theory of Work Adjustment can be used to provide a systematic analysis of these (vocational rehabilitation) problems.

In the first place, a "problem" can be defined, in the context of the Theory of Work Adjustment, as an undesirable outcome. The "undesirability" of the outcome can, in turn, be defined with reference to the individual person or to the work environment, or both, as being outcome levels lying below the minimum acceptable levels. Problems, therefore, are of varying magnitudes, and their seriousness depends on how far they are below acceptable levels.

Ordinarily, one would speak of undesirable satisfaction outcomes with reference to the individual person (i.e., one defines his/her minimum acceptable level of satisfaction). Likewise, undesirable satisfactoriness outcomes are ordinarily defined with reference to the work environment (the work environment defines the minimum acceptable levels of satisfactoriness). However, it is also possible to consider a satisfactoriness problem from the perspective of the individual person, and likewise a satisfaction problem from the perspective of the work environment. Obviously, undesirable tenure outcomes can be considered from both perspectives.

Undesirable outcomes are problems in themselves, whether they be realized (i.e., existing) or potential (i.e., predicted, expected, or anticipated). Undesirable outcomes are problems also in terms of their effects on the morale and behavior of the person or the work environment. Undesirable outcomes may produce feelings of anxiety, frustration, and other negative feelings besides dissatisfaction, and, in addition to the unsatisfactory behavior, may lead to inappropriate and often self-defeating behavior intended to minimize or eliminate the undesirable outcomes. Analogous "side effects" may be described for the work environment. These "side effects" (of undesirable outcomes as problems) may occur whether the outcomes be realized or potential, existing or anticipated.

In addition, potential undesirable outcomes may be problems to the extent that the predicted outcomes are inaccurate. Inaccuracy in predicted outcomes, according to the Theory of Work Adjustment, would reflect inaccurate assessments of the individual person and/or the work environment. Such inaccurate assessments are often labeled "inaccurate perceptions" when speaking of the person. ("The individual has inaccurate perceptions of himself/herself or of the work invironment.") However, the work environment, too, may have "inaccurate perceptions" of people and of itself, especially because "work environments" are made up of people.

If an outcome were a problem (i.e., undesirable), the Theory of Work Adjustment would locate the source of the problem in the discorrespondence between the individual and the work environment. Two strategies are logically available: 1) minimize the discorrespondence, or 2) consider alternative work environments (in the case of the individual) or individuals (in the case of the work environment). The discussion that follows is from the perspective of the individual person, because vocational rehabilitation is about people. (An analogous discussion can, of course, be made from the work environment's perspective.)

With respect to minimizing the discorrespondence, "intervention" can take place on either the individual or the work environment side. ("Intervention" is an appropriate term because it denotes a coming-in-between the individual and the environment.) Intervention on the individual side can take the form of modifying the expression of a person's abilities, as in, for example, the acquisition of new skills founded on the residual abilities of the disabled person. This form of intervention is probably the most familiar to, and the most utilized by, vocational rehabilitation workers. Most rehabilitation facilities are set up to provide this form of intervention. Public (and also private) rehabilitation agencies consider vocational training as the most basic approach to vocational rehabilitation.

Intervention on the individual side can take the form of modifying perceptions and attitudes. In a sense, this can be seen as modifying the manifestation of the person's needs. Thus, some needs may be emphasized over other equally important ones. Furthermore, the person's perceptions of himself/herself and the work environment may be modified. For instance, some abilities may be emphasized over others equally as strong. Some features of the work environment (reinforcers, requirements) may be emphasized over other features equally as prominent. This form of intervention is familiar to vocational rehabilitation workers as counseling or the part of counseling that is most similar to psychotherapy. In any event, the counseling interview is the tool most frequently used to effect these modifications of perception. In recent years, group work has been used to achieve these objectives.

Intervention on the work environment side can take the form of modifying the ability (skill, response) requirements and/or modifying the reinforcer system. While, in practice, a change in skill requirements affects the reinforcer system, and vice versa, it is conceptually possible to effect significant changes in one (requirements or reinforcers) without necessarily effecting significant changes in the other. Modifications of this sort are involved in what might be called "job redesign." It is conceivable that not only the jobs and the work would need redesigning, but also the employing organization and even ultimately the economy and the society. This is because these other job-transcending entities will determine, in the final analysis, the skills required and the reinforcers provided in jobs.

If intervention via minimizing discorrespondence were not feasible or productive, then consideration of other, potentially more correspondent, work environments (or nonwork environments, in the case of some) would be the logical alternative. In some instances, this alternative would be the more economical or more efficient. In other instances, this alternative should be considered last. When to do which would be facilitated by more and better information as required by the Theory of Work Adjustment. That is, better assessment of individual persons, work environments, and work adjustment outcomes will provide the essential information needed to make rational (i.e., cost-benefit) decisions of the sort called for above, whether the costs and benefits be reckoned from the viewpoint of the person, the employing organization, or society in general.

The preceding discussion illustrates the usefulness of the Theory of Work Adjustment in the conceptualization of a field of application, vocational rehabilitation. The theory may similarly be used to conceptualize other fields of study or application, e.g., school adjustment or the training of counselors. This is, indeed, a long way from the simple problem with which it all began. But the theory's future is, in a manner of speaking, still ahead of it. Much testing and confirmation remain to be done; better instruments and measures need to be developed; more explication is required; better specification of assumptions is needed. When all of these are accomplished, the theory will have to be modified—or overthrown. In the nature of scientific progress, the theory is no more than a way station, a stepping stone, to be used to achieve the next advance, and thereby to succeed by its very failure.

REFERENCES

Anastasi, A. 1958. Differential Psychology. Macmillan, New York.

Anderson, L. M. 1969. Longitudinal changes in level of work adjustment. Unpublished doctoral dissertation, University of Minnesota, Minneapolis.

Borgen, F., D. J. Weiss, H. E. A. Tinsley, R. V. Dawis, and L. H. Lofquist. 1968a. The measurement of occupational reinforcer patterns. Minnesota Studies in Vocational Rehabilitation, No. XXV. Industrial Relations Center, University of Minnesota, Minneapolis.

Borgen, F., D. J. Weiss, H. E. A. Tinsley, R. V. Dawis, and L. H. Lofquist. 1968b. Occupational reinforcer patterns. Vol. 1. Minnesota Studies in Vocational Rehabilitation, No. XXIV. Industrial Relations Center, University of Minnesota, Minneapolis.

Dawis, R. V., G. W. England, and L. H. Lofquist. 1964. A theory of work adjustment. Minnesota Studies in Vocational Rehabilitation, No. XV. Industrial Relations Center, University of Minnesota, Minneapolis.

Dawis, R. V., G. W. England, L. H. Lofquist, and D. Hakes. 1958. Research plan and bibliography. Minnesota Studies in Vocational Rehabilitation, No. I. Industrial Relations Center, University of Minnesota, Minneapolis.

Dawis, R. V., L. H. Lofquist, and D. J. Weiss. 1968. A theory of work adjustment: A revision. Minnesota Studies in Vocational Rehabilitation, No. XXIII. Industrial Relations Center, University of Minnesota, Minneapolis.

Fox, H., W. S. Albers, and A. Hellweg. 1954. Triple audit: Employee Attitude Scale development and preliminary norms. Industrial Relations Center Mimeograph Release, No. 6. Industrial Relations Center, University of Minnesota, Minneapolis.

Gay, E., D. J. Weiss, D. D. Hendel, R. V. Dawis, and L. H. Lofquist. 1971. Manual for the Minnesota Importance Questionnaire. Minnesota Studies in Vocational Rehabilitation, No. XXVIII. Industrial Relations Center, University of Minnesota, Minneapolis.

Ghiselli, E. E. 1960. The prediction of predictability. Ed. Psych. Meas. 20:3–8.

Ghiselli, E. E. 1966. The Validity of Occupational Aptitude Tests. Wiley, New York.

Gibson, D., D. J. Weiss, R. V. Dawis, and L. H. Lofquist. 1970. Manual for the Minnesota Satisfactoriness Scales. Minnesota Studies in Vocational Rehabilitation, No. XXVII. Industrial Relations Center, University of Minnesota, Minneapolis.

Lofquist, L. H., and R. V. Dawis. 1969. Adjustment to Work: A Psychological View of Man's Problems in a Work-oriented Society. Appleton-Century-Crofts, New York.

Murray, H. 1938. Explorations in Personality. Oxford University Press, New York.

Rosen, S., D. J. Weiss, D. D. Hendel, R. V. Dawis, and L. H. Lofquist. 1972. Occupational reinforcer patterns. Vol. II. Minnesota Studies in Vocational Rehabilitation, No. XXIX. Industrial Relations Center, University of Minnesota, Minneapolis.

Saunders, D. R. 1956. Moderator variables in prediction. Ed. Psych. Meas. 16:209–222.

Schaffer, R. H. 1953. Job satisfaction as related to need satisfaction in work. Psych. Mono. No. 364.

Schuh, A. J. 1967. The predictability of employee tenure: A review of the literature. Pers. Psych. 20:133–152.

Scott, T. B., R. V. Dawis, G. W. England, and L. H. Lofquist. 1960. A definition of work adjustment. Minnesota Studies in Vocational Rehabilitation, No. X. Industrial Relations Center, University of Minnesota, Minneapolis.

Taylor, K. E., and D. J. Weiss. 1972. Prediction of individual job termination from measured job satisfaction and biographical data. J. Vocat. Behav. 2:123–132.

Tyler, L. E. 1965. The Psychology of Human Differences. Appleton-Century-Crofts, New York.

U.S. Department of Labor. 1970. Manual for the USTES General Aptitude Test Battery, Section II: Development. Washington, D.C.

Weiss, D. J., R. V. Dawis, G. W. England, and L. H. Lofquist. 1967. Manual for the Minnesota Satisfaction Questionnaire. Minnesota Studies in Vocational Rehabilitation, No. XXII. Industrial Relations Center, University of Minnesota, Minneapolis.

Weiss, D. J., R. V. Dawis, L. H. Lofquist, and G. W. England. 1966. Instrumentation for the theory of work adjustment. Minnesota Studies in Vocational Rehabilitation, No. XXI. Industrial Relations Center, University of Minnesota, Minneapolis.

14

Psychological Evaluation of the Blind Client

MARY K. BAUMAN

Previous chapters have discussed the development, use, and significance of norms. To be acceptable, a standard test must provide statistical studies and compilations of the results of use of that test with one or more well defined and presumably typical groups. Without these "norms," psychologist and counselor would be at a loss to interpret the test scores of any individual client.

APPLICABILITY OF NORMS FOR THE SIGHTED

In the interpretation of test results of blind clients, norms developed on sighted groups can be used only with utmost caution.

A simple definition of a test might be that it is standard material, used in a standard way, yielding scores that measure only, or chiefly, what that test claims to measure; these scores are then compared with similarly obtained scores of a standard or well defined population.

In testing blind clients it may be necessary to deviate from one or all parts of this definition. The material itself may be changed, for example, by putting ink print into braille or using blocks with rough and smooth sides instead of red and white sides. The test materials may not be used in a standard way; for example, the test may be read to the client instead of read by him, extra practice time may be allowed, time limits may be varied or discarded, etc. In many cases the purity of what the test is supposed to

249

measure is greatly muddied; for example, on a dexterity test, the totally blind client must distinguish by touch which end of a bolt should be inserted into a nut, must orient himself tactually in the work space, etc. The dexterity test therefore measures not only his speed and manual coordination, but his tactual discrimination and his ability to keep his place in the work space.

Blind people are never part of a typical group. Their life experiences have been so different from those of typical sighted people that the norms provided with tests for the sighted are frequently totally unsuitable for use with the blind. Yet in most cases there is no alternative. The psychologist must make a judgment with regard to how, and how much, he should change the test materials and the testing procedure, how and how much the blind client differs from the normative group, and put all these immeasurable factors together into a prediction for that client.

NORMS FOR THE BLIND

A natural question would be, "Why not develop norms for the blind?" For some tests this has been done rather successfully. However, it is not easy, and some of the so-called norms available in the literature are questionable because they are established on very small groups of blind people, or because the blind population used has doubtful claim to being representative.

Except in a large population center, it is difficult to find enough blind people to form a normative group. This is especially true because roughly half of all blind people are more than sixty years of age, and, if rehabilitation is defined by potential employability, their age often disqualifies them. To develop norms, the research worker needs a fairly homogeneous group, and the preceding pages show how lacking in homogeneity any geographically available group of blind people is likely to be. Therefore, much time, patience, and a fairly wide and/or well populated geographical area are required in order to develop large enough groups of blind people with similar amounts of vision, education, and other qualities that may be important to a specific kind of test. Needless to say, considerable financial support is also necessary to reach and to test such a normative population.

When the test involves concrete materials, as performance measures of mental ability or measures of dexterity do, it is absolutely necessary to develop norms in relation to amount of useful vision because vision has a great effect on speed, orientation, ease of learning, and smoothness of handling unfamiliar materials. At the student level, norms should always include both residential and day school populations, although reaching enough of the latter is often very difficult. At the adult level, it is important to include people with both sheltered and competitive work experience, although, again, it is often very difficult to reach the latter. For some kinds of tests, age of visual loss could also be a significant variable.

All of these considerations have slowed the development of tests for blind people. However, there is also some philosophical question about the value of norms based on blind people, especially if they are to be used in a rehabilitation program where the goal is competitive employment. To tell a potential employer that the client did well compared with blind people may tell him nothing; he may already be convinced that no blind person could do the work of his company. The counselor should be able to express the abilities of clients in terms that prove their capacity to compete with sighted workers. Far more effective than saying, "This girl is the best blind typist we have ever tested," is saying, "This girl can type at 60 words per minute." Norms give the counselor useful information, but in placement he should, as much as possible, describe his client in terms of practical measures appropriate to that client's field of specialization.

ADJUSTMENTS IN TESTING PROCEDURES

Staff newly assigned to work with blind clients will profit by training in how to guide a blind person and how to explain to him details of the environment. There are several brief illustrated brochures that might help with learning these skills, and the American Foundation for the Blind can provide not only brochures but also a film (Blechman, 1970; Dickman, 1972).

Within the testing situation the blind client should be told all pertinent information that a seeing person would naturally obtain by sight. Unless the object of the testing is to learn whether the client can distinguish objects by touch, the psychologist should describe the test materials, at the same time encouraging the client to explore them by touch. If the client hesitates, the psychologist may appropriately guide his hands, with particular emphasis on the characteristics of the test that will affect good performance. To plan how he will present each test, the psychologist must first decide exactly what he wants to learn from the test. He should tell the client everything except what the test is intended to measure.

Questionnaire types of tests are easily adapted by reading them to the blind client, either in person or through a tape recording. For those clients who are proficient in braille, the tests may be brailled, but the psychologist should determine the braille reading ability of each client before he uses much in the way of brailled material. Except among those who lost their vision early in the school years, good braille reading is rare.

If tests are read individually to each client, the answers can be given orally and recorded by the examiner. Where a single decision is required, such as "True" or "False," this is a very efficient procedure. In multiple choice tests, such as the Miller Analogies Test and some tests of judgment, aptitude, and achievement, the blind person's score may be reduced by the requirement that he hold in mind, very accurately, each of four or five alternative answers. Reading the possible answers at least twice improves accuracy; for clients who read braille, it is very helpful to have the possible answers put into braille so that the client may refer to them as he makes his choice. In the case of the Miller Analogies Test, braille sheets of possible answers are available from the Psychological Corporation.

While individual reading and oral answering of a test may be efficient, it does deprive the blind person of that privacy that a sighted person has when he reads for himself and records his decisions on an answer sheet. One way to overcome this is to have the client record his answers by typing or braille; carefully handled, this would also make possible the testing of more than one client at a single reading of the test.

Another procedure for answering is the use of tickets that may be placed by the client into several piles, one for "True," another for "False," or whatever the decisions involved are. These tickets may be small pieces of cardboard that the psychologist has numbered to correspond to the test items and placed in a box from which the client can take them one by one as he wishes to make his responses. Such cards can be used over and over, but they do have the disadvantage that someone must put them back into numerical order after each use.

It is also possible to buy strips of tickets that are already numbered, the kind of tickets frequently used for selling chances or for admission to various events. A roll of such tickets can be prepared so that it contains the correct number of tickets for the planned test; in addition, each tenth (or other designated) ticket can have a hole punched through it, and the recording can state when the next ticket should have a hole through it. The client can be instructed that these holes will help him know that he is in the right place in his roll of tickets and that if he finds he is out of place he is to call the test administrator. Thus, errors can be avoided.

INTELLIGENCE AND GENERAL ABILITY TESTS

Verbal Measures of Mental Ability

Bauman's (1968) study of tests used with blind clients showed that some form of the Wechsler (WAIS, WISC, WB II) was used in far more evaluations than was any other test. When the client retained useful vision, both Verbal and Performance scales were often given, but major emphasis was placed upon the Verbal Scale. Its great value lies in the fact that it is administered to the blind client exactly as it is to the seeing, so neither client nor psychologist is at a disadvantage. Regular Wechsler norms are used. They must be interpreted in the light of the client's educational history and life experience, but that would be true for sighted clients as well. The reason for the client's limited experience may be blindness, but the effects do not greatly differ from the effects of deprivation from other causes.

Certain subtest patterns are frequently met. Digit Span is often high because blind people must exercise memory more than most sighted people do; much of their learning is done by listening very carefully. On the other hand, they are as subject to test-taking anxiety as are seeing people, so the Digit Span subtest reduced by tension is just as frequently found among the blind as among the seeing. Another subtest that tends to run low is Arithmetic because facility with numbers is relatively difficult to achieve without vision; braille and mathematics do not mix easily! The client who could not fully profit by schooling because of poor vision tends to register low subtest values for Information, Arithmetic, and Vocabulary, the three subtests most likely to be affected by formal schooling. Young blind people who have lived a very sheltered life may rate low on the Comprehension subtest, apparently part of a general inability to reason in practical ways because such thinking has too often been done for them by protective family and friends.

A very small number of psychologists still use an adaptation of the Binet made by Hayes (1941) by combining selected verbal items from Forms L and M of the Stanford-Binet. Never very useful for teenagers or adults, its content now seems outdated even for children, although it might be useful as a double check where the WISC yields doubtful results.

Various Wechsler Performance Scales

If the client has fairly useful vision at the near point, some or all subtests of the various Wechsler Performance Scales (WAIS, WISC, WB II) may be used, but some psychologists feel that the results are probably inaccurate even when they seem to be good. Their argument is that it cannot be known how much better those scores would have been had the client had normal vision. This is true, but if, as sometimes does occur, the client obtains a higher Performance than Verbal IQ, one can be reasonably sure that he will function more comfortably and effectively with concrete than with verbal materials on the job.

Thus, use of the several Wechsler Performance Scales is not outruled. If the picture material includes details too small for his visual discrimination, the Block Design and Object Assembly subtests may be used as some supplement to the Verbal IQ, with the Scaled Score providing a rough evaluation of the results.

When the Performance IQ is much lower than the Verbal IQ it is extremely difficult to determine whether the Performance IQ is measuring lack of ability or lack of vision; under these circumstances it should probably be discarded.

Nonlanguage Learning Test

An early effort to find some task that would give information about performance functioning regardless of amount of vision was Bauman's (1947) Nonlanguage Learning Test (NLL). Adapted from the old Dearborn Formboard, Bauman regards it as a clinical instrument rather than as a test because she varies administration with amount of vision and, to some extent, with the mental ability of the client; she is less interested in a numerical score (although norms are available) than in observing the client's reactions and his improvement from trial to trial.

Although primarily intended for use with adults it can prove too easy for an adult with a great deal of useful vision; a few very capable preschool children have, given training, done it well. In the hands of an experienced clinician it can thus assist with the understanding of a wide age spread of visually handicapped and totally blind clients. It has the advantage of allowing the psychologist to watch the reactions of the client far better than many tests do, and changes in manner of presentation can considerably vary the levels of difficulty. However, its clinical nature can become a disadvantage in the sense that the psychologist must use it for a while to develop skill in its interpretation.

The NLL board contains eight holes, two of oval shape, two diamonds, two rectangles, and two hexagons. These holes are filled, in some cases by two blocks, in some cases by three blocks that may be interchanged between holes of the same shape. The test administrator removes four blocks, a half-block of each shape, and so rearranges the remaining blocks so that moves that follow certain rules readily return the half-blocks to the board.

Clients with enough vision to distinguish the shapes of the blocks may be told merely to get the blocks back into the board, with the suggestion that they try to remember how they manage this so that they can, on a later trial, do it faster. A totally blind client of average ability is taught, step by step, just how to get the blocks in, and if he fails to do this independently he is retaught for each of three trials. Between these extremes of no and intense training, the clinician may use variations that give more or less help.

Interpretation includes factors such as ability of the client to apply the rules, ability to react flexibly to an error, tendency to repeat incorrect moves that have not been effective, planfulness versus trial and error behavior, evidences of frustration or tendency to give up, and initiative in departing in useful ways from the procedures originally taught.

Haptic Intelligence Scale for the Adult Blind

As reported by the Shurragers (1964), the Haptic Intelligence Scale (HIS) is a refinement and further development of work begun by the Shurragers and S. B. Watson 10 years earlier. Four of its six subtests listed below are essentially adaptations of WAIS Performance Scale subtests.

Digit Symbol Digit Symbol consists of a large plastic plate embossed with simple geometric forms in random arrangement and a smaller plastic plate that presents one sample of each of the six forms used. On the samples, one to six raised dots show the number with which each form is to be associated. Exploring with his preferred hand and checking the samples with his nonpreferred hand, the subject is asked to state aloud the number associated with each shape, reading in order across the large plate. The score is the number correctly identified within the time limit.

Object Assembly Object Assembly consists of a block, doll, hand, and ball, each dissected into several pieces. Speed and accuracy of assembly result in scores for the four objects.

Block Design Block Design consists of four 1.5-inch cubes, each of which has two smooth sides, two rough sides, and two sides diagonally bisected into half rough, half smooth. With these blocks, the client is asked to form patterns identical to those on seven plates. Scores again depend upon accuracy in copying the plate patterns and upon speed.

Object Completion Object Completion presents 16 familiar objects from which one important part has been removed, such as a comb with a missing tooth. Score depends upon the number of missing parts correctly named.

There is no parallel to the Picture Completion subtest of the WAIS, but two new tasks have been added:

Pattern Board   Pattern Board consists of a 7.5-inch square with five rows of five round holes, except for the center, which contains a fixed peg. The examiner makes patterns of varying complexity by inserting wooden pegs into the open holes; he allows the subject to examine briefly each pattern, then removes the loose pegs and asks him to replicate the pattern. Score depends upon speed and accuracy.

Bead Arithmetic   Bead Arithmetic consists of a large abacus with five beads below the divider and two beads above. Test items vary in difficulty from reading one-digit numbers entered by the examiner to solving addition problems entered by the client.

Because it was assumed that the HIS would often be used in conjunction with the WAIS Verbal Scale, the HIS normative population was chosen to match the WAIS normative population in age and geographical location. It was felt that this would make possible a more direct comparison of scores on the two scales.

Much excellent professional effort went into the development of the HIS, and for totally blind clients more than 16 years of age it probably provides the best available evaluation of performance ability, although intercorrelations of HIS subtests are high, ranging from 0.53 to 0.71, and their correlations with the HIS Total Score range from 0.69 to 0.82. This implies that a common factor is contributing strongly to all HIS subtests and that they are less effectively measuring a variety of performance abilities than the WAIS subtests do (Shurrager, 1961).

In practice the test has not found wide use for at least some of the following reason. 1) Administration time can easily require over 1 hour, sometimes over 2. Unless the client is readily available to the psychologist over several days (as in a rehabilitation facility or other institution) it may be inappropriate to spend so much of the evaluation time on the measurement of one limited segment of the client's total abilities and interests. 2) Norms are not available for clients less than age 16. 3) Norms are based entirely upon persons without useful vision. In most rehabilitation settings, such persons make up only about 25 percent of the clients. 4) Many schools are now teaching arithmetic to visually handicapped students through use of the abacus. The Bead Arithmetic subtest is invalidated and must be omitted if the client has been taught to use the abacus. 5) For some years the HIS testing kit was not available, and now its cost is almost prohibitive. 6) Clear research evidence is not yet available to show that the HIS does measure the same abilities measured by the Wechsler Performance Scale; interpretation of the results is clouded by this lack.

Stanford-Kohs Block Design Test

Kohs' original work with block designs has inspired a number of psychologists, of whom the best known is probably Wechsler. Ohwaki adapted the test for use with blind persons by covering each color with a different textile. His norms, based on Japanese subjects, have not proven useful in the United States, but Suinn and Dauterman first developed United States norms on the cloth-covered blocks, then made more durable blocks from rough and smooth plastic with only two colors, black and white. Their report (1966) based on the use with 425 legally blind persons more than 16 years of age, provides norms for groups with varying amounts of functional vision. Although the lowest age in the normative group is 16, informal communication indicates that a number of psychologists have used it with youths below that age with quite successful results. For a few clients the test proves very time-consuming, but in general it requires less time than does the HIS. The disadvantages of the Stanford-Kohs are chiefly that its norms provide a rather limited spread in IQ and that it involves only one type of mental operation, the copying of patterns. A few otherwise very competent blind people prove unable to work with this concept so it proves to be no real measure of their total performance ability.

The Vocational Intelligence Scale
for the Adult Blind, and the Tactual Reproduction Pegboard

As part of a complex project under Tiffin (1960), Jones and Gruber developed the Vocational Intelligence Scale for the Adult Blind (VISAB) and the Tactual Reproduction Pegboard (TRP). Again, norms are not available for clients less than age 16, but they are available for both the totally blind and the partially sighted. The VISAB consists of a series of plastic plates on which groups of figures are embossed; the client is asked to choose, in each group, the figure that is least like the others. The TRP is a double pegboard; the examiner places peg designs of increasing complexity on one side, and the client tries to reproduce them accurately on the other side.

Neither test has had a great deal of acceptance, and neither is currently available for purchase. A few psychologists who happen to have the tests include them in batteries of clients with primarily nonverbal vocational goals.

Other Nonverbal Tests of Mental Ability

Although some of them represent many years of research effort, the other performance, or nonverbal, tests within the broad area of general mental ability have seen little use and information about them appears only in research reports.

Among these are Anderson's adaptations of the Raven Progressive Matrices, called the Tactual Progressive Matrices (Curtis, 1972); the Blind Learning Aptitude Test by Newland (1969); measures of form perception by Weiner (1963); measures of form discrimination by Crandell et al. (1968); and an adaptation of an abstract reasoning test by Morse (1970).

A specialized test chiefly relating to mobility but probably relevant in any situation where imagery is important is the Stanford Multi-Modality Imagery Test by Dauterman (1972). This involves a brief training period during which the client is instructed in how to make three-sided or four-sided figures with rubber bands on a fiberboard rectangle, an exercise in "Conceptualizing Spatial Relations" and, finally, the test itself. The test phase requires constructing images of geometric patterns from verbal instructions without the use of any physical paraphernalia. Dauterman believes that the test has some potential for assessing rehabilitation potential.

Nor can we overlook the contribution that might be made by the various tests involving drawings. A psychologist already very skilled in evaluating drawings would probably find them useful even with clients of quite limited vision, although it is constantly necessary to make judgments about whether unusual productions result from poor vision or from other causes. Koppitz (1964) gives an excellent discussion of the Bender Gestalt Test as a test of intelligence. However, because blindness is often part of a multiple handicap in which brain damage is either definitely known or strongly suspected, the more familiar use of the Bender for evaluation of brain damage is probably its most productive application in work with visually handicapped clients.

APTITUDE AND PROFICIENCY TESTS

Measures of Manual Dexterity

World War II gave great impetus to rehabilitation and, especially, to the use of psychological testing in rehabilitation. Because a large percentage of jobs then available were factory jobs, measures of speed and dexterity were very important. An early study by Bauman (1946) compared test results for employed and unemployed blind people, and disclosed that test intercorrelations tend to be higher for blind than for sighted subjects. This tendency toward higher intercorrelations appears repeatedly in various studies of use of tests with blind clients, and appears to tap some "G" factor of blindness, possibly made up of orientation, tactual discrimination, and kinesthetic memory.

Bauman's (1958) later work provides norms for clients with and without useful vision on five dexterity tests. It is emphasized that these tests give far more information than the mere measure of manual speed. They provide an opportunity to observe the client in action, doing rather than verbalizing. His reaction to difficulties and his response to training can be observed. Orientation in a work space, ability to follow patterns of movement, ability to maintain attention and effort at what he may perceive as a dull and repetitive task, and sheer motivation are demonstrated. Without these action tests, the psychologist would see a less complete picture of his client. Used for these purposes, dexterity tests may have a contribution to make in the evaluation of even those clients whose goals are college and the professions.

Minnesota Rate of Manipulation Test The Minnesota Rate of Manipulation Test consists of a long, narrow board into which round holes have been cut, four from top to bottom and 15 from one end of the board to the other. Into these 60 holes identical round blocks fit. The test has two parts, Displacing and Turning. In Displacing, the client moves the blocks, one by one, in a pattern that is simple, yet, for some persons, difficult to follow. Thus, orientation in the work space and following directions of movement can be measured. Turning requires that each block be turned over with a standard movement sequence involving the hands and also alternation in the hand movements at the end of each row. Again, learning, particularly to reverse hand movements on each row, is demonstrated in action.

Penn Bi-Manual Worksample The Penn Bi-Manual Worksample is a board with 10 rows of 10 holes each in the center and a pan at each end. One pan contains bolts, the other nuts. The task requires picking up a bolt with one hand, a nut with the other, twisting them together just enough to catch, and placing them into the holes. A second part of the task requires picking up the assemblies, one by one, unscrewing nut from bolt, and returning each part to its correct pan. The test results in two scores, the number of minutes and seconds required to complete each of the two activities.

Of the various dexterity tests, the Bi-Manual Worksample probably involves the most comprehensive and varied sampling of manual activities, and it has shown better relationship to success in manipulative jobs. It is, in fact, a familiar test for the selection of sighted workers in manual jobs; the blind person does exactly the same task using tactual rather than visual cues and is allowed more practice time.

Crawford Small Parts Dexterity Test   The Crawford Small Parts Dexterity Test, also designed to test sighted persons, has two parts. With blind clients only the second part, Screwdriver Dexterity, is used. The task involves placing small set screws in a metal plate by hand, then turning each one with the small screwdriver until it is level with the top of the metal plate. Again, extra practice time is allowed for the totally blind client to become accustomed to his materials and to develop orientation in the work space.

Some studies have been made with the Purdue Pegboard and the tool dexterity tests but significant normative groups have not been reported. A psychologist who is familiar with a particular dexterity test not listed here would do well to try it with his blind clients. He may find that it has no significant visual component and that the visual handicap does not, therefore, reduce the client's score very much.

Other Aptitude Tests

Some ink print aptitude tests have been put into braille or large type, and many have been used by reading them aloud. Aptitude for sales, supervision, etc., can thus be used as long as there are safeguards so that the blind person's score is not reduced because he is a poor reader or because he cannot accurately keep in mind the multiple alternative answers so often characteristic of these tests.

Such special aptitudes as that for music received early attention in the work of Kappes (1931) and Merry (1931). Bigman (1950) developed a clerical aptitude test that has been of some use. Gardner's (1965) adaptation of the Foreign Language Aptitude Test had a brief popularity in the 1960s. Dexterity and mechanical aptitude tests have been developed by Curtis (1950) and Clawson (1968).

A number of rehabilitation centers also use "worksamples," a term that covers tasks of varying length and complexity, often developed on the basis of the job content of local industries. In a few of these, statistical studies have been made and at least rough standards set; the value of others depends upon the familiarity of the administrator with industrial standards. There is an urgent need to pull this potentially helpful information together into a form that could be shared with other psychologists.

One of the most frequently used aptitude tests, the Scholastic Aptitude Test (SAT), has been adapted for use with blind students by braille-plus-recording with answers typed by the student. Administered under the same highly controlled conditions required for the SAT's use with sighted students, this is scored and reported from Princeton in the standard way. Each year it plays a significant part in the admission of blind youth to colleges.

PERSONALITY EVALUATION

Questionnaires

Psychologists who are already comfortable with the interpretation of a particular personality inventory with seeing people may very effectively use that same inventory by reading it to blind clients. It is wise, however, to review the items carefully to be sure that few, if any, would have a different meaning for a blind person; indeed, it would be well to have a competent blind psychologist involved in such a review. The Minnesota Multiphasic Personality Inventory has a long history of being used in this way since the early reports of Cross (1947) and Potter (1950).

During the late 1940s Bauman developed the Emotional Factors Inventory that was largely validated by the Study of Adjustment to Blindness (Bauman, 1954). Later this was adapted for teenagers in the Adolescent Emotional Factors Inventory (Bauman 1963, 1964). Most of the items for both inventories came from discussions by blind adults or adolescents of their own problems or of problems they observed in companions; thus, content is highly relevant to the problems of blindness. Subscales relate to sensitivity, social competency, adjustment to home, school, and boy-girl relationships, morale, independence, and attitudes regarding blindness.

Less widely used are several inventories devised for specific purposes, such as those of Cowan et al. (1962) and Hardy (1968). These evaluate too narrow an area for general use but could be very helpful in research or as supplementary scales.

Projective Tests

For the many clients with at least moderately effective near vision, the psychologist can use his favorite projective materials even though they are ink blots, pictures, incomplete sentences, etc. Sentence or story material can even be used with totally blind clients by oral presentation.

A number of efforts have been made to develop tactual and auditory projective materials specifically for the blind. In most cases they have no real research basis and little recorded use. Two auditory projective tests listed below do have a record of moderate acceptance.

Auditory Projective Test   The Auditory Projective Test (Braverman and Chevigny, 1952) includes a number of types of auditory stimuli, but the most interesting section provides a series of conversations in nonsense syllable form. These parallel the interpersonal relationships suggested by some of the TAT cards, and stories given in response to each of these conversations can be interpreted very much as TAT stories would be.

Sound Test   The Sound Test includes stimuli of varying complexity and length, some rather simple sounds, such as footsteps, other combinations of music, sounds, and voices. Palacios (1964) provides suggested scoring categories, and reports the use of this test with the same group of clients who participated in the Purdue research that resulted in the VISAB and the TRP. Although there are no norms in the statistical sense, her categories of sample responses help to standardize analysis of protocols.

MEASURES OF INTEREST

It is easy to adapt almost any interest inventory for blind clients by reading it to them, and because interest choices have less loading of personal privacy than do personality inventory responses, there is little objection to the examiner recording the client's choices. The psychologist may, therefore, use those inventories with which he is most familiar although, again, it is wise to review items for heavy visual components and to avoid the inventory that has too many of these.

In practice, the Kuder Preference Record, the California Occupational Interest Inventory (Lee-Thorpe), and the Strong Vocational Interest Blank have had wide acceptance. For the Kuder, Howe Press makes a raised dot answer sheet, and it is also possible to test several persons together by having them type their responses. When giving the instructions for any of these inventories, it is well to ask the blind client to try to imagine that he can do all of the items, that he has ample ability and vision to do all; emphasize that this is an interest inventory, not a request that he evaluate his ability to do each item.

Bauman (1973) has developed an interest inventory from content of job descriptions of blind workers and from their choices of recreation. Because test items were taken from the reports of successful blind workers the test has face validity, but it has appeared too recently for any follow-up studies. However, Bauman (1973) says:

> In the area of interest, interpretation of results may be more challenging than problems of administration. There is a marked tendency, among visually handicapped persons, to make many choices in the social service area and, to slightly less extent, in music. The first

of these tendencies seems, often, to result from the fact that blindness tends to enforce dependence upon others, and the individual would like to repay this and also might find ego satisfaction in playing the role of the helper. He had admired those who have helped him and would like the experience of being the person to whom others are grateful. The interest in music arises in part from the fact that the blind person, of necessity, turns to sound as a source of pleasure, and perhaps in part from some extra emphasis on music in many schools for the Blind (p. 112).

INTERPRETATION OF TEST RESULTS

Effects of Variations in Procedure

Tests are merely tools, and while standard procedure has great value, there are times when quite unstandard procedure is the only thing that makes sense. The psychologist is trying to understand and evaluate people, not give tests for their own sake.

In adaptation of test materials or test procedures for blind persons, the psychologist must carefully think through what kind of information he is trying to obtain. To the best of his ability, he must leave intact those aspects of the test that relate to what he is trying to measure; all other aspects should be so adjusted that the blind person's time and energy are spent chiefly on demonstrating the ability the psychologist wishes to measure. For some tests this may result in a very good sample of the measured ability, but it may so change procedures that the original norms are useless. The reading aloud of printed test materials that have time limits in printed form is a good example of this. When read aloud, without time limit, the test becomes a power test and must be so interpreted.

These differentiations are particularly tricky on worksamples and similar use of concrete materials because a test of mechanical aptitude, for example, may in fact become a measure of tactual discrimination for a blind person. If mechanical aptitude is to be evaluated it is necessary to eliminate almost completely all need to discriminate one part from another by touch.

Coping with Inadequate Norms

The best way to meet the constantly recurring problem of inadequate norms for blind people is by experience—lots of experience—on the part of the psychologist or counselor. However, there are inevitably professionals who are new to work with the blind, and they carry a considerable burden of responsibility for doing the best they can with admittedly poor material.

If the only norms available for a particular test are based on seeing people, the applicability of those norms to blind clients depends largely upon how much vision, and/or its side effects, would be likely to affect performance on this test. It has already been noted that the great value of the various Wechsler Verbal Scales lies in the belief that all of the mental operations measured by those scales can be accomplished at no disadvantage by those without vision. Consequently, Wechsler norms are used without adjustment and without apology.

If the test provides norms on a blind population, the psychologist must carefully consider the nature of that population. Did it include totally blind and partially seeing and, if so, are there separate norms for tasks where vision contributes to success? Is the normative group made up, as so often it is, of people with narrow life experience, such as sheltered shop workers or residential school students? If so, the psychologist working with a person whose work history has been competitive and/or whose educational history has been in public day schools must recognize certain potential differences between his client and the normative group, and his interpretation must take these into account.

Another kind of normative group, found all too often in the literature of tests for the sighted as well as the blind, is the student group. When adults are being evaluated the only available norms may be on student groups, but if the test could be much affected by greater age or greater life experience such norms must be applied with caution.

Importance of Observations

The psychologist working with blind clients must make far more use of observations during testing than is usually necessary in working with seeing clients. Indeed, some centers test seeing people almost entirely, or entirely, with paper-and-pencil tests that are placed before them by clerks or by graduate students and no observations are recorded. This is impossible with blind clients for whom a knowledgable person must constantly make adjustments to suit each client's specific characteristics and needs.

Each of those adjustments should be a matter of record and, perhaps even more important, the reasons for making the adjustments should be recorded. Was the client unable to see the large print despite an ophthalmological report that implied useful vision? Did the client have trouble hearing questions and instructions so that he constantly requested that they be repeated? Did he seem to shield his eyes from the glare of the testroom lighting, yet function well in a dim light? Did he show anxiety or frustration at certain kinds of test materials or certain parts of the interview?

A list of suggested kinds of observations could go on indefinitely. The best procedure is to record everything, even if it seems unimportant, when it occurs. Later, that point may help pull together test findings that do not seem to integrate into a meaningful whole.

Importance of the Interview and History

No report should merely record test scores and their bare interpretation; rather, the report should integrate the meaning of those scores and the observations of the testing session with what the client says about himself and his known history. Unless the psychologist makes a real effort to understand the history, background, and wishes of the client, with consideration for all the possible peculiarities of history and background discussed in earlier sections of this chapter, he will lack a well rounded picture of the client and may say some very foolish things about him. At times, the history almost contradicts the test findings; when this is true, the psychologist should try to determine how this could happen. Both history and test scores are facts; how can it be that they do not mesh? At times the answer is found in factors that are quite difficult to measure, such as the client's rejection of his own blindness or his motivation to overcome the handicaps and differences that blindness imposes. An understanding of such factors may be the key to rehabilitation process.

The Psychologist as a Member of the Rehabilitation Team

The psychologist will be most useful to counselor, agency, and client if he can function as a member of the rehabilitation team. This implies a good level of communication between the referring agency and the psychologist.

In making a referral, agency staff should provide the psychologist with a brief but complete statement of all information about the client that is already known to the agency. Some psychologists, based in agencies and with ample time, will prefer simply to study the complete client record. For the psychologist based outside the agency, transfer of the very important and confidential record might be impractical if not impossible. Also, the psychologist in private practice may not have time to seek details in an agency record which, in many cases, is inches thick. It is well for the psychologist to develop a form or an outline that makes clear just what information will be helpful but that is not so complex that filling it out for each psychological examination is a burden. The point is that, no matter how it is managed, there should be good communication between agency and psychologist, and this should invariably include giving the psychologist basic ophthalmological, medical, educational, family, and work history.

It is also extremely helpful if the staff member making the referral rather specifically states what information he would like to receive as a result of the psychological examination. This will ensure that the psychologist uses the tools and interpretation that are most likely to produce the required information.

On the other hand, it is the responsibility of the psychologist to help in keeping communication open between himself and the referring agency and to try to address his evaluation and subsequent report to the needs of that agency. His report should be written in terms that are easily understood by counselors, and its recommendations should be practical and oriented to action that is feasible for that agency. The psychologist, therefore, must know, at least in a general way, the functions and potential services of the agency, and he should know the schools, training centers, rehabilitation services, etc., that are available.

The psychologist should be available, perhaps by telephone, for at least some consultation so that the puzzled counselor can ask just what was meant by a less than clear diagnosis or recommendation. He should also participate in in-service training and similar activities designed to give counselors and other agency staff a better understanding of the psychologist's functions and the content of his reports.

Finally, both agency staff and psychologist will probably grow if there is some feedback to the psychologist about the clients he has evaluated. He cannot be expected to improve in his understanding of blind people if he drops his reports into the mail and never again hears anything of that client. He may even appropriately participate in agency staffing concerning clients with rather complex records.

Such a circle of communication, making the psychologist a true member of the rehabilitation team, will not only serve the blind client but also will enrich the professional experience of counselor and psychologist alike.

REFERENCES

Bauman, M. K. 1946. Studies in the application of motor skills techniques to the vocational adjustment of the blind. J. Appl. Psych. 30:144–154.

Bauman, M. K. 1947. Report on a nonlanguage learning test. AAWB Proceedings, pp. 99–101. American Association of Workers for the Blind, Washington, D.C.

Bauman, M. K. 1954. Adjustment to Blindness: A Study as Reported by the Committee to Study Adjustment to Blindness. State Council for the Blind, Harrisburg, Pa.

Bauman, M. K. 1958. Manual of Norms for Tests Used in Counseling Blind Persons. American Foundation for the Blind, New York.

Bauman, M. K. 1964. Group differences disclosed by inventory items. Intern. J. Ed. Blind 13:101–106.

Bauman, M. K. 1968. Tests Used in the Psychological Evaluation of Blind and Visually Handicapped Persons, and A Manual of Norms for Tests Used in Counseling Blind Persons. American Association of Workers for the Blind, Washington, D.C.

Bauman, M. K. 1973. An interest inventory for the visually handicapped. Ed. Visually Handicapped 5:78–83.

Bauman, M. K., H. Platt, and S. Strauss. 1963. A measure of personality for blind adolescents. Intern. J. Ed. Blind 13:7–12.

Bigman, G. T. 1950. A clerical test for the visually handicapped. New Outlook for the Blind. 44:80–83.

Blechman, R. O. 1970. What Do You Do When You See A Blind Person? American Foundation for the Blind, New York.

Braverman, S., and H. Chevigny. 1952. The Auditory Projective Test. American Foundation for the Blind, New York.

Clawson, L. E. 1968. A study of the Clawson Worksample Tests for measuring the manual dexterity of the blind. New Outlook for the Blind 62:182–187.

Cowen, E. L., R. P. Underberg, R. T. Verrillo, and F. G. Benham. 1961. Adjustment to Visual Disability in Adolescence. American Foundation for the Blind, New York.

Crandell, J. M., D. D. Hammill, C. Witkowski, and F. Barkovich. 1968. Measuring form-discrimination in blind individuals. Intern. J. Ed. Blind 18:65–68.

Cross, O. H. 1974. Braille adaptation of the Minnesota Multiphasic Personality Inventory for use with the blind. J. Appl. Psych. 31:189–198.

Curtis, J. W. 1950. Administration of the Purdue Pegboard test to blind individuals. Ed. Psych. Meas. 10:329–331.

Curtis, W. S. 1972. The Development and Application of Intelligence Tests for the Blind: A Research Utilization Conference. University of Georgia, Athens.

Dauterman, W. L. 1972. Manual for the Stanford Multi-Modality Imagery Test. American Foundation for the Blind, New York.

Dickman, I. R. 1972. Living with Blindness. American Foundation for the Blind, New York.

Gardner, R. C. 1965. A language aptitude test for blind students. J. Appl. Psych. 49:135–141.

Hardy, R. E. 1968. A study of manifest anxiety among blind residential school students. New Outlook for the Blind 62:173–180.

Hayes, S. P. 1941. Contributions to a Psychology of Blindness. American Foundation for the Blind, New York.

Kappes, M. 1931. Measures for musical talent. Teachers Forum 4:2–7.

Koppitz, E. M. 1964. The Bender Gestalt Test for Young Children. Grune and Stratton, New York.

Merry, R. V. 1931. Adapting the Seashore Musical Talent Tests for use with blind pupils. Teachers Forum 3:15–19.

Morse, J. L. 1970. The adaptation of a non-verbal reasoning test for use with the blind. Ed. Visually Handicapped 2:79–80.

Newland, T. E. 1969. The Blind Learning Aptitude Test. U.S. Department of Health, Education and Welfare, Washington, D.C.

Palacios, M. H. 1964. The Sound Test: An Auditory Technique. Privately published by the author, Marion, Ind.

Potter, S. S. 1950. A method for using the Minnesota Multiphasic Personality Inventory with the blind. *In* W. Donahue and D. Dabelstein (eds.), Psychological Diagnosis and Counseling of the Adult Blind. American Foundation for the Blind, New York.

Shurrager, H. C. 1961. A Haptic Intelligence Scale for Adult Blind. Illinois Institute of Technology, Chicago.

Shurrager, H. C., and P. S. Shurrager. 1964. Manual for the Haptic Intelligence Scale for Adult Blind. Psychology Research, Chicago.

Suinn, R. M., and W. L. Dauterman. 1966. Manual for the Stanford-Kohs Block Design Test for the Blind. Stanford University School of Medicine, Stanford.

Tiffin, J. 1960. An Investigation of Vocational Success with the Blind. O.V.R. Grantee Designation-PRF 1588. Purdue Research Foundation, Purdue University Press, Lafayette, Ind.

Weiner, L. H. 1963. The performance of good and poor Braille readers on certain tests involving tactual perception. Intern. J. Ed. Blind 12: 72–77.

15

Psychological Evaluation of the Deaf Client

EDNA S. LEVINE

A person who is born deaf is caught in the clash between two discordant environments: a silent one fashioned by the inability to hear, and a dominating one set by the conventions of a hearing culture. To effect conciliation and integration of these conflicting worlds is the major goal of rehabilitation. What the outcome may be in a given case depends in large measure upon what the deaf person himself can contribute to the goal. This chapter will explore the strategies used by psychology in making the judgment.

THE DEAF DEFINED

Despite the relatively small size of the deaf population, approximating under half a million in the United States (Schein and Delk, 1973), there is an overwhelming abundance of divergent definitions, as many, in fact, as there are disciplines in the rehabilitation picture (Public Health Service Publication No. 1,227, 1964). Each views the deaf from the perspective of its own particular specialty, while to the general public, the deaf are still thought of as "deaf-mute" or "deaf-and-dumb."

To bypass the definition issues, the writer offers the following compromise in the form of a summary of factors that characterize the life situation of the large majority of persons termed "deaf."

The deaf constitute a minority group of persons of potentially normal mental and psychological attributes whose *physical impairment* lies in severe irreversible damage to the sensori-neural and/or cortical structures necessary for normal hearing, a condition that is present from birth or from the formative years and is not amenable to current medical or surgical treatment; whose *disability* is a loss of functional hearing of such severity that the ability to hear conversational speech as well as most informational messages transmitted through sound, both vocal and nonvocal, is lost to them even with the use of a hearing aid; and whose *major handicaps* stem from the resultant break in the lines of auditory communication with the world, such as to: 1) limit the input of information mainly to visual channels; 2) prevent the normal acquisition of all forms of verbal language: spoken, written, read; 3) block the acquisition of knowledge; 4) impair the establishment of normal communicative relations with society; and 5) obstruct the processes of enculturation and adaptation. In short, the world of the deaf is a place that is visible to the eye but incomprehensible to the ear.

THE LINGUISTIC IMPACT

To build verbal lines for one who from birth has never heard the sounds of spoken language is considered one of the most complex undertakings in the annals of education. The methods and issues involved are dealt with elsewhere in the literature. Briefly summarized, the problem involves teaching the meaning of every single word that is being learned; teaching how to recognize unheard language by watching the lips and face of a speaker (lip- or speech-reading); teaching how to put words together to form sentences and express thoughts; teaching how to speak a word that the pupil has never heard and cannot hear; and, in certain systems of instruction, teaching how to spell out and to read back verbal language when expressed in standard hand and finger positions (fingerspelling). The task is slow and laborious, without any great motivation for the burdened learner whose maturational needs soon outstrip the sparse information potential of his small store of painfully acquired verbal language.

The deaf, however, have not permitted their linguistic problems to dampen their communicative drive. The deaf are lively people and lively communicators. Their main and beloved method of communication is the language of signs, a nonverbal mode of communication in which words and concepts are ideographically expressed through established gestures and conventional positions of hands and arms accompanied by "body language" and facial expression (Fant, 1964; Riekehof, 1963). As used by the deaf in everyday communication, the language is nongrammatical by English standards, and it does not lend itself to verbatim transposition to or from statements in straight English. It is, however, a vivid and vigorous message conveyor. Furthermore, it is easily learned and seemingly requires none of the special abilities such as are required by the deaf in the learning of speech and speech reading. Although traditionally banned from classroom instruction in the belief that its nongrammatic form would impair the learning of straight language, it is now included in the system of instruction known as Total Communication (O'Rourke, 1972).

Finally, to illustrate something of the range and variety of the linguistic outcomes of the complex educational picture, the following samplings, taken from personal communications to this author, are presented here as examples of the kinds of language expression a service worker with deaf persons is apt to encounter:

1. Exceptional linguistic facility:

> I am deaf
>   That is true
> And yet I can hear.
> I can hear with my eyes
>   And with my eyes I can hear
> Music, sound, harmony.
> See yonder robin soaring
>   It is music in motion.
> Look over there, children playing at tag,
>   That is sound at play.
> Read this poem by Shelley
>   That is harmony to my eyes.
> With all the sounds I can hear
>   With my eyes
> How can I be deaf?
>
> Naomi Leeds

2. A typical teen-ager:

> Dear Dr. L.
> How are you? I am feeling so hot. I am glad that I receive your letters.
> I have no news for you. I have many news because I don't know to language and what's call.
> When I come home with you then I will explain.

I am glad that it will be very soon to see you on Wednesday.
Much love always
Guess who????

3. Functionally illiterate:

Dear:
(I "forget" too letter sorry "O.k.")
I learn "gone" picture book A,B,C,D, for.
I know not look pictures.
I mean the notice see answer for confusion write to paper "o.k."
I ask me wait, that office you, and conversation sings Language that office for.
the you write "himself" you write bring I.
    Thank you

It is obvious even from this highly abridged discussion and these few illustrations that deafness does not reduce all so affected to one common denominator. Of far greater influence in determining outcomes is the complex of surrounding circumstances including factors such as family acceptance and management, school experiences, special abilities and disabilities, motivation, intellectual endowment, experiential outlets, psychological defenses, health, and above all communicative fulfillment.

SPECIAL CONSIDERATIONS IN PSYCHOLOGICAL PRACTICE

A complex task faces psychological examiners whose practice takes them into the psychologically uncharted area of the deaf. Space permits only highlight problems to be discussed. The two considered in this section deal with the heterogeneity of the deaf client population and with the special competencies needed by psychological evaluators of the deaf.

Deaf Client Heterogeneity

The "deaf and dumb" stereotype follows most deaf people into many rehabilitation settings. While there may be greater proportion of certain linguistic levels as compared with others for rehabilitation service, psychological examiners must nevertheless be prepared for a heterogeneous practice. For example, there are among deaf rehabilitation clients deaf persons who can speak and read the lips with amazing skill; others who can speak but who have trouble reading the lips; still others who can read the lips but whose speech is incomprehensible; and some who can do neither. There are deaf persons who are masters of all forms of communication, and others who are masters of none. There are those whose speech is incomprehensible but whose linguistic abilities are exceptional, and conversely others with good speech but limited concepts.

There are also deaf persons whose educational experiences have been an enrichment, and more whose education has been a failure. There are deaf persons whose school life contacts with their families and with hearing communities have been restricted to weekend or holiday visits home, and others who have lived at home all their school days, whether for better or worse. There are some deaf people who seldom see another deaf person whether because of family censures or lack of opportunity, and others who have a full, rich life with both the deaf and the hearing. There are deaf persons who cannot communicate with other deaf persons because of a lack of a mutually understood method of communication, and many who cannot communicate with members of their own families for the same reason.

Finally, there are the emotionally healthy and the emotionally ill; the mature and the unbelievably immature; those of high mental endowment and those of limited capacity; the sick and the well; and the multiply handicapped. Within the range of these extremes are countless combinations and variations of achievement, ability, and adjustment.

To reduce this heterogeneity to manageable proportions is extremely difficult. The following is a rough attempt at categorization.

Exceptional There are deaf people with superior functioning intelligence, outstanding achievement, and superior linguistic abilities. They may or may not have intelligible speech, although the best oral communication among the deaf is to be found in this category. So too is the finest manual communication. They may or may not have good lipreading ability. In this group are deaf clients who have succeeded in regular schools as well as in schools for the deaf and are college bound for professional preparation.

Above Average There are deaf people with good functioning intelligence and generally good life adjustment, but with substantially less than equivalent linguistic and scholastic attainments. Their verbal language as measured by reading achievement is generally at about sixth through ninth grade. Those with college ambition cannot meet the admission requirements of colleges for the deaf. Nevertheless, many are leaders among their peer groups and active in extracurricular or community activities. They may or may not have intelligible speech or good lipreading ability; however, they possess sufficient fluency in verbal language for good written communication.

Average These are deaf people with markedly retarded scholastic attainments despite mental potential for better achievement. Their verbal language level as measured by reading achievement is generally at fourth grade and often at third grade. Intelligible spoken communication is uncommon, and written communication is often incomprehensible to the uninitiated. Nevertheless, many such persons are capable of good life adjustment and of acquiring a variety of vocational skills at which they may be as good as or better than their hearing peers.

Below Average—Marginal People in these closely overlapping categories function at severely retarded levels whether because of actual mental retardation, an exceptionally late school start or no schooling at all, brain impairment, or serious long-time psychological problems. Linguistic resources are drastically limited; in fact, most are functionally illiterate at best. Numbers in the marginal category have no ability whatsoever to read, write, sign, or communicate in other than pantomime and self-devised gestures. Psychologically, they are isolated beings with only the self to draw upon and with drastically impoverished concepts of social reality. Nonetheless, a surprising proportion are animated, lively persons and some are well motivated to rehabilitation efforts.

In connection with the foregoing categories, it is important to emphasize that they are based on *functioning* rather than on potential intelligence. For example, there are people in the marginal category who are potentially of average or even better than average intelligence but who function as retarded. There are people in the "average" category who are of potentially superior mental endowment. However, the weight of educational and other life circumstances and communicative deficiencies depresses the development and optimum expression of original endowment.

Hard Core Deaf Finally, another category needs to be mentioned that is common enough in rehabilitation practice and that is designated as the "hard core deaf" by DiFrancesca and Hurwitz (1969). These are deaf clients who have been failures in school, work, and society, not through lack of intelligence or the ability to work in competitive employment, but rather through deficient social and emotional functioning. The authors observe that these "clients differ from other rehabilitation populations in that they appear more disposed to relate and solve problems of life on the basis of their feelings or affect." Among their distinctive attributes are lessened ability to see beyond the personal frame of reference, unreflective response to problems that is based more on immediate need and gratification than on objective reality, and living for the immediate present rather than for the planned future. Examples in this author's experience are the woman who would not take a good job on 34th Street because she had established a fixed boundary line that did not extend below 42nd Street for her place of employment; and the man who left a good job because the exit door was several more feet away from his desk than suited his convenience. Needless to add, both suffer chronic unemployment.

Special Competencies of Examiners

To carry out the psychological imperative "to protect the right of each individual to be soundly evaluated . . . " (American Psychological Association, 1970) requires exceptional competencies on the part of examiners of the deaf.

First are the usual professional competencies expected in all psychological practice. These are summarized by Terman and Merrill (1960) as follows:

> The competent examiner must possess, in high degree, judgment, intelligence, sensitivity to the reactions of others, and penetration as well as knowledge of and regard for scientific methods and experiences in the use of psychometric techniques. No degree of mechanical perfection of the tests themselves can ever take the place of good judgment and psychological insight of the examiner (p. 47ff.).

In addition, there are the special competencies required in the psychological evaluation of deaf clients. Important as the regular professional accreditations are, the special competencies, particularly in regard to communication and the use of tests, are more important. It is an ironic fact that psychology's "chiefest tool," the word, and principal instrument, the test, are major problems in examining the deaf. Such was the judgment of over 100 respondents to a survey of psychological tests and practices with the deaf conducted by the writer (Levine, 1974).

The following is a space-limited digest of the two foremost problems involved in psychological practice with the dear: communication and psychological testing.

Communication It is a cardinal rule of psychological practice that the method of communication between examiner and subject is determined by the needs and wishes of the subject. With the "exceptional" deaf client this usually presents no problems. Both client and examiner can communicate in the verbal mode, whether spoken or written. But with the large majority of deaf clients, examiners should be prepared to follow the client's manual communicative lead. What this entails, as well as various cautions that must be observed in oral communication, are summarized below.

A. Manual Communication: Method An examiner is prepared to communicate with manually oriented clients when he can use as many as possible of the distinctive methods of communicating as are used by the deaf—invariably, the language of signs, and, hopefully, fingerspelling, as well as the language of pantomime, gestures, and facial expression. The ability to use these modes suffices for *expressive* communication.

However, expressive communication is only one side of the coin of interpersonal exchange; the other is *receptive* communication. Not only must an examiner be able to use the languages of the deaf, he must be able to *understand* messages and statements that a client conveys to him in these modes. To "read back" manual messages is the hardest part of the communicative assignment for nondeaf examiners, for such persons must become accustomed to an entirely new form of language input as well as the many different ways deaf clients have of using their languages. And even after the examiner has mastered these skills, he has only completed the initial phase of his total communicative task.

Language The next phase of an examiner's communicative skills deals with his ability to convey a fluent message in the sign language. To do this requires more than the ability to sign. It requires the ability to arrange the signs in the way that is the habitual pattern for discourse in the language. This is often likened to telegraphic writing, consisting mainly of key words set up in a kind of order-of-priority arrangement.

To illustrate, an examiner addresses the following WAIS question in meticulous signs to a sign oriented deaf youth: "What should you do if while in the movies you were the first person to see smoke and fire?" The client understands most of the signs but is completely baffled by the question. What's movies got to do with getting a job, he wonders. After all, he's here for a job. Or maybe it's a job in the movies. But fire? A fireman?

The communicative defect in the examiner's message is that he has made a long verbatim transposition of a verbal statement into its signed equivalent. Furthermore, the question concerns an imaginary situation, and the "pretend" element has not been made clear to the literal-minded client. Finally, by the time the examiner has reached the end of his long statement, the client is confused as to what the original question was.

In all likelihood, the client would have understood the question if it had been signed and punctuated by the examiner's facial expression something as follows: "You. Movies go? (smile) Movies like? (smile) Imagine here movies. Imagine, same play. Here movies. (It often takes some time to get this "pretend" idea across and some actual playacting, with the examiner conveying pleased antitipation the while. When the "pretend" idea has finally registered, the examiner continues.) O.K. here movies. You sit, watch. (Rapt expression as if watching a movie, slowly turning to puzzled expression.) Smoke! (alarm) See fire! (Alarmed, look at floor to indicate the fire is not in the picture but in the movie house.) You. What do? (pointedly questioning, look at client)." In passing, it is not to be wondered that examiners customarily employ performance scales in testing the deaf.

In any event, an examiner's preparation to communicate with his sign oriented clients requires him to use and to understand the manner of discourse in which signed statements are ordinarily expressed, and to acquire sensitivity in the use and understanding of the facial expressions and body language that accompany the signed message.

Concepts When the examiner has finally mastered the methods and language to reach the minds of his deaf subjects, he must now prepare himself to understand the concepts he finds when he arrives at this psychological destination.

To make sense of the complexities of modern reality is often a challenge to the nondeaf. For minds entrapped in linguistic and cultural impoverishment, reality is often a jumble of fragmented events, and the derivative concepts express the attempts of the deaf person to piece them together, to make some sense of what he sees but does not really know. Often the resultant concepts strike the uninitiated as weird if not downright pathologic. They are not necessarily so. They simply indicate how the deaf person sees himself and the world from his experientially deformed perspective.

The culminating phase of an examiner's psycho-communicative skills involves his ability to grasp the fundamental meaning of the concepts a deaf client is trying to express no matter how defective the language or how off-beat the concept may appear. Finally, the examiner must learn how to express himself not only in the same style as his subject, but also at the same conceptual level, or else he is in danger of talking over the head of his client. Once these abilities are mastered, the examiner is well on his way to "knowing" the deaf and knowing his deaf clients. He is ideally prepared for most communicative eventualities.

Where the ideal is not possible, a trained interpreter is called upon to establish the communicative linkage between examiner and client. Skill is required in using an interpreter to avoid take-over of the psychologist's role as well as to guard procedural objectivity (Levine, 1960). Services of interpreters can be obtained through the local chapters of the Registry of Interpreters for the Deaf.

B. Oral Communication For most examiners, a great burden is lifted from their shoulders when communication can take place in the verbal mode. But even here, the examiner must be aware of certain problem situations that may arise. In lipreading, for example, to ease the pressures on clients who are under the strain of having to see rather than to hear conversation, the following cautions are observed:

1. Examiner and client should always face one another at a distance of not more than four feet apart.

2. Light should not glare the client's vision but should come from behind him and be directed onto the examiner's face.

3. Examiner should speak carefully and naturally and avoid mouthing, grimacing, shouting, speaking without voice, excessive slow-down in speech, smoking or chewing while speaking, as well as turning his head away or moving about.

4. Examiner should watch for signs of fatigue on the part of the lipreader or signs of puzzlement indicating difficulty in comprehension. When fatigue sets in, a rest period or coffee break are in order. With difficulties of comprehension, the statement should be reworded in simpler, more visible forms, or written aids should be used with difficult key words and proper names.

5. Pads and pencils should always be available, one set for the examiner and another for the client.

In certain cases, examiners experience difficulty in understanding the speech of a client even after listening for awhile to become accustomed to its tones and rhythms. The examiner himself may have to resort to lip-reading and supplement what he hears by watching the client's lip movements. If he still cannot understand what the client is saying, written communications will have to be used, or if the client prefers and the examiner is able, manual communication.

Psychological Testing As in communication so in psychological testing, few if any special difficulties are encountered when testing deaf clients in the "exceptional" category. Although they have not been reared in the same psychological settings as have the nondeaf, they have nevertheless managed to create such environments for themselves and so can be exposed to the same psychological instruments as the hearing without doing excessive violence to standardization theory.

Serious testing problems may arise in regard to much of the remaining deaf rehabilitation-client population, and the greater the linguistic and sociocultural impoverishment, the greater the problems. The root difficulty in psychological examination lies in the fact that for deaf adults there are no mental or personality tests devised for their distinctive psychological environments or standardized on their unique life experiences. In effect, this is an "unstandardized" population with which examiners are obliged to use hearing-standardized tests in the absence of more appropriate instruments.

Birch (1958) declares that traditional tests "were never designed to answer the questions that arise in a rehabilitation setting" (p. ix). Probably the sharpest attack on the use of standardized tests with unstandardized groups comes from the area of the culturally disadvantaged minority groups. Anderson and Smith (1969) sum up the situation by stating that the "evidence suggests that in evaluating the disadvantaged, predictive instruments developed on one population may be inappropriate when used on a population with differing characteristics" (p. 27).

How inappropriate such tests can be is illustrated by the following items taken from personality measures that have at one time or other been used with the deaf: "My hearing is apparently as good as that of most people," taken from the Minnesota Multiphasic Personality Inventory; or, "While in trains, busses, etc., I often talk to strangers," taken from the same source; or, "Do you prefer traveling with someone who will make all the necessary arrangements to the adventure of traveling alone?" taken from the Bernreuter Personality Inventory.

When a deaf person answers items such as these factually, providing of course he can understand the test language, he generally "deviates from the norm." Since deviations in personality measures suggest maladjustment, the deaf subject runs the risk of being scored maladjusted simply because his answers to standardized test items are based on his distinctive and unstandardized life experiences. Even when a conscientious examiner carefully pores over the test, eliminates the most obviously inappropriate items, and simplifies the test language, the principles on which the remaining items were selected still remain: they are based on hearing life experiences and reactions; hence, they may be just as inappropriate for the deaf as are the eliminated items, albeit less obviously so.

This lack of appropriate instruments in evaluating deaf clients places a whole new burden of special competencies upon an examiner's shoulders. Not only must he acquire the complex communicative skills needed for work with the deaf, he must also become a highly proficient test expert. Out of the many hundreds of traditional tests, he must be able to judge which offer least penalties to a given deaf client, how best to administer the test under varying communicative conditions, what adaptations and modifications need to be made in a particular case, how to evaluate a client's responses in the absence of appropriate norms, and how to realistically interpret what the test findings signify with a subject who is deaf.

Over and above these special problems is the cloud of dissatisfaction hovering over psychological tests in general. As expressed by Cronbach (1970):

My overall impression of today's practical tests is that they are obsolescent. Tests that saw the light of day before 1949, with new norms and new scoring procedures, are in many areas the best we have today . . . I cannot escape the feeling that the things actuarially scored tests cannot do are more important that the things they can do (p. xxvii).

This expresses the general feeling of respondents to the writer's previously cited survey of psychological tests and practices with the deaf, namely that the things most hearing-standardized tests cannot do in regard to deaf subjects outweigh the things they can do. As expressed by one respondent: "Because of the many problems of validity arising when testing the deaf, results of any test should never be considered as meaningful unless they are viewed as part of the pattern of information about the individual."

In effect, examiners of the deaf do the best they can with the tests available to them. As a rule, the soundness of test findings and interpretations rests more with an examiner's competencies than with the test capability.

PSYCHOLOGICAL EXAMINATION OF DEAF REHABILITATION CLIENTS

Frame of Inquiry

Although the focus of every psychological examination is always on the subject, the procedures involved are additionally determined by the intended purpose of the examination. In a rehabilitation setting, the frame of inquiry is identified by the acronym SKAPATI (Pinner, 1970), in which the letters represent the following information areas:

S—Skills: The applicant's use of knowledge to execute or perform effectively and readily

K—Knowledge: His background, adequacy of job related information, "know-how"

A—Ability: His proficiency in any kind of work or activity

P—Physical: His physical and emotional capacity to do the job

A—Aptitudes: His potential or undeveloped abilities

T—Traits: His personal characteristics, which include primarily appearance, attitude, manner

I—Interests: Choice of vocation, the kind of work he is interested in doing

The same broad SKAPATI areas are involved in the examination of deaf clients. However, there are a number of specifically significant items of inquiry that arise from the ramifications of the disability and that need particular attention. A number are summarized below.

1. Communicative status
   A. What are the client's resources in expressive communication, particularly in speech and written language?
   B. What are the client's resources in receptive communication, particularly in reading and speechreading?
   C. What is the fit between the client's communicative resources and the communicative requirements for proposed vocational training, placement, occupational advance?
   D. What is the fit between a client's communicative resources and his intellectual potential and motivation for profiting from tutoring in communication?
   E. What broadened vocational areas might be feasibly opened to the client if he were to attain increased communicative facility? How great an increase would be required? Is this within the realm of possibility?
2. Vocational factors
   A. What are the client's vocational aspirations and how realistic are they?
   B. What is his level of know-how in regard to such matters as applying for a job; work conditions; labor unions; taxes, social security, insurance; shop language; salaries; the job market; etc.?
   C. What are his objectively determined vocational interests, aptitudes, skills?
   D. What are the nature, quality and duration of his previous work experiences; his principal problems?
   E. How does the client's communicative status affect vocational planning?
   F. What are the client's motivations and assets for improving his abilities and for learning new skills?
3. Intellectual status
   A. What is the relationship between the client's intellectual potentials and his actual functioning intelligence as indicated by life and school achievements?
   B. What are the speed, sharpness, relevance of his mental operations; how good a learner is he; how acute an observer?
   C. What is the fit between the client's functioning intelligence and his vocational aspirations, preferences, selection?
   D. What is his degree of insightful reasoning?
   E. What is his mental capability to handle such symbol systems as numerical, graphic, etc.?
4. Adjustment status
   A. How does the client get along with deaf people? hearing people?

B. What are his preferred group settings?

C. How flexible is the client; how great is his tolerance to frustration, stress, sustained effort; concentration?

D. What is his self-image; what are his principal motivations; how does he react to authority figures?

E. What is his independence/dependence "quotient?"

F. Does he present a neurotic disturbance, eccentric behavior? If so, how incapacitating is it so far as employment is concerned? Should he be referred for psychiatric appraisal?

5. Socioeconomic and family factors

A. Is the client a member of a deaf or hearing family?

B. What is his marital status; his domestic responsibilities?

C. What is his role in family decision-making; in personal decision-making?

D. How realistic are family aspirations in regard to the client? How persuasive is family influence on his thinking?

E. How supportive or obstructive is the family to the client's rehabilitation?

6. Social participation

A. What are the client's chief social outlets?

B. What is the extent of his participation in the activities of his deaf peer group; hearing peer group?

C. What are his organizational or club memberships? Has he ever been an office-holder; a group leader?

D. What is the extent of his sociocivic awareness?

7. Physical and health status

A. What other physical conditions and/or disabilities are present that must be considered in vocational planning and placement?

B. In particular, what is the condition of the client's visual ability; what is the likelihood of deteriorating vision (Vernon, 1969)?

Techniques of Examination

The principal techniques for obtaining answers to questions such as the foregoing are the same for the deaf as are used in all examination inquiry: personal history, interview, and psychological testing, with observation providing concomitant data. Details concerning the use of these techniques in case of hearing handicapped persons and a comprehensive history guide are presented elsewhere in the literature (Levine, 1960). The discussion below summarizes some of the key functions of each technique.

Personal History   Personal history has evaluative meaning only insofar as an examiner is able to recognize a significant history item when he sees it and to relate its influence to the total picture. In the case of clients who are deaf, this requires considerable familiarity with the deaf sub-culture and with the circumstances, deprivations, and experiences characterizing the lives of deaf persons. Such knowledge is another essential qualification for examiners of the deaf.

To an examiner so prepared, a deaf client's personal history indicates: 1) the principal life areas requiring remediation in the service of vocational rehabilitation; 2) the amount of remediation a given client is likely to achieve in each area; 3) the areas of remediation that warrant highest service-priority on the basis of practical gains a client is apt to make; and 4) the nature and possible influence of the mental, psychological, and physical assets and liabilities a deaf client brings to rehabilitation efforts.

To briefly illustrate, "knowing" the deaf can provide the following sampling of guides in interpreting history information:

1. A deaf client is of at least average mental ability if history shows a true reading achievement level of fourth grade.

2. A deaf client may be of at least average mental ability even if history shows a reading level below fourth grade.

3. A deaf client is probably of above-average mental ability even if history shows an arithmetic achievement score of sixth grade no matter how low his reading level.

4. A deaf client presents a good intellectual and adjustment picture if history shows good vocational, domestic, and social functioning regardless of test scores.

5. Where history indicates a client's inability to speak or read the lips, he may nevertheless be of any intellectual or scholastic achievement level. Oral communicative inability is no reflection on mental ability or linguistic achievement.

6. Where history indicates that a client's inability to speak or to read the lips is present in youth and adulthood, remediation in these areas will not result in significant gains.

7. Where history indicates that the causes for long-term, stubborn learning negativisms and disabilities are to be found in such factors as brain damage, deeply rooted psychological disorders, or adverse and inappropriate school experiences, spectacular remediation gains are not to be anticipated.

In reviewing a client's personal history, it is safest to conclude that the information indicates the basic minimum of the deaf person's abilities and to assume that the client will respond to wise rehabilitation planning and management regardless of how deficient his present level of functioning may be.

Interview To see the world through the eyes of experientially impoverished deaf clients is an extraordinary experience for nondeaf examiners. Unfortunately, not many can take advantage of the opportunity. There is the communication barrier that stands in the way: the previously discussed communicative factors of method, language, and concepts.

Regardless of the barriers, the first obligation of examiners is to put the client at ease by informing him of the purpose of the interview. An examiner should master sufficient signs to inform the sign-oriented client that the examiner wants to be of help, and that to do so it is necessary to know something about the client, his vocational interests, his abilities and aptitudes. Hence, the interview. Without such explanation, the deaf client may attribute the procedure to sheer nosiness and become doubly uncommunicative. This is not an uncommon reaction.

In the event the examiner and the client cannot communicate satisfactorily beyond this point, the embarrassment of the impasse is overcome by simply using the time for administering achievement tests. This fulfills a practical need for the examiner in establishing the client's level of linguistic and scholastic function. An interpreter can be obtained for the next interview session.

Communicative exchange may be difficult even with an interpreter. Apart from lacking the language, many deaf clients also lack the introspective ability to tell their own story even in their own way. In such instances, the examiner uses some simple projective tests to break the ice. The interview can then proceed based ostensibly on the client's test responses. Skillful handling can lead the client into discussing more personal matters relating to his own experiences and feelings.

In interpreted interviewing, a number of cautions need to be observed. Deaf clients are often as loathe to unburden themselves before interpreters as before members of their own families. The interpreter should therefore be acceptable to the client, and the client should be doubly assured of the confidential nature of all aspects of examination including interview.

The following excerpt illustrates something of the course of interview with a sign-oriented deaf client on completion of the course study in a school for the deaf and as conducted by a manually skilled interviewer:

Interviewer	"Tell me about when you were little. Could you hear when you were young?"
Client	"What mean?"
Interviewer	"Before. Little. Hear can you?"
Client	"No. Dumb me. Hear nothing little me."

Interviewer	"Become deaf how?"
Client	"I deaf since small—still deaf."
Interviewer	"How deaf? sick? accident? what?
Client	"Vomited, ear hurt, stomach hurt, was twisted, sick, very hot, hurt, other different things."
Interviewer	"How old sick?"
Client	"Not remember."
Interviewer	"Mother, father, deaf?"
Client	"No Father hearing but signs. Mother hearing not signs, talks."
Interviewer	"Brothers? sisters?"
Client	"Sister nothing, Brother one."
Interviewer	"How old brother?"
Client	"Old thirteen."
Interviewer	"Deaf brother?"
Client	"Hearing."

Further interview dealt with various school problems of the client; after discussing them the client said his arms were tired and he wanted to stop. When asked to sum up his school problems in written communication, the client quite willingly wrote: "I teased in the dormitory. I don't like . . . school. I knew troubling in the . . . School for the Deaf. I didn't never to tease. I am very quiet." The word "tease" was supplied by the interviewer in response to the client's request to tell him how to spell the verbal equivalent for the sign "tease."

For a communicatively handicapped examiner, the frustrating element in interview is his awareness of the willingness of most deaf clients to impart all kinds of personal information to a trusted interviewer, and the examiner's inability to get at this vital data.

Psychological Testing Psychological testing of deaf clients takes place in the frame of communicative problems and test limitations previously discussed. Nevertheless, testing represents an additional source of much needed and hard to come by data, and as such it is not to be lightly dismissed because of the problems involved. When wisely used and with the application of sound clinical judgment, psychological testing can prove a helpful ally to examiners of the deaf.

Pre-test Preparation In psychological testing, as in the interview, the deaf client should be given preliminary explanation of the purpose of the testing procedure and orientation as to what is involved. To be exposed to unknown procedures for undisclosed reasons is as exasperating or as threatening to a deaf person as it would be to anyone.

Test Selection Unless otherwise indicated, it is best to begin the test procedure with reading achievement tests and some samples of the client's written productions. In this way, the examiner can judge which types of tests (verbal, nonverbal, nonlanguage, paper-and-pencil, or performance) will best suit a client's expressive, responsive, and conceptual styles. Once having determined the types, the examiner then selects the specific tests or test items he plans to use in examination.

Test Administration The first prerequisite in administering a test to a deaf client is to make absolutely sure that the client understands what he is expected to do with each task. Unless this is done, the examiner has no way of knowing whether failure on a particular item was the result of the client's inability to perform the task or to his inability to understand the examiner's instructions. In the case of certain tests, adaptations will have to be made in standard directions as illustrated previously with the WAIS question. Occasionally, sample tasks may have to be devised to illustrate what the directions mean. Both adaptation and sample-tasking, when carefully done, can be accomplished without harming objectivity.

If an understanding of test directions is still not achieved despite adaptation of standard directions and sample tasks, an interpreter is called upon. The procedure in administering a test through an interpreter is rather awkward because the examiner must keep one eye on the interpreter and the other on the client, while at the same time trying to maintain objectivity and guard against the natural inclination of many interpreters to give a little help to the client through suggestive signing and facial expression.

Tests Used with Deaf Clients Listings and comments regarding psychological tests used with the deaf are presented elsewhere in the literature (Donoghue, 1968; Eddington, 1973; Levine, 1960, 1963, 1971, 1974; Stewart, 1968; Vernon and Brown, 1964). By and large, the tests mentioned in these and other sources cover the same ground. Preferred tests are those that require a minimum of verbal language, and test selection is generally guided by ease of administration and scoring. The tests used are generally individual tests, or if not, are usually individually administered.

In the previously cited survey of tests and practices (Levine, 1974), over 90 different tests reported by the respondents are used in whole or by item in the areas of intelligence, personality, achievement, vocationally related attributes, and for special clinical purposes, for the age range from 6 through 18 years. Omitting the tests used with the very young, the highest ranking tests were:

1. Intelligence: Performance sections of the Wechsler scales; the Leiter Intelligence Tests; Hiskey–Nebraska Test of Learning Aptitude; Goodenough-Harris Drawing Test; the Arthur adaptation of the Leiter; and the Columbia Mental Maturity Scale

2. Achievement: Wide Range Achievement Test; Stanford Achievement Tests

3. Personality: Bender-Gestalt; House-Tree-Person; Thematic Appercep-tion Test; Rorschach Technique (for psychopathy)

Because the population on which the survey was based was not a rehabilitation population, there was limited reference to vocational tests. However, those frequently used in rehabilitation settings include the following:

4. Vocational: Minnesota Paper Formboard; Crawford Small Parts Dex-terity; O'Connor Finger Dexterity; DAT Mechanical Reasoning, Spatial Relations; Minnesota Clerical Aptitude; California Picture Interest Inven-tory; Geist Picture Interest Inventory; and tests in more specialized aptitude areas, such as art, engineering, physical sciences, and college potential as indicated.

The administration of most verbal-vocational tests is contingent upon a sixth grade reading level. Otherwise, the picture and manipulative tests are used.

Descriptions and reviews of the tests mentioned above can be found in the Buros *Mental Measurement Yearbook* volumes, with an interesting evaluation of the Geist Picture Interest Inventory-Deaf Form, Male, sup-plied elsewhere by Bolton (1971).

To tease out as much information as possible from intelligence tests and to account for the wide differences in functioning intelligence often found among clients with similar performance tests scores, the current shift is in the direction of using verbal sections of the Wechsler Scales or verbal items from the scales in addition to the performance portions. To illustrate the differences in functioning intelligence between two deaf clients with similar WAIS Performance scores, a sampling of responses is presented in Table 1, which were taken from this author's files and made by two deaf teenagers with strikingly similar backgrounds in all respects save linguistic proficiency. The test was administered manually to both subjects, and in the case of linguistically inferior Subject A, adaptations were made to ensure comprehension of the questions asked.

Obviously, there is more to be considered in the mental evaluation of deaf clients than performance IQ. The latter points to the client's mental potential; but it is through feasible verbal test inquiry that the examiner can estimate the conceptual level of a client's mental functioning and the level of understanding for rehabilitation.

As for the use of personality tests with the deaf in rehabilitation settings, responses are not generally scored but rather are content scruti-

Table 1. A sample of responses to verbal items of the Wechsler Adult Intelligence Scale[1]

	Subject A	Subject B
Comprehension		
Finding envelope	Take stamp off; save it	Mail it
Bad company	Easy spoil me	Learn bad things from them
Pay taxes	Don't know	Support government
Born deaf	Don't know	Cannot hear how to talk
Similarities		
Orange-banana	Both yellow, good to eat, healthy	Both fruits
Coat-dress	Both pretty	Both are to wear
Dog-lion	Both brown, have mouths	Both animals
Air-water	Both windy	Cannot live without air or water
Eye-ear	Eye can open and shut, ear wakes up when you hear	Both parts of body

[1] From this author's files.

nized. Their chief value is in sparking interview exchange, and not infrequently in indicating symptoms of gross psychopathology.

The practical usefulness of achievement tests has been previously noted, particularly in reading achievement. Another useful finding in rehabilitation situations is the client's arithmetic achievement level, which serves as a valuable index of a client's potentials in mastering vocational operations involving measurements of various kinds.

Interpreting Test Findings With all but the exceptional deaf, interpreting intelligence and personality test findings is more a clinical than a measurement procedure. Each of a client's responses is studied in the light of: 1) the process the item is designed to tap; 2) the client's particular background of experiences and deprivations; and 3) the norm system of the given test. Weaving the information together results in a response pattern that is then examined for rehabilitative assets and liabilities.

If the pattern is in line with the client's life circumstances, it is an expected outcome from a particular background. Deviant from hearing norm patterns though it may well be, it cannot be considered deviant in the true pathological sense. It simply indicates the deformity of the client's environment of which he is the outcome. While this does not make life any easier for him, it opens the door a little wider for rehabilitation understanding and management.

Observation Previously discussed handicaps to formal psychological examination of deaf clients place a high premium on the value of observation in filling some of the gaps. Although the examiner seeks the same kinds of observational leads with the deaf as with the nondeaf, in the case of the deaf certain leads possess particular evaluative significance. All else being equal, possibly the most important relate to the client's communicative drive, his capacity for independent action, and his capacity for concentration and levels of tolerance for stress and frustration. For example, in regard to communicative drive the examiner should consider: how sharp is the client at picking up communicative clues in the face of difficulty; how responsive is he to the examiner's efforts to make himself understood; how persistent and ingenious is he in making himself understood; or does he remain passive to the whole interpersonal exchange effort?

During test procedure, how quickly does the client grasp test directions, and how accurately; does he continually look to the examiner's face for hints, praise, encouragement, or is he capable of proceeding on his own until the task is satisfactorily completed? In working on a task, for how long a period can he labor over it to get it done; is he aware when it is correctly completed; does he see and correct his errors, or does he reach an impasse and simply give up in disgust or repeat the same approach and the same errors over and over?

At the conclusion of the test procedure, is the client interested in knowing how he did, indifferent, hostile, discouraged? Does he seem to consider the whole operation a silly waste of his time, or does he look on it as a challenging experience? Does he want to know when he can come again, or is he glad the whole thing is over and done with?

With communicatively handicapped clients in particular, clues such as these are exceptionally useful in gauging how willingly the client will meet life in a hearing world half way, and what impression he is apt to make on the authority figures he meets en route. These and other observational details, such as manner, appearance, general attitude, behavioral "deafisms," all are involved in predicting a deaf client's success or failure in finding his niche in a hearing society.

Evaluation

With clients whose examination procedures are as handicapped with difficulties as are the severely disadvantaged among deaf clients, evaluation

---

cannot be conducted solely on the basis of a single examination. The implications derived from a first examination need to be tested in life as the client undergoes rehabilitation remediation. Improvement in the client's condition may be sufficiently striking to cast new light on his abilities and potentials, and require a consequent shift in rehabilitation remediation and expectation. As a client's condition changes, it is necessary to know the amount and direction of change; to review the changes in the light of the nature of the remediation approaches; to appraise past recommendations in view of the changed situation; and to decide what the next phase of rehabilitation should be. This involves a continuing process of examination and evaluation until the client is optimally set on the right road.

SUMMARY

A psychological evaluator of deaf clients must be prepared to deal with a total range of human abilities and potentials that, in a majority of instances, are hidden behind a unique communicative barrier. To penetrate the barrier and to get to the person demands unusual skills and exceptional competencies. Experienced psychological examiners consider the challenge that the deaf person presents worth the effort of acquiring the skills.

For many uninitiated examiners, the picture of defects and deficits in the examination findings of many deaf clients is apt to cast a pall of pessimism over the deaf in general and over rehabilitation efforts in their behalf in particular. This is a mistake. Irremediable defects and deficits are certainly present, much to the frustration of concerned field personnel. But the client is also frustrated. A surprising number of communicatively disadvantaged deaf clients demonstrate unexpected bursts of motivation and the will to accomplish when accomplishment lies with the realm of possibility, and when they know that someone has faith in their abilities.

REFERENCES

American Psychological Association. 1970. Psychological assessment and public policy. Amer. Psych. 27:266.
Anderson, W., and A. Smith. 1969. Personality characteristics of the disadvantaged. In J. T. Kunce and C. S. Cope (eds.), Rehabilitation and the Culturally Disadvantaged, p. 27. University of Missouri—Columbia.
Birch, H. G. 1958. Introduction. In E. Haeussermann (ed.), Developmental Potential of Preschool Children, p. ix. Grune and Stratton, New York.
Bolton, B. 1971. A critical review of the Geist Picture Interest Inventory: Deaf form: Male. J. Rehab. Deaf 5:21–30.

Cronbach, L. J. 1970. Essentials of Psychological Testing. 3rd Ed., p. xxviii. Harper & Row, New York.

Donoghue, R. J. 1968. The deaf personality—A study in contrasts. J. Rehab. Deaf 2:37—52.

DiFrancesca, S. J., and S. N. Hurwitz. 1969. Rehabilitation of the hard core deaf: Identification of an affective style. J. Rehab. Deaf 3:34—41.

Eddington, G. 1973. The school psychologist and the hearing impaired child. Highlights 52:8—11.

Fant, L. 1964. Say It with Hands. American Annals of the Deaf, Washington, D.C.

Levine, E. S. 1960. The Psychology of Deafness. Columbia University Press, New York.

Levine, E. S. 1963. Studies in the psychological evaluation of the deaf. Volta Rev. 65 (special issue): 496—512.

Levine, E. S. 1971. Mental assessment of the deaf child. Volta Rev. 73:80—97.

Levine, E. S. 1974. Psychological tests and practices with the deaf: A survey of the state of the art. Volta Rev. 76:298—319.

O'Rourke, T. J., ed. 1972. Psycholinguistics and total communication: The state of the art. Amer. Ann. Deaf.

Pinner, J. 1970. General employment: The responsibility of an employment interviewer. J. Rehab. Deaf Monograph No. 2, p. 45.

Public Health Service Publication No. 1,227. Proceedings: Conference on the Collection of Statistics on Severe Hearing Impairments and Deafness in the United States. Washington, D.C.

Riekehof, L. 1963. Talk to the Deaf. Gospel Publishing House, Springfield, Mo.

Schein, J. D., and M. Delk. 1973. How many deaf people? Rehab. Rec. 14:36—38.

Stewart, L. G. 1968. The vocational rehabilitation process. In A. B. Crammatte (ed.), Multiply Disabled Deaf Persons (Workshop Report). Rehabilitation Service Administration, Washington, D.C.

Terman, L. M., and M. A. Merrill. 1960. Stanford-Binet Intelligence Scale: Manual for the Third Revision, Form L-M, p. 47ff. Houghton-Mifflin, Boston.

Vernon, M. 1969. Usher's syndrome. J. Chronic Dis. 22:133—151.

Vernon, M., and D. W. Brown. 1964. A guide to psychological tests and testing procedures in the evaluation of deaf and hard of hearing children. J. Speech Hearing Disord. 29:414—423.

16 | Psychological Evaluation of the Mentally Retarded Adult

MARVIN ROSEN and MARVIN S. KIVITZ

The history of psychological testing is closely related to concerns about identifying and educating the mentally retarded. The first intelligence test is usually attributed to Alfred Binet, who was commissioned to identify "mental defectives" before their entrance into French normal schools. Fertile ground for the development of psychological measurement procedures had already been cultivated by the monumental studies of individual differences by Sir Francis Galton, the faculty psychology of the eighteenth century Scottish philosopher Thomas Reid, the phrenology movement originated by Gall, the pedigree investigations of the Jukes (Dugdale, 1900) and Kallikaks (Goddard, 1914), and the pioneering "mental tests" of James McKeen Cattell (1948), first published in 1890.

However, it was not until Binet conceived the idea of arranging tests in order of difficulty that the potential utility of tests was recognized, and not until much later that they achieved general acceptance. The original Binet-Simon Scales first appeared in 1905 and were used for classification of "feeblemindedness." The 1908 revision of the scales introduced the concept of mental age. These developments subsequently led to the introduction of the Binet Scales in the United States by Goddard, the Stanford revision by Terman in 1916, and the large scale testing of draftees during World War I. Later developments included the use of more sophisticated statistical procedures, such as factor analysis in identifying homogeneous tests of abilities and personality traits (Cattell, 1957; Eysenck, 1960; Guilford, 1959, 1967; Thurstone, 1938), the development of the Wechsler Scales, and the deviation IQ. During the last three decades there has been a rapid proliferation of projective tests of personality, more widespread use of tests in industry and personnel work, and reliance upon behavioral and situational measures suitable for behavior analysis and behavior modification.

FUNCTIONS OF PSYCHOLOGICAL EVALUATION

Although Binet tests were intended primarily for classification, tests are now applied to broad goals of clinical diagnosis and prediction. They are used to assess not only intellectual behavior but also social and emotional responses and more subtle dynamic processes involving both conscious and unconscious motivation. The introduction of psychoanalytically oriented procedures by Rorschach (1942), Murray (1938), Rappaport (1945), and others has changed the evaluation process from a purely objective psychometric procedure to a more subjective, intuitive, and highly personalized endeavor.

These drastic changes in the purpose and process of assessment have aroused heated controversy and contention among psychologists so that the use of tests and their interpretation varies greatly according to differences in theoretical or even philosophical orientation. Those who view testing as a holistic, broad-band clinical process look with disdain at the more objective paper and pencil procedures, despite their claims of higher reliability and factorial validity. Others advocate a "cookbook" (Meehl, 1956) approach to testing, offering evidence that the accuracy of clinical judgment is, by definition, inferior to actuarial approaches (Meehl, 1954). Meehl has gone so far as to suggest that the worst thing a clinician may do in evaluating a client is to personally interact with him or even think about his responses. With that controversy largely unresolved, psychological testing was subjected to attack from another quarter by those who attack intelligence testing as discriminatory, culturally biased, and unfair to the economically disadvantaged. Fuel has been added to the fire by a revival of the ageless and insoluble nature-nurture controversy with proponents of genetic factors (Jensen, 1969) attributing as much as 80 percent of the variance in IQ scores to heritability components.

Despite this furor over testing, some areas of general agreement may be found. Most psychologists would agree that psychological tests, whether interpreted by clinical or actuarial means, must have an established predictive validity with meaningful criteria in order to be useful. Whatever the genetic contribution to the variance of IQ tests, they are valid predictors of one important criterion, school achievement.

The structure and nature of this volume impose two constrictions upon the scope of this chapter. First, that the evaluation be limited to adults rather than to children; second, that the focus be evaluation for use in rehabilitation facilities. However, this problem is treated from a broader vantage point reflecting current philosophy and research findings in the field of mental retardation, and the conclusions drawn should have more general applicability.

The successful application of psychological tests in the evaluation process rests upon several factors: 1) the selection of assessment procedures relevant to the functioning or adjustment of the mental retardate; 2) the reliability of the instruments selected; 3) their validity as predictors of relevant criteria; 4) proper administration of the procedures according to standardized conditions of testing; 5) use of normative information relevant to the client being evaluated; and 6) organization and interpretation of test scores according to the conceptual model of mental retardation held by the examiner. The reader is referred to standard texts of tests and measurements for a fuller discussion of concepts of reliability, validity, norms, and standardization. The importance of a conceptual model, linking test constructs to personality and behavioral constructs, is emphasized below.

Benton (1964) has listed the purposes of psychological evaluation of the mentally retarded as: 1) differential diagnosis, including the determination of whether or not the individual belongs in the category labeled mental retardation and his subcategory designation, and 2) statement of an expected prognosis in response to educational or therapeutic measures. Benton (1964) points out that diagnosis rests firmly upon the concept of mental retardation held by the examiner.

> The diagnostic procedures and judgments which are covered by the collective term "psychological evaluation" bear a reciprocal relationship to fundamental theory in the field of mental retardation. In clinical work, diagnostic practice is dependent upon, and, in large measure, determined by, prevailing theoretical assumptions about the nature of mental retardation. Thus the decision, on the basis of a psychological evaluation, that a given individual is or is not mentally retarded ultimately depends as much on the clinician's fundamental conception of the nature of mental retardation as it does on the specific findings of the examination (p. 16).

Consequently, one purpose of this chapter is to expound a conceptual model concerning mental retardation that can serve as a theoretical underpinning for the use of psychological tests in evaluating this population. Without such a model, evaluation becomes a smorgasbord of conceptually unrelated test procedures, even when the test constructs have meaningful referents in the overt behavior of the subject. Of course, it is rare that an examiner does not employ such a model, although the process may be an implicit one. In the use of an intelligence test, for example, the examiner knowingly or unknowingly assumes that the mental tasks sampled by the IQ test chosen bear some relation to the domain of behaviors relevant to the purposes of the evaluation. As will be brought out later, if the purpose of the assessment is the prediction of competence in social or vocational situations, this assumption is probably unwarranted.

A conceptual model for evaluation must be sufficiently flexible to accommodate changing ideas in the field. With increased experience in educating and training the mentally handicapped and with greater emphasis upon research, much of the previously accepted dogma of retardation is no longer acceptable. That mental retardation is an irreversible process was once widely believed. Another prevalent notion concerned the constancy of the IQ and its utility as a measure of "innate capacity." Both of these assumptions led to the general acceptance of another idea termed "pseudo-retardation." This term was applied to persons once diagnosed as mentally retarded but who, over time, demonstrated IQ increments to nonretarded levels. Since retardation was considered irreversible and IQs stable, such an occurrence implied error in the diagnostic judgment at time of the original evaluation. More recent interpretation regards the IQ function as a measure of current intellectual functioning rather than as an index of capacity. Longitudinal studies provide a basis for expecting IQ change over time either because of unreliability in the testing procedure, irregularities in the development of intelligence (Bayley, 1949, 1955, 1968), or as a response to changes in environmental conditions (Butterfield, 1967; Clarke and Clarke, 1954; Heber et al., 1968; Rosen et al., 1968; Skeels and Dye, 1939; Skeels, 1941). Reasoning from these findings, the concept of pseudoretardation is unnecessary.

CONCEPTUAL MODEL

A useful model for the psychological evaluator is presented below. It is consistent with current understanding of the retarded and provides a workable basis for both evaluation and programming. The model is based upon the following points:

1. Irrelevance of etiological systems of classification and the need for a nosology based upon current, observable behaviors or constellations of behavior

2. Statistical deviation as a necessary but insufficient criterion of mental retardation

3. The importance of social criteria of functioning and performance (coping and adaptive behavior) in evaluation and classification

4. The low utility of the disease model of mental retardation; the need to deal with retarded behavior rather than with mental retardation

5. Recognition of the humanitarian and legal principle of normalization in programming but not as a factor in evaluation or classification

6. Consideration of more subjective variables, such as attitudes, feelings, and conflict, in evaluation

7. Recognition of the effects of motivational, social, and emotional variables upon behavior

8. Recognition of the effects of expectations of others in influencing behavior of mental retardates and the sometimes deleterious effects of labels.

Psychiatric nosological systems may be traced to Kraepelin (1925) who first classified psychoses into that type with a cyclical course and a good prognosis versus that originating during adolescence and showing a progressive deterioration. Kraepelin labeled the first condition that of manic depression and the second, dementia praecox. This designation was based upon presumed ideology, prognosis, and response to clinical diagnostic systems. An etiological model was also later applied to classification of the mentally retarded. Zigler and Phillips (1961) have criticized the use of such classification systems as being poorly related to symptomatic behavior and have argued instead for a classification system based upon current observable behaviors and constellations of symptoms. In keeping with this criticism, the current emphasis in psychological approaches to mental retardation has been placed upon retarded behavior rather than upon the construct "mental retardation" (Bijou, 1963; Throne, 1970).

The need for criteria of current behavior in defining and in identifying mental retardation is further underscored by an appreciation of the inadequacy of definitions based solely upon statistical deviation from the mean. Geneticists agree that intelligence is polygenic in origin, so that the distribution of this variable follows the normal bell-shaped curve. IQ tests have been constructed according to this assumption, and IQ scores are computed to "normalize" any irregularities in the distribution of scores obtained in the standardization of the test. Because "normal" functioning represents a range along this distribution rather than a single IQ point (e.g., IQ = 100), relatively small deviations must still be regarded as normal. An IQ of 75, for example, is no more abnormal than an IQ of 125. Both represent normal variation around a mean. Zigler (1967) has made this point in a description of the familial retarded as qualitatively similar to normal intelligence groups in that they represent the lower end of the normal distribution curve of intelligence. Psychologists have emphasized the importance of social and motivational factors in determining the performance of these people (Bijou, 1963; Cromwell, 1963; Zigler, 1966), who may vary greatly in their actual functioning in society. Whether or not those persons should be labeled mentally retarded must depend on factors other than IQ.

There has also been found, however, a slightly elevated frequency of very low IQs centering around a mean of about 30. The obtained frequencies of these scores represent a higher incidence than would be predicted from the normal distribution curve. These scores are obtained from persons suffering severe organic deficiencies, and they are interpreted as representing a second distribution of intellectual functioning superimposed upon the bell-shaped curve and representing people who *are* qualitatively different from most of the population. Evaluation of such persons is usually not feasible by standard intelligence tests, which are insensitive to small differences at that low IQ level and require a degree of comprehension and verbal proficiency beyond that of the subject population. These persons frequently require the structure and supervision of a sheltered residential and work setting.

While degree of statistical deviation is important in determining how a person functions in relation to a normative group, it is insufficient in estimating the degree or nature of his social deficits because wide variation in social competence exists at all IQ levels.

According to the latest definition accepted by the American Association on Mental Deficiency (Grossman, 1973), mental retardation refers to those cases involving a developmental and intellectual growth occurring at birth or shortly thereafter, and adversely affecting a person's ability to adapt to his environment. Although clinical medical classification is acceptable, the manual also describes the criteria for behavioral classification based upon both functioning IQ and adaptive behavior, i.e., the ability to cope with environmental demands at various levels of functioning. Thus, social areas of functioning are now considered an important factor in the diagnosis and classification of mental retardation.

These variables should include dimensions that reflect the client's capacity to cope with environmental demands at home, on a job, in the community, or in education and training programs. The evaluator must also consider the type of environmental setting in which the client is being evaluated, e.g., a sheltered workshop, a group home, a competitive job in the community, or in a hospital. In making this determination the clinician must be able to go beyond the traditional IQ concept and evaluate the client's capacity for vocational functioning at sheltered or independent, competitive levels, as well as his ability to deal with ordinary social, interpersonal relationships without appearing inappropriate or bizarre.

Szasz (1960) has been the most vocal critic of the medical or disease model of "mental illness." He points out that while physical illness is diagnosed in terms of deviation from some physical norm (e.g., a fever), so-called mental illness represents deviation from normative psychosocial, legal, or ethical behavior. Accordingly, it is logically inconsistent to evoke concepts of physical causality upon behaviors that may represent problems in living. Those who endorse these ideas have criticized the use of drug therapies in treating mental disorder, have attacked the nosological system based logically on etiological consideration (Zigler and Phillips, 1961), and have generally advocated treatment strategies based upon social learning techniques (Bandura, 1969; Ullman and Krasner, 1966). This approach has also been applied with the mentally retarded. Behavior modification techniques have been markedly influential in areas such as toilet training (Dayan, 1964; Ellis, 1963; Hundziak et al., 1965); self-help (Bensberg et al., 1965; Blackwood, 1962; Roos, 1965; Watson, 1967); academic instruction (Birnbrauer et al., 1965); language (Bricker and Bricker, 1970; Lovaas, 1966); and the structuring of living or work environments as "token economies" (Giradeau and Spradlin, 1964).

While attacks upon the "disease model" need not have a direct impact upon the evaluation process in mental retardation, they serve as reminders that psychological assessment procedures sample behavioral repertoires, not cerebral functioning or genetic endowment; that concerns should be focused upon socially relevant behavior, rather than events occurring at conception, during pregnancy, delivery, or early infancy. The view of mental retardation as maladaptive social functioning, whatever the IQ, should guide the examiner in his choice of assessment procedures and his emphasis in presenting his findings.

Nirje (1969) has described the principle of normalization as necessary to provide the mentally handicapped with their full rights and benefits as citizens. Normalization refers to the desire "to let the mentally retarded obtain an existence as close as normal as possible . . . the normalization principle means making available to the mentally retarded patterns and conditions of everyday life which are as close as possible to the norms of the mainstream of society" (p. 181). This principle has been adapted for the standards for residential facilities by the Joint Commission of Accreditation of Hospitals (1971). A psychologist testing the mentally retarded must be aware of the rights of the mentally retarded for as normal a living situation as possible whether or not they reside in sheltered or living situations.

Classification of even severe levels of mental retardation must not carry with it the implication of denial of basic human rights. However, it should be clearly understood that normalization is a humanitarian rather than a psychological principle (Rosen and Kivitz, 1973). It does not bear upon personal attributes relevant to level of functioning, and it is not a substitute for sound criteria of personal and emotional adjustment. It does not imply that all mentally retarded persons can be equated psychologically, and it does not deny the existence of differences between the retarded and the intellectually average or superior populations, or the absence of real problems of coping behavior. Individual differences among the mentally retarded as well as between retarded and nonretarded populations must dictate the manner of applying the normalization principle. Adequate selection and training of persons for independent living situations must still be the major emphasis of normalizing procedures. For those judged incapable of independent living situations, environmental changes within sheltered living and work situations should be dictated by the desire to make living as normal as possible.

While criteria of adaptive behavior are essential in diagnosis and classification, it would be a disservice to ignore more subjective variables, such as personal adjustment, in evaluating the mentally retarded. Rosen and Kivitz (1973) have suggested that at least seven dimensions should be considered in understanding the personal adjustment of the mentally handicapped. These include areas of self-concept, attitudes and motivation toward independence and initiative, perception of reality according to societal norms, the adequacy of mechanisms for emotional expression, purposive or goal-directed behavior, interest in other people and the ability to engage in interpersonal relationships, and the capacity for heterosexual relationships and behaviors.

The importance of motivational variables affecting the performance of the mentally retarded has been well documented. Cromwell (1963) predicts that retarded children will have a lower generalized expectancy of success than normals as a result of having had fewer successes in past situations. This is substantiated by studies demonstrating differential effects, in normals and retarded subjects, of failure in experimental situations (Heber, 1957). It has also been shown that lowered expectations for performance are consistently linked to actual performance in both normal and retarded persons (Diggory, 1966; Rosen, Diggory, and Werlinsky, 1966; Rosen et al., 1971). The examining psychologist must be aware of the close link between performance and motivation, not only on psychological tests, but also in classrooms and on a job. His evaluation of "levels" of retardation must be tempered by a knowledge of the variance in performance as a function of motivational variables, regardless of intellectual level.

Finally, the powerful effect of expectations placed upon retarded persons because of their level of intellectual and social functioning should be acknowledged. Rosenthal and Jacobson (1968) have demonstrated this effect with normal children who respond differentially to expectations about their abilities. The likelihood of underevaluating the potential of a retarded person because of a diagnostic label must be recognized by those engaged in the evaluation process. Older labels such as "trainable" and "educable" have limited usefulness and may actually be detrimental to the retarded because of the preconceived expectations they connote about performance levels. With appropriate motivational conditions and sound and well proven curricula, retarded persons have been shown to be capable of academic attainment (Birnbrauer et al., 1965) and fine perceptual discriminations (Sidman and Stoddard, 1966), previously judged impossible.

RELATIONSHIP BETWEEN
EVALUATION PROCESS AND EVALUATION GOALS

Because testing strategies vary according to the nature of the referral, all psychological evaluations are not alike. An evaluation conducted for one purpose (e.g., classification and screening) serves poorly for other purposes (e.g., planning for educational needs). The choice of testing instruments and procedures will be determined largely by the specific evaluation needs, and it is rare that a given set of procedures will serve more than one purpose. Three major goals are accomplished by psychological evaluation: 1) diagnosis and classification, 2) prediction of future functioning in specific behavioral areas, and 3) prescriptions for remediation or treatment based upon measured needs of the client.

Psychologists are continually called upon to classify the mentally retarded in terms of intellectual functioning or levels of adaptive behavior. Such demands may arise because of state or federal regulations for funding or as an aid in educational planning. In addition to classifying intellectual functioning, the psychologist may also desire to identify specific areas of strength or weakness and to provide a qualitative description of the client's style of thinking, his characteristic approach to novel situations, and the rigidity or concreteness of his thought processes. These embellishments to the evaluation are often subjective and personal and do not have the established reliability and validity of the IQ.

Prediction is one major purpose of psychological evaluation because the validity of any test refers to its correlation with a relevant criterion. As indicated earlier, the criterion used for validating IQ tests has traditionally been school performance, and the IQ is not a good predictor of other criteria. Validation of tests of personality is more difficult, and there are few well established procedures for predicting social or interpersonal behavior from test scores. Even the manual dexterity and perceptual-motor tests traditionally used in vocational evaluation of the mentally retarded are of dubious validity in predicting work behaviors.

Ideally, psychological testing should be useful for prescriptive teaching or treatment. This involves the identification of individual cognitive strengths and weaknesses to be used in choosing training or educational strategies. Immediate or eventual prescription is implicit in classification and prediction procedures. Classification is presumably accomplished in order to implement treatment strategies that represent the closest match between a person's intellect and personality and the available programs. Similarly, the valid prediction of a criterion behavior has only academic interest unless the predictive relationship, once established, is used in selection for a particular purpose. For example, if it can be shown that persons who score well on the Porteus Maze are likely to succeed in independent living situations after discharge from an institution, while low scorers have high failure rates, then the Porteus could be used for selection for discharge. That psychological tests should have a purpose beyond description or classification is an idea frequently overlooked or misunderstood (Renner, 1962).

SYSTEMS OF CLASSIFICATION AND DIAGNOSIS

The Manual on Terminology and Classification of the American Association on Mental Deficiency (Grossman, 1973) provides standards for classification and diagnosis according to medical, intellectual, and behavioral criteria. As indicated earlier, medical diagnosis is based upon etiological considerations. Tredgold and Soddy (1956) define endogenous retardation as encompassing all cases of retardation without some known external causative agent. The term is reserved for retardation determined on the basis of heredity, i.e., the broad classification of familial retardation with a high incidence of sibling involvement and traceable historical origins in previous generations.

Exogenous retardation is so labeled because of a known or presumed causative agent. Exogenous retardation would be inferred from a negative family history for retardation, a history of brain injury or conditions that are suggestive of injury, such as anoxia during delivery, and positive neurological findings for brain damage including an abnormal electro-encephalogram. The exogenous category is further subdivided into those cases associated with infective causation (e.g., congential syphilis, Rubella); toxic causation (e.g., lead poisoning, Thalidomide); endocrine disturbances (e.g., cretinism); or traumatic causation (as by anoxia, hemmorrhage); and the deprivative deficiencies associated with deprivation of nutritional elements or cultural deprivation.

Intellectual functioning, as measured by standardized IQ tests, is meaningful in terms of the comparisons they allow with reference groups of the same chronological age as the person being evaluated. It is customary to delineate classification categories according to the person's position relative to such a reference group. It is important that the reference group be appropriate (as similar as possible) to the person being tested. IQs can be expressed in terms of deviation units representing the standard deviation of the particular test utilized. The limits accepted by the American Association on Mental Deficiency are listed in Table 1 for the Stanford-Binet and the Wechsler Intelligence Scales. It is important to realize that identical IQs obtained on tests having different standard deviations are not equivalent in meaning.

Persons functioning about two or more standard deviations below the mean (about 2.5 percent of the population) are considered Mentally Retarded; persons functioning between two and three standard deviations below the mean are labeled Mildly Retarded. This represents approximate IQ values between 50 and 70. Persons with IQs between 30 and 50 are labeled Moderately Retarded. Those with IQs between 20 and 30 are labeled Severely Retarded, while persons with IQs below 20 (essentially untestable by standardized procedures) are termed Profoundly Retarded.

Adaptive Behavior

The sole use of the IQ in classification and diagnosis of mental retardation has been criticized because it is not predictive of levels of independent functioning or of specific behavioral problems. The Manual on Terminology and Classification (Grossman, 1973) specifies that the diagnosis of mental retardation must rest upon the demonstration of deficiencies along two general dimensions, measured intelligence and adaptive behavior. Adaptive behavior refers to the success of a person in adapting to the natural and social demands of his environment. The level of adaptation is

Table 1. IQ scores according to standard deviation values

| | | Obtained intelligence quotient | |
Standard deviation units	Levels	Stanford-Binet and Cattell[1]	Wechsler Scales[2]
−2.01 to −3.00	Mild	68−52	69−55
−3.01 to −4.00	Moderate	51−36	54−40
−4.01 to −5.00	Severe	35−20	39−25
⩾−5.0	Profound	19 and below	24 and below

[1] Standard deviation = 16.
[2] Standard deviation = 15.

Modified from Grossman, H. J., ed. 1973. Manual on Terminology and Classification in Mental Retardation, Revision, p. 18. American Association on Mental Deficiency.

assessed in terms of the degree to which a person is able to function and to maintain himself independently, and the degree to which he satisfactorily meets the culturally imposed demands of personal and social responsibility. Adaptive behavior is classified into four levels according to adequacy in meeting societal demands at each age level. Broad criteria of the four levels of adaptive behavior for preschool age, school age, and adult age levels have been described. The Adaptive Behavior Scale (Nihira et al., 1969) published by the American Association on Mental Deficiency is gaining acceptance as a measure of these behaviors.

INSTRUMENTATION FOR CLASSIFICATION

Evaluating Intelligence and Cognitive Areas

Although numerous measures of intelligence have been published, there is little question that the most frequently used test is the Wechsler Adult Intelligence Scale (WAIS) (1955). This procedure has the most extensive adult norms which are arranged in age groupings of 5-year intervals. The test provides separate estimates of verbal and nonverbal (performance) functioning and consists of 11 separate subtests. The availability of the Performance IQ as a means of evaluating relatively nonverbal or inarticulate persons affords the WAIS a decided advantage over the Stanford-Binet which is highly loaded with verbal items and often places the adult retarded at a decided disadvantage. The items of the WAIS are also more suitable to an adult population, while the Binet items are juvenile at the lower age levels. The same limitations that hold in general for the WAIS also hold with a retarded population. The verbal and performance categorizations are not factorially pure, nor are the subtests. Factor analyses of the WAIS yield Verbal, Memory, Perceptual, and g factors (Cohen, 1957). Furthermore, the reliability of the subtests (Rosen et al., 1968) and the reliability of difference scores between individual subtests may be low (McNemar, 1957), making profile analysis hazardous, except from extreme subtest differences.

Tests of specific cognitive abilities may be used for classification or diagnosis. Where the client is deficient in expressive language skills it is advisable to use a nonverbal intelligence measure to substitute for the WAIS verbal scale or to supplement it. The Peabody Picture Vocabulary Test (Dunn, 1970) provides an assessment of mental age determined solely by receptive language. The client responds by identifying one of four pictures for each vocabulary item. The test is limited by restricted norms and the sole reliance upon receptive language as a measure of comprehension. The procedure has the advantages of having been developed for retarded and language deficient populations and for ease of administration.

The Leiter International Performance Scale (1952) was developed for nonhearing clients but may be used for less verbal clients even with normal hearing. However, the items are highly abstract in nature, and the test is long and cumbersome.

The Illinois Test of Psycholinguistic Ability (McCarthy and Kirk, 1961) provides a basis of describing language function according to three dimensions derived from Osgood's (1957) language model: 1) channels of communication (auditory input, vocal output, and visual input, motor output); 2) levels of organization (automatic-sequential and representational); and 3) psycholinguistic process (decoding, association, encoding). Nine subtests tap these dimensions. However, the reliability of the subtests is low, and the test is useful only when specific educational programs exist with curricula based upon this model.

A variety of tests exist for evaluating perceptual-motor functioning (Frostig, 1966) but, here again, evaluation must feed into specific training programs to be useful, and the procedures are not typically used with adults in rehabilitation programs.

Testing for Organicity

Because of the tenacity of etiological systems of diagnosis in mental retardation, the diagnosis of organic brain damage is a frequent reason for referral to a psychologist.

Two broad approaches to this problem have been applied. The psychologist may use the same clinical signs as the medical practitioner in diagnosing organicity from behavioral signs of hyperactivity, motor problems, impulsivity, and poor attention span. Such cases are usually diagnosed as minimal brain damage, Strauss syndrome, or hyperkinetic child, terms used when the child appears to have at least normal intelligence. In this syndrome perceptual problems, communication deficits, dyslexia, or other specific learning disability and neurological evidence may or may not be exhibited. When intelligence scores fall within a mentally retarded range (IQ less than 70) these signs may be indicative of exogenous mental retardation.

The second approach to the diagnosis of organic impairment is by the use of psychological tests of perceptual, cognitive, or language functioning. A variety of psychological assessment procedures have been used for this purpose. Tests of organicity have their origin in the conceptual tests devised by Goldstein in assessing the psychological effects of traumatic war injuries during World War I (Goldstein and Scheerer, 1941). The tests are based on the assumption that there is a loss of capacity for abstract reasoning and rely heavily upon sorting procedures, such as the Color Form Sorting Test. Wechsler also concerned himself with this problem and suggested that organicity produces effects similar to those of senility. The Deterioration Index included in the scoring procedure of the original Wechsler Bellevue Scales diagnosed organicity on the basis of a ratio between tests of "old learning" such as Information and Vocabulary that allegedly "held" despite organic processes of deterioration, and tests of "new learning" that "didn't hold," i.e., reveal decrements as a result of organic damage. Wechsler also developed a memory scale for the same purpose (Wechsler, 1945).

Although the Deterioration Index has not withstood attempts at cross validation, the difference between Verbal IQ and Performance (perceptual-motor) IQ on the Wechsler tests is generally accepted by clinicians as indicative of organicity. This inference rests upon a presumed association of perceptual and perceptual-motor deficits and organicity. A variety of clinical tests and procedures have subsequently been applied to detect organic pathology. A few of the most commonly used are the Porteus Maze Tests (Porteus, 1959), reportedly sensitive to frontal lobe damage resulting in deficiencies in foresight and planning ability; the Bender Visual-Motor Gestalt Test (Bender, 1938; Koppitz, 1958; Pascal and Suttell, 1951), associated with disturbances in recognition or reproduction of complex figural configurations; and numerous physiological procedures such as phi phenomenon, spiral visual aftereffect, and reversible figures (Spivack and Levine, 1957). Even the Rorschach has been utilized for this purpose by a sign approach in which organicity is inferred from indices such as an unusually small record, delayed reaction time for responses, distortions in reality testing (% F−), the absence of human movement responses, and color naming (Piotrowski, 1936, 1937).

The Neuropsychology Laboratory of the Indiana University Medical Center has developed a psychological test battery for the evaluation of adults and children. This battery was designed to identify patterns of brain damage for individual diagnosis according to variation in type, lateralization or location, and duration of cerebral lesions. The tests were devised to measure pure motor functions, sensory-perceptual functions, and more complex psychomotor performances. The adult battery consists of Halstead's battery of neuropsychological tests (Halstead, 1947), the Wechsler-Bellevue Scale (Form I) (Wechsler, 1944), the Trail Making Test (Armitage, 1946; Reitan, 1955, 1958), a modification of the Halstead-Wepman aphasia screening test (Halstead and Wepman, 1949), various tests of sensory-perceptual functions, and the Minnesota Multiphasic Personality Inventory (Hathaway and McKinley, 1943). A considerable amount of research has provided validating data for individual tests in the battery using neurological reports or criteria. The inferences derived from the total test battery are difficult to validate because they apply to individual diagnosis rather than to group differences. In general, validity attempts have been positive, but test procedures and neurological procedures show a great deal of overlap so that a truly independent criterion does not exist. Furthermore, the generalization of results from one organic group to another is questionable. As Reed states:

> For some of the work, however, formal cross-validation studies have not been possible, this being particularly true of the work focusing specifically on how one interprets a set of psychological test results . . . The problem of cross-validating interpretive procedures is a particularly nasty one for two reasons: it is technically difficult to do so because only a very few investigators have had sufficient training and experience to enable them to make reasonable interpretations of the specific battery of tests that Reitan, et al. have employed. An additional dimension of nastiness is added by the fact that clinical interpretive procedures are probably extremely vulnerable to the biased characteristics of the sample on which the procedures were learned (Unpublished paper, p. 28).

Despite the promise of such research, numerous literature reviews have concluded that the validity of such procedures for detecting organicity has not been established (Maher, 1963; Sarason, 1949; Yates, 1954).

The case against using psychological tests for the diagnosis of organicity rests upon several arguments: first, the absence of a sound theoretical model of brain functioning and its relation to measured intelligence.

Numerous clinical observations suggest that structural damage to the brain need not be accompanied by lowered intellectual functioning. Furthermore, it is naïve to assume that structural damage to the brain will have uniform effects regardless of extent, locus, time of lesion, or individual differences between patients.

Second, criterion problems in validating tests of organicity: the unreliability of psychiatric diagnosis makes it difficult to find a stable criterion to use in validating psychological tests of organicity. When tests are validated against clear-cut cases of organicity, their use in diagnosing cases where organicity is subtle or minimal results in prediction errors.

Third, the general failure of validated tests of brain damage to withstand empirical tests of cross validation: one reason for this finding is a lack of specificity of organic signs. Many of the indices associated with organic conditions are also correlated with functional syndromes. Because of these problems, Yates (1954) lists several criteria that should be accepted as minimal standards in validating a test of organicity. 1) The external criteria should consist of several clinical groups: a brain damaged group, a group of patients diagnosed as functionally psychotic, and a group of normal controls; 2) the test should present data for adequate samples of the above mentioned groups; 3) the data should be presented in such a way as to enable the clinician to estimate the degree of possible error when assigning patients to one of these groups diagnostically (e.g., the probability of making false positive and false negative errors by using different cutting scores); 4) cross validation data should be available with new criterion groups; 5) the influence of various factors such as age, sex, and intelligence level should be controlled. Yates concludes that most tests purporting to be measures of brain damage do not meet these criteria; hence, their validity has not been evaluated.

One summary of this area (Maher, 1963) concludes that "attempts to apply tests, constructed within current concepts of intelligence, to the detection of biological phenomenon such as brain damage have been largely unsuccessful" (p. 250). Maher believes that the solution of clinical problems related to brain damage will best be furthered by the development of an experimental science of neuropsychiatry.

Because of these problems the construct of organic brain damage has little meaning for psychological or educational programs. Nevertheless, the psychologist is often called upon to make such a diagnosis, especially when supportive test results are required for funding the person to participate in special education or rehabilitation programs for the brain damaged. In these situations it is wise to gear testing toward the evaluation of perceptual, cognitive, or educational deficits, where they exist, that are often associated with organic dysfunctioning and to confine the evaluation to the description of the operational components of the syndrome without dealing with the knotty problems of predicting organicity.

Evaluating Social Functioning

The importance of evaluating social functioning, in addition to IQ level, in the diagnosis of mental retardation has created a need for valid measures of adaptive behavior. The Vineland Social Maturity Scale (Doll, 1965) has traditionally been used to assess the client's competence at performing according to expectations of performance for each chronological age level. A parent is usually used as the informant and the scale has been validated against the Stanford-Binet as a criterion measure. A social age, comparable to the mental age, and a social quotient, comparable to the IQ, are derived. Unfortunately, the scale is poorly suited to the evaluation of adults. The items themselves are far too few in number, and narrow in scope to allow meaningful discriminations between people.

The Adaptive Behavior Scale (Nihira et al., 1969) represents an attempt to correct this deficiency. The scale attempts to evaluate the coping behavior of the mental retardate in relation to the demands and requirements of his environment. The original scale was developed by Leland et al. (1967), and numerous item analysis and validity studies (Nihira and Shellhaas, 1970; Nihira, 1969; Foster and Nihira, 1969) have been conducted.

The classification system provided by the Adaptive Behavior Scale ranges from Level I, mild negative deviation from population norms, to Level V, the extreme lower limit of adaptive behavior. Part I of the Adaptive Behavior Scale is designed to measure the client's skills and abilities in the following behavior areas: independent functioning, physical development, economic activities, language development, number and time concepts, occupation (domestic), occupation (general), self-direction, responsibility, and socialization. Part II of the Scale is intended to measure behaviors considered unacceptable by those having daily contact with the retardate. The areas covered include: violent and destructive behavior, antisocial behavior, rebellious behavior, untrustworthy behavior, withdrawal, stereotyped behavior and odd mannerisms, inappropriate interpersonal manners, unacceptable vocal habits, peculiar or eccentric habits, sexually aberrant behavior, self-abusive behavior, hyperactive tendencies, and psychological disturbances.

The Adaptive Behavior Scale represents the most systematic attempt to develop a reliable instrument that will survey a comprehensive (though certainly not exhaustive) set of observable behavior significant for day-today functioning. However, as will be elaborated later, the assessment of adaptive behavior should not substitute for more traditional measures of emotional adjustment and personality.

Another approach to the assessment of social functioning concerns basic information and skills in handling everyday problem solving and decision making. While the Vineland and Adaptive Behavior Scales involve ratings by a knowledgeable informant, a more direct approach is to measure such skills directly. It is important to evaluate basic social skills such as social sight vocabulary, ability to tell time, monetary knowledge, and skills in using public transportation in programs preparing persons deficient in such skills by remedial adult education. A scale that shows promise for this purpose is the Fundamental Achievement Series (Bennett and Doppelt, 1968). This test is conveniently administered by cassette tape recorder, and it includes both verbal and numerical items in areas such as recognition of signs and common objects, understanding of transportation, menus, addresses and telephone numbers, comprehension and utilization of basic numerical concepts and relationships, understanding of numerical and monetary values, calendars, bills and checks, and telling time. Rosen and Hoffman (1974b) evaluated one hundred mentally retarded persons at a residential school and rehabilitation center, and found the Fundamental Achievement Series to be a reliable and useful diagnostic tool for the identification of specific social learning deficiencies, especially when used in conjunction with standard IQ and school achievement tests.

Emotional Functioning and Personality

It has been pointed out (Rosen and Kivitz, 1973) that normalization has been misinterpreted as a psychological rather than as a humanitarian principle and that adaptive behavior, while useful for identification of behavioral deficiencies requiring training or modification, is not a substitute for basic constructs of emotional health and adjustment. Adaptive behaviors do not represent dimensions of personality but of performance. Furthermore, they are neither positive in perspective, representing only minimal standards of functioning at each level, nor consistent with standards of adjustment typically applied to nonretarded populations.

Nor do orthodox psychoanalytic conceptions of development provide a useful model for studying personality in mental retardation. Structural models based upon psychosexual development, closely linked to concepts of fixation and regression to oral, anal, and phallic stages of development, seem to cling to outmoded views of the retarded as infantile, childlike, unsocialized, and amoral. There seems little utility in such an approach for the psychological evaluator concerned with assessment of competence in work or community living situations.

Attempting to define a model of emotional adjustment that is "beyond normalization," Rosen and Kivitz (1973) have specified seven dimensions along which the personal adjustment of the mentally retarded should be evaluated:

1. Self-concept: A recognition of one's learning problems and limitations along with a recognition that self-esteem need not be contingent upon learning deficits; the ability to set realistic goals and to realistically evaluate one's own capacity to achieve these goals.
2. Independence: An orientation to life in which there is acceptance of responsibility for one's own achievement. Rotter (1966) has termed this an internal locus of control, and the phenomenon has been studied in the retarded (Bialer, 1961; Cromwell, 1963; Shipe, 1971).
3. Reality testing: A perception of reality that is sufficient to allow awareness of behavior considered as the norm by society.
4. Emotional development: The ability to express appropriate affect when the situation demands, or to control affect when expression is inappropriate.
5. Goal-directed behavior: Demonstration of purposive striving toward some meaningful goal, such as an occupational choice. The ability to realistically visualize such a goal and to persevere in its pursuit.
6. Interpersonal relationships: The flexibility required for successful day-to-day interactions with people, including the ability to empathize with others and to express interest in their problems.
7. Sexual development: Possession of a sufficient degree of information and coping skills so as to perform adequately in both casual and intense sexual relationships with enjoyment and without anxiety or guilt.

This model is not intended to replace adaptive behavior in evaluation but to supplement it. These authors have found it to be a more meaningful conceptualization of personality of the mentally retarded than more traditional "dynamic" models based on levels of psychosexual development. The latter approach, unnecessarily pessimistic, makes little allowance for the possibility of improved adjustment.

Despite the need to evaluate the mentally retarded along dimensions relative to their emotional adjustment, few measures exist that the clinician may use confidently. Standardized, empirical tests of personality, such as the Minnesota Multiphasic Personality Inventory (MMPI) (Hathaway and McKinley, 1943), require a degree of reading comprehension and capacity for self-report that is usually far beyond the ability of the mentally retarded client. Projective tests of personality, such as the Rorschach and Thematic Apperception Test, are highly verbal in nature. It is likely that the major component of response variance obtained with the use of such procedures will be a function of verbal or intellectual competence, rather than of personality factors.

An alternative approach is to develop assessment measures reflecting empirical evidence about the behaviors of the retarded that is most pertinent to the daily functioning and coping of this population. Clark, Kivitz, and Rosen (1968) have been conducting a long-term longitudinal investigation of a large group of mental retardates discharged from Elwyn Institute over the past 10 years, and they have published numerous studies dealing with areas such as marriage, employment satisfaction, sociosexual problems, and other criteria of community functioning. Attempts to predict such functioning from standard psychometric tests have been unfruitful. Rosen, Floor, and Baxter (1971) have suggested that the development of such prognostic procedures should sample areas of personality where there is pre-established construct validity of the measures chosen and meaningful criteria of community functioning. For example, if exploitation is a phenomenon frequently occurring to the mentally retarded in the community, its relation to personality variables such as helplessness and acquiescence should be determined. Once construct validity for relevant personality dimensions in the retarded is established, it will be possible to construct reliable and valid measurement procedures.

Reasoning from studies of mentally retarded adults living in the community, Rosen, Floor, and Baxter (1971) speculated about five components of the "institutional personality." These included helpless and dependent behaviors, over-compliance or acquiescence, inadequate self-concept and related motivational deficits, inappropriate behavior, and sociosexual inadequacies.

Floor and Rosen (1975) have operationally defined helplessness as a seeming inability to deal with emergency situations or reversals and an absence of independent problem solving behavior. They present normative data for several situational tests of helplessness with mentally retarded and control populations.

Acquiescence to institutional rules, regulations, and authority may make for good institutional residents but may interfere with self-assertion and independent decision making in the community. It has been suggested that acquiescence as a personality trait is directly related to susceptibility to exploitation. Rosen, Floor, and Zisfein (1975) have investigated acquiescence as a personality measure with the mentally handicapped.

Inappropriate and bizarre behaviors may be largely institutional in nature. An inventory for identifying students demonstrating such behaviors as over-friendliness, belligerence, and childishness has been described by Rosen and Hoffman (1974a).

One variable that is central to all aspects of behavior of the mentally retarded is self-concept. Epstein (1973) has pointed out that, while disagreement about the self-concept as an explanatory construct still exists, " ... there can be no argument but that the subjective feeling state of having a self is an important empirical phenomenon that warrants study in its own right" (p. 405). The relevance of self-concept to performance decrements in mentally retarded populations has been well recognized (Cromwell, 1963; Rosen et al., 1966; Rosen et al., 1971; Zigler, 1966) and numerous investigations have studied the effects of subjective awareness of capabilities, expectancies for success, internalized responsibility for behavior, and other indices of self-perception and self-evaluation. Most models of psychotherapy and rehabilitation developed for retarded populations (Bialer, 1967; Hannon, 1968; Sternlicht, 1966) have alluded to changes in self-concept as desirable outcome criteria.

Despite the importance of self-concept as a personality dimension, there has been little application of self-concept measures as clinical tools. Zisfein and Rosen (1974) report the clinical use of four self-concept measures with a retarded population: 1) a general self-evaluation scale; 2) a level of aspiration procedure; 3) a risk-taking choice; and 4) a self-comparison scale in which the subject is asked to compare himself with "other people." Classification of subjects according to levels of self-concept determined by laboratory procedures appeared promising in sorting subjects in a manner similar to that accomplished using projective testing procedures.

The area of personality evaluation of the retarded is one of great need but little progress. There is still a large gap between personality research and available personality measures with proven clinical utility. Future development of personality tests for the retarded will need to draw heavily from research investigations that provide construct validation of personality dimensions that can be reliably assessed from overt behavior.

Academic Level

Standardized measures of academic achievement typically used with normal intelligence populations also may be used with the mentally retarded. The Wide Range Achievement Test (Jastak and Jastak, 1965) is a quick screening procedure to evaluate spelling, arithmetic skills, and work recognition. More thorough procedures such as the Metropolitan Achievement Tests (Hildreth et al., 1948), providing more specific information, also may be utilized. However, while these tests were developed to be administered in a group setting, individual administration with the mentally handicapped client is strongly advised. A new test has been designed specifically for the mentally handicapped and reduces the necessity for detailed and complicated instructions. The Peabody Individual Achievement Test (Dunn and Markwardt, 1970) appears to be a promising procedure for the mentally retarded. Wilson and Spangler (1974) have recently reported its reliability for a multihandicapped population.

Vocational Competence

In evaluating the mentally retarded client for rehabilitation planning it is usually desirable to assess vocational competence and potential. Because there is little correspondence between intellectual functioning and the ability to function within a work setting, separate estimates of vocational competence should be included in the evaluation. Two broad levels of vocational functioning can be specified. At the highest level the client is capable of successful performance at a competitive work situation. At this level, occupational skills are usually in unskilled or semiskilled operations such as unskilled factory work or service occupations (e.g., janitorial service, kitchen worker, hospital orderly, or nurses' aide). In such settings, the client must be able to function with minimal supervision. A second level of functioning requires the ability to perform in a sheltered work situation. The sheltered contract workshop provides meaningful work experiences for many mentally retarded persons. In such settings, there is a great deal of supervision, and demands made upon the client are below those in competitive employment. The individual client must be capable of performing repetitive, packaging, and subassembly tasks. He may or may not be required to be capable of transporting himself to and from the workshop, depending upon the location of the shop.

In making vocational evaluations, a distinction is usually drawn between the client's present level of vocational functioning and his potential after receiving appropriate training. A number of evaluation scales are available to be completed by the immediate work supervisor or vocational counselor acquainted with the client's day-to-day functioning. The Work Evaluation Scale (Taylor, 1961) was developed by Goodwill Industries of Tacoma, Washington. It consists of a short rating form used in describing on-the-job behavior of handicapped persons. Forty-four statements can be answered "True," "False," or "Don't know" by the work supervisor. A total work competence score is derived, as well as seven subscales of Work Enthusiasm, Work Adequacy, Supervision Needed, Rebellious Attitude, Personal and Social Difficulties, Overt Anxiety and Confusion, and Medical Problems. It is recommended that scores be derived from the averages of ratings given the client by four work supervisors. Under these conditions Taylor reports the reliability of the total score to be 0.82.

The Scale of Employability for Handicapped Persons (Gellman, 1960) was developed at the Jewish Vocational Service of Chicago, to predict successful and unsuccessful vocational outcome. The rating procedure consists of three separate scales: 1) a Counseling Scale completed by a vocational counselor and consisting of items relating to past performance and the ability of the client to meet employer expectations; 2) a Psychology Scale completed by the psychologist after administration of the psychological test battery and reflecting behavior in the test situation; 3) a Workshop Scale completed by vocational counselors acting as foremen in a rehabilitation workshop program.

The three scales may be treated independently. Inter-rater reliability for the Workshop Scale was reported as 0.52, while predictive validities with outcome criteria were statistically significant but extremely low at two different agencies (r = 0.23 and 0.43, respectively).

Both the Taylor and the Gellman Scales are long and cumbersome to administer. A study at Elwyn (Rosen et al., 1970b) found that a simple Global Rating Scale utilizing one question, "How do you evaluate the client's chances to live and work in the community?" was as reliable and valid a predictor as the longer, multidimensional scales. However, earlier validities obtained with the scale were not replicated in a cross validation (Rosen et al., 1972).

The Minnesota Scales of Employment Satisfaction (Carlson et al., 1962) is the most useful procedure available for measuring work satisfaction. The Scales, which were derived from a cluster analysis of all the items sampled, include general job satisfaction and satisfaction with working conditions, supervision, compensation, and coworkers. An additional scale rates sensitivity of social status of the job. The Scale provides published norms for eight different comparison groups consisting of a total of 1,168 skilled and unskilled, blue and white collar, handicapped and nonhandicapped persons. Clark, Kivitz, and Rosen (1968) used the Minnesota Scales of Employment Satisfaction with a mentally retarded population and found it to be a useful and reliable procedure, provided the scale was individually administered and the more difficult questions were paraphrased when necessary (Rosen et al., 1970a).

It is customary in a vocational evaluation to use well accepted tests of perceptual-motor and manual dexterity because of their alleged relation to many job activities, their historical association with vocational counseling, and their face validity for assessing work performance. The tests that are most commonly employed include the Purdue Pegboard (Tiffin, 1948), the Minnesota Rate of Manipulation Test (Ziegler, 1949), the Bender Visual-Motor Gestalt Test (1938), the O'Connor Finger Dexterity

Test (1938), and numerous others. The validity of these procedures for predicting vocational success either during training or after completion of training, is poorly established. Their use for vocational prediction, in the absence of such necessary validating data, is discouraged. This is not to deny the importance of a criterion analysis of necessary job behaviors and the use of procedures that sample elements of this criterion. It is likely that for some work tasks, traditional vocational tests are sufficiently similar to the job to warrant their inclusion in the test battery. The Jewish Employment and Vocational Service of Philadelphia (Work Samples, 1968) has pioneered in the development of work samples consisting of the same occupational skills for which the client is being trained. However, the uncritical use of even work samples, except for predicting specific success at vocational tasks, is unwarranted without established validation procedures. At Elwyn Institute it has been found that the best prediction of work competence derives from training and tryout in the work situation itself.

Evaluation of Community Functioning

The importance of deriving meaningful measures of community functioning of the mentally retarded is underscored by the recent trend in rehabilitation philosophy placing emphasis upon training and discharge for institutions. Numerous follow-up studies have been conducted to study the community adjustment of mentally retarded persons first identified in public schools or within institutions. In general, these results have been positive, indicating that the majority of mentally retarded persons between and IQs of 50 and 80 are capable of independently living and working in the community. Dating from the prototype report of Fernald (1919), through more recent studies of Fairbanks (1933), Baller (1936), Charles (1953), Dinger (1961), Kennedy (1966), and Miller (1965), the investigators have been consistent in revealing satisfactory adjustment of many previously institutionalized persons or those first identified in the public schools.

Masland, Sarason, and Gladwin (1958) have pointed out that the majority of people in those studies have made an adequate social adjustment, most being self-supporting. Criteria for evaluation have consisted of the more obvious indices of community functioning, including such variables as welfare assistance, service in the armed forces, self-support, competitive or sheltered employment, savings accounts, voting, occupational level, periods of unemployment, social activities, civic and recreational activities, marriage, divorce, having children, job tenure, economic status, housing, antisocial behavior, and work performance. This aspect of evaluation of the retarded is extremely important, and should not be overlooked. Available scales are published in most of the follow-up studies reported. The reader is referred particularly in the studies of Baller (1936), Charles (1953), and Kennedy (1966) for this purpose.

Clark, Kivitz, and Rosen (1968) have been conducting a long-term longitudinal investigation of a large group of mental retardates discharged from Elwyn Institute over the past 10 years and have published numerous studies dealing with employment satisfaction, sociosexual problems, and exploitation.

Prediction of Community Functioning

Follow-up studies mentioned previously leave little doubt that there is a large proportion of the population classified as mentally retarded who are capable, from a social viewpoint, of adequately coping with society's demands during their adult years. This being the case, it is important to be able to specify the probability of such an outcome associated with various subgroups, treatments, or personal characteristics of the client. Because the value of any psychological test procedure necessarily rests upon its predictive validity for relevant criteria, the issue is a crucial one in performing psychological evaluation. The point has been put succinctly by Heber (1959): "There is a great need for research directed toward a determination of the significant variables related to the ultimate personal, social, and vocational adjustment of the mentally retarded. Then, and only then, will we be in a position to carry out research evaluations of various kinds of educational treatments designed to accomplish favorable modifications on these significant variables" (p. 1,018).

Windle (1962) has reviewed the literature dealing with prognostic studies up to 1962. Reviews have also been supplied by Eagle (1967), Goldstein (1964), and Tizard (1958). The conclusions of these authors are extensive, and the reader is referred to them for a more thorough discussion. In general, there is agreement that research studies have been poorly designed, have not used comparable criterion measures, and thus results have been contradictory. Few variables have been isolated that bear known relationships to meaningful criteria of functioning in the community. Many of the predictive variables that have been identified relate to the likelihood of release but bear no relationship to adjustment after discharge from an institution, thus reflecting institutional policy rather than meaningful factors affecting behavior. Windle concludes that there is no meaningful relationship between diagnosis (e.g., endogenous versus exogenous) and outcome. Age at discharge may have a curvilinear relation to outcome with greater likelihood of success accruing from older clients up until some limit. Overall IQ and a superiority of Performance IQ over Verbal IQ seem to relate to probability of discharge but are not prognostic for adjustment after release. No general conclusions may be drawn concerning personality variables and later adjustment.

Rosen et al. (1970b) reported a group of modest correlations between perceptual-motor scores and work adjustment during institutional training programs and later criteria of community functioning. However, none of these relationships withstood the scrutiny of cross validation (Rosen, Floor, and Baxter, 1972).

Thus, despite the vital need for evaluative procedures that will predict community functioning, there is little justification for the assumption that available tests of client abilities and disabilities have proven prognostic relationships with meaningful criteria of community functioning of the mentally retarded client. Rosen, Floor, and Baxter (1971) have suggested that the development of such procedures should sample areas of personality where there is pre-established construct validity of the measures chosen and meaningful criteria of community functioning. For example, if exploitation is a phenomenon occurring frequently to the mentally retarded in the community, its relationship to personality variables such as helplessness and acquiescence should be determined. Once construct validity for relevant personality dimensions in the retarded is established, it will be possible to construct reliable and valid measurement procedures.

FUTURE TRENDS

Changing needs in the field of rehabilitation have greatly strained existing models and the practice of psychological evaluation. In previous decades psychologists were content to classify levels of mental retardation. There was little concern about prediction. IQs were considered stable, and mental retardation irreversible.

As concepts about the retarded become more optimistic, demand increases for accurate estimates of capabilities (not deficits) and potential for training. Although psychological procedures have been placed under general attack from many quarters, the most useful criticism has been leveled by psychologists themselves. McClelland (1973) has urged that competence, not capacity, be tested. Sidman and Stoddard (1966) have pointed out that there exists no valid measure for predicting the rate of learning other than an actual teaching program. Lindsley (1970) has indicated that children are not mentally retarded but that their behavior in average environments may be retarded. Lindsley concentrates on exceptionalizing the circumstances under which children function so as to increase the frequency of normal behavior.

Bricker (1970), Throne (1970), and others have called for a diagnostic strategy based upon treatment, and the choice of categories of evaluation criteria that derive meaning only from the specific behavioral objectives to be achieved by treatment. Bricker (1970) writes: " . . . The primary method for studying and understanding developmental retardation is to develop a process to teach such children or adults to behave 'normally' " (p. 16). ". . . Only the failure of a perfectly valid, perfectly reliable, perfectly efficient program of training will convince me that the identification of the deficit is sufficient reason to stop trying to educate the child. Somehow, I cannot feel that we have reached perfection in the development of training programs" (p. 20).

So let it be, in evaluating the mentally retarded adult for rehabilitation goals. As valid programs are developed for teaching independence, psychologists will become increasingly disenchanted with traditional classification and diagnostic goals and will find methods for evaluation in terms of realistic training programs and realistic vocational and social opportunities for the mentally retarded. Behavioral measurement should be increasingly relied upon for evaluating areas requiring modification and the results of treatment. Competency tests for basic vocational and social learning areas will replace traditional IQ determinations and tests of vocational "potential." Hopefully, expertly sequenced training-evaluation programs will be developed in all areas of personality, emotional, and social functioning according to this model. The role of psychological evaluator, in the traditional static sense, will be replaced by that of the diagnostician-programmer.

REFERENCES

Armitage, S. G. 1946. An analysis of certain psychological tests used for the evaluation of brain injury. Psych. Mono. 60:No. 1 (Whole No. 277).
Baller, W. R. 1936. A study of the present social status of a group of adults who, when they were in elementary schools, were classified as mentally deficient. Gen. Psych. Mono. 18:165–244.
Bandura, A. 1969. Principles of Behavior Modification. Holt, Rinehart and Winston, New York.
Bayley, N. 1949. Consistency and variability in the growth of intelligence from birth to eighteen years. J. Gen. Psych. 75:165–196.
Bayley, N. 1955. On the growth of intelligence. Amer. Psych. 10:805–818.
Bayley, N. 1968. Behavioral correlates of mental growth. Amer. Psych. 23:1–17.
Bender, L. 1938. A Visual-Motor Gestalt Test and Its Clinical Use. American Orthopsychiatric Association Research Monograph, No. 3.
Bennett, G. K., and J. E. Doppelt. 1968. Fundamental Achievement Series. Psychological Corp., New York.

Bensberg, G. J., C. N. Colwell, and R. H. Cossell. 1965. Teaching the profoundly retarded self-help activities by behavior shaping techniques. Amer. J. Ment. Defic. 69:674–679.

Benton, E. L. 1964. Psychological evaluation and differential diagnosis. In H. A. Stevens and R. Heber (eds.), Mental Retardation: A Review of Research. University of Chicago Press, Chicago.

Bialer, I. 1961. Conceptualization of success and failure in mentally retarded and normal children. J. Personal. 29:303–320.

Bialer, I. 1967. Psychotherapy and other adjustment techniques with the mentally retarded. In A. A. Baumeister (ed.), Mental Retardation: Appraisal, Education, and Rehabilitation. Aldine, Chicago.

Bijou, S. W. 1963. Theory and research in mental (developmental) retardation. Psych. Rec. 13:95–110.

Birnbrauer, J. S., M. M. Wolf, J. D. Kidder, and C. E. Tague. 1965. Classroom behavior of retarded pupils with token reinforcement. J. Exper. Child Psych. 2:219–235.

Blackwood, R. O. 1962. Operant Conditioning as a Method of Training the Mentally Retarded. Doctoral dissertation, Ohio State University. University Microfilms, Ann Arbor, Mich.

Bricker, W. A. 1970. Identifying and modifying behavioral deficits. Amer. J. Ment. Defic. 75:16–21.

Bricker, W. A., and D. D. Bricker. 1970. A program of language training for the severely language handicapped child. Except. Children 37:101–111.

Butterfield, E. C. 1967. The role of environmental factors in the treatment of institutionalized mental retardates. In A. A. Baumeister (ed.), Mental Retardation: Appraisal, Education, and Rehabilitation. Aldine, Chicago.

Carlson, R. E., R. V. Davis, G. W. England, and L. H. Lofquist. 1962. The measurement of employment satisfaction. Minnesota Studies in Vocational Rehabilitation, XIII. Bulletin No. 35. University of Minnesota, Minneapolis.

Cattell, J. M. 1948. Mental tests and measurements. In W. Dennis (ed.), Readings in the History of Psychology, pp. 347–354. Appleton-Century-Crofts, New York.

Cattell, R. B. 1957. Personality and Motivation Structure and Measurement. Harcourt, Brace, and World, New York.

Charles, D. C. 1953. Ability and accomplishment of persons earlier judged mentally deficient. Genet. Psych. Mono. 47:3–71.

Clark, G. R., M. S. Kivitz, and M. Rosen. 1968. A Transitional Program for Institutionalized Adult Retarded. Vocational Rehabilitation Administration, Project No. RD-1275P. Department of Health, Education and Welfare, Washington, D.C.

Clarke, A. D. B., and A. M. Clarke. 1954. Cognitive changes in the feebleminded. Brit. J. Psych. 45:173–179.

Cohen, J. 1957. A factor analytically based rationale for the WAIS. J. Consult. Psych. 21:451–457.

Cromwell, R. L. 1963. A social learning approach to mental retardation. In N. R. Ellis (ed.), Handbook of Mental Deficiency, pp. 134–158. McGraw-Hill, New York.

Dayan, M. 1964. Toilet training retarded children in a state residential institution. Ment. Retard. 2:116–117.

Diggory, J. C. 1966. A Study of Self-Evaluation. Wiley, New York.

Dinger, J. C. 1961. Post-school adjustment of former educable retarded pupils. Except. Children 27:353–360.

Doll, E. 1965. Vineland Social Maturity Scale. Condensed Manual of Directions. American Guidance Service, Circle Pines, Minn.

Dugdale, R. L. 1900. The Jukes: A Study in Crime, Pauperism, Disease and Heredity. 6th Ed. Putnam, New York.

Dunn, L. M., and F. C. Markwardt. 1970. Peabody Individual Achievement Test: Manual. American Guidance Service, Circle Pines, Minn.

Eagle, E. 1967. Prognosis and outcome of community placement of institutionalized retardates. Amer. J. Ment. Defic. 72:232–243.

Ellis, N. R. 1963. Toilet training the severely defective patient: An S-R reinforcement analysis. Amer. J. Ment. Defic. 68:98–103.

Epstein, E. 1973. The self-concept revisited: Or a theory of a theory. Amer. Psych. 28:404–416.

Eysenck, H. J. 1960. The Structure of Human Personality. Methuen, London.

Fairbanks, R. 1933. The subnormal child: Seventeen years after. Ment. Hygiene 17:177–208.

Fernald, W. E. 1919. After-care study of the patients discharged from Waverly for a period of twenty-five years. Ungraded 5:25–31.

Floor, L., and M. Rosen. 1975. Investigating the phenomenon of helplessness in the mentally subnormal. Amer. J. Ment. Defic. 79:565–572.

Foster, R., and K. Nihira. 1969. Adaptive behavior as a measure of psychiatric impairment. Amer. J. Ment. Defic. 74:401–404.

Frostig, M. 1966. Administration and Scoring Manual. Developmental Test of Visual Perception. Consulting Psychologists Press, Palo Alto.

Gellman, W. 1960. A Scale of Employability for Handicapped Persons. Office of Vocational Rehabilitation, Project No. 64-57. Jewish Employment and Vocational Service, Chicago.

Giradeau, F. L., and J. E. Spradlin. 1964. Token rewards in a cottage program. Ment. Retard. 2:345–351.

Goddard, H. H. 1914. The Kallikak Family: A Study in the Heredity of Feeblemindedness. Macmillan, New York.

Goldstein, K., and M. Scheerer. 1941. Abstract and concrete behavior: An exploratory study with special tests. 53, Psych. Mono. (Whole No. 2).

Goldstein, M. 1964. Social and occupational adjustment. In H. A. Stevens and R. Heber (eds.), Mental Retardation: A Review of Research. University of Chicago Press, Chicago.

Grossman, H. J., ed. 1973. Manual on Terminology and Classification in Mental Retardation. American Association on Mental Deficiency, Washington, D.C.

Guilford, J. P. 1959. Three faces of intellect. Amer. Psych. 14:469–479.

Guilford, J. P. 1967. The Nature of Human Intelligence. McGraw-Hill, New York.

Halstead, W. C. 1947. Brain and Intelligence. University of Chicago Press, Chicago.

Halstead, W. C., and J. M. Wepman. 1949. The Halstead-Wepman aphasia screening test. J. Speech Hearing Disord. 14:9—15.

Hannon, R. W. 1968. A program for developing self-concept in retarded children. Ment. Retard. 6:33—37.

Hathaway, S. R., and J. C. McKinley. 1943. Manual for the Minnesota Multiphasic Personality Inventory. University of Minnesota Press, Minneapolis.

Heber, R. 1957. Expectancy and Expectancy Changes in Normal and Mentally Retarded Boys. University Microfilms, Ann Arbor, Mich.

Heber, R. 1959. Promising areas for psychological research in mental retardation. Amer. J. Ment. Defic. 63:1014—1019.

Heber, R., R. Dever, and J. Conry. 1968. The influence of environmental and genetic variables on intellectual development. In H. J. Prehm, L. A. Hamerlynch, and J. E. Crosson (eds.), Behavioral Research in Mental Retardation, pp. 1—23. University of Oregon Press, Eugene.

Hildreth, G. H., R. D. Allen, H. H. Bixler, W. L. Connor, and F. B. Graham. 1948. Metropolitan Achievement Tests: Manual for Interpretating. World Book Company, Yonkers-on-Hudson, N. Y.

Hundziak, M., R. A. Maurer, and L. S. Watson. 1965. Operant conditioning in toilet training for severely mentally retarded boys. Amer. J. Ment. Defic. 70:120—124.

Jastak, J. F., and S. R. Jastak. 1965. The Wide Range Achievement Test. Guidance Associates, Wilmington, Dela.

Jensen, A. R. 1969. How much can we boost IQ and scholastic achievement? Harvard Ed. Rev. 39:1—123.

Joint Commission on Accreditation of Hospitals. 1971. Standards for Residential Facilities for the Mentally Retarded. JCAH, Chicago.

Kennedy, R. J. R. 1966. A Connecticut Community Revisited: A Study of the Social Adjustment of a Group of Mentally Deficient Adults in 1948 and 1960. Project No. 655, Office of Vocational Rehabilitation, U.S. Department of Health, Education and Welfare, Washington, D.C.

Koppitz, E. 1958. The Bender-Gestalt Test and learning disturbances in young children. J. Clin. Psych. 14:292—295.

Kraepelin, E. 1925. Dementia Praecox and Paraphrenia. Translated from Eighth German Edition. Livingston, Edinburgh.

Leiter, R. G. 1952. Part II of the Manual of the 1948 Revision of the Leiter International Performance Scale. Psychological Service Center Press, Washington, D.C. (Test now published by C. H. Stoelting Co.)

Leland, H., M. Shellhaas, K. Nihara, and R. Foster. 1967. Adaptive behavior: A new dimension in the classification of the mentally retarded. Ment. Retard. Abstr. 4:359—387.

Lindsley, O. R. 1970. Direct measurement and prosthesis of retarded behavior. In C. A. Fargo, C. Behrns, and P. A. Nolen (eds.), Behavior Modification in the Classroom. Wadsworth, Belmont, Calif.

Lovaas, O. I., J. P. Berberich, B. F. Perloff, and B. Schaeffer. 1966. Acquisition of imitative speech by schizophrenic children. Science 161:705—707.

Maher, B. M. 1963. Intelligence and brain damage. In N. R. Ellis (ed.), Handbook of Mental Deficiency, pp. 224—252. McGraw-Hill, New York.

Masland, R. L., S. B. Sarason, and T. Gladwin. 1958. Mental Subnormality: Biological, Psychological and Cultural Factors. Basic Books, New York.

McCarthy, J. J., and S. Kirk. 1961. Illinois Test of Psycholinguistic Abilities: Experimental Edition. Institute for Research on Exceptional Children, University of Illinois, Urbana.

McClelland, D. C. 1973. Testing for competence rather than for "intelligence." Amer. Psych. 28:1–14.

McNemar, Q. 1957. On WAIS difference scores. J. Consult. Psych. 21:239–240.

Meehl, P. E. 1954. Clinical vs. Statistical Prediction. University of Minnesota Press, Minneapolis.

Meehl, P. E. 1956. Wanted—a good cookbook. Amer. Psych. 11:263–272.

Miller, E. L. 1965. Ability and social adjustment at midlife of persons earlier judged mentally deficient. Genet. Psych. Mono. 72:139–198.

Murray, H. A. 1938. Explorations in Personality. Oxford University Press, New York.

Nihira, K. 1969. Factorial dimensions of adaptive behavior in mentally retarded children and adolescents. Amer. J. Ment. Defic. 74:130–141.

Nihira, K., R. Foster, M. Shellhaas, and H. Leland. 1969. Adaptive Behavior Scales. American Association on Mental Deficiency, Washington, D.C.

Nihira, K., and M. Shellhaas. 1970. Study of adaptive behavior: Its rationale, method and implication in rehabilitation programs. Ment. Retard. 8:11–16.

Nirje, B. 1969. The normalization principle and its human management implications. In R. B. Kugel and W. Wolfensberger (eds.), Changing Patterns in Residential Services for the Mentally Retarded, pp. 179–195. President's Committee on Mental Retardation, Washington, D.C.

O'Connor, J. 1938. Administration and Norms for the Finger Dexterity Test. Tech. Rep. Human Engineering Lab, No. 16. (Test now published by C. H. Stoelting Co.)

Osgood, C. E. 1957. Motivational dynamics of language behavior. Nebraska Symposium on Motivation. University of Nebraska Press, Lincoln.

Pascal, G. R., and B. J. Suttell. 1951. The Bender Gestalt Test. Grune & Stratton, New York.

Piotrowski, Z. A. 1936. Organic lesions. Rorschach Research Exchange 1(2):23–39.

Piotrowski, Z. A. 1937. The Rorschach ink-blot method in organic disturbances of the central nervous system. J. Nervous Ment. Dis. 86:527–535.

Porteus, S. D. 1959. The Maze Test and Clinical Psychology. Pacific Books, Palo Alto.

Rappaport, D., M. Gill, and R. Schaefer. 1945. Diagnostic Psychological Testing. (2 vols.) Year Book Publishers, Chicago.

Reed, H. B. C. Biological intelligence. Unpublished paper based on a research program supported in part by grants NB 01468, NB 05211, and CD 00015 from the Public Health Service to Ralph M. Reitan.

Reitan, R. M. 1955. The relation of the Trail Making Test to organic brain damage. J. Consult. Psych. 19:393–394.

Reitan, R. M. 1958. The validity of the Trail Making Test as an indicator of organic brain damage. Percept. Motor Skills 8:271–276.

Renner, K. E. 1962. Comment on: "Must all tests be valid?" Amer. Psych. 17:507–508.

Roos, P. Development of an intensive habit-training unit at Austin State School. Ment. Retard. 3:12–15.

Rorschach, H. 1942. Psychodiagnostics. Verlag Hans Huber, Berne.

Rosen, M., J. C. Diggory, L. Floor, and M. Nowakiwska 1971. Self-evaluation, expectancy and performance in the mentally subnormal. J. Ment. Defic. Res. 15:81–95.

Rosen, M., J. C. Diggory, and B. E. Werlinsky. 1966. Goal-setting and expectancy of success in institutionalized and noninstitutionalized mental subnormals. Amer. J. Ment. Defic. 71:249–255.

Rosen, M., L. Floor, and D. Baxter. 1971. The institutional personality. Brit. J. Ment. Subnorm. 17(Part 2):1–8.

Rosen, M., L. Floor, and D. Baxter. 1972. Prediction of community adjustment: A failure at cross-validation. Amer. J. Ment. Defic. 77:111–112.

Rosen, M., L. Floor, and L. Zisfein. 1974. Investigating the phenomenon of acquiescence in the mentally handicapped: I. Theoretical model, test development and normative data. Brit. J. Ment. Subnorm. 20(Part 2, No. 39):58–68.

Rosen, M., L. Floor, and L. Zisfein. 1975. Investigating the phenomenon of acquiescence in the mentally handicapped: II. Situational determinants. Brit. J. Ment. Subnorm. 21(Part 1, No. 40):6–9.

Rosen, M., R. Halenda, M. Nowakiwska, and L. Floor. 1970. Employment satisfaction of previously institutionalized mentally subnormal workers. Ment. Retard. 8:35–40.

Rosen, M., and M. Hoffman. 1974a. An inventory of inappropriate behavior. Train. School Bull. 71:179–187.

Rosen, M., and M. Hoffman. 1974b. Use of the Fundamental Achievement Series with a mentally retarded population. J. Spec. Ed. Ment. Ret. 11(2):87–93.

Rosen, M., and M. S. Kivitz. 1973. Beyond normalization: Psychological adjustment. Brit. J. Ment. Subnorm. 19(37):64–70.

Rosen, M., M. S. Kivitz, G. R. Clark, and L. Floor. 1970b. Prediction of post-institutional adjustment of mentally retarded adults. Amer. J. Ment. Defic. 74:726–734.

Rosen, M., L. Stallings, L. Floor, and M. Nowakiwska. 1968. Reliability and stability of Wechsler IQ scores for institutionalized mental subnormals. Amer. J. Ment. Defic. 73:218–225.

Rosenthal, R., and L. Jacobson. 1968. Pygmalion in the Classroom: Teacher Expectation and Pupils' Intellectual Development. Holt, Rinehart and Winston, New York.

Rotter, J. B. 1966. Generalized expectancies for internal versus external control of reinforcement. Psych. Mono.: Gen. Appl. 80:1.

Sarason, S. B. 1949. Psychological Problems in Mental Deficiency. Harper & Row, New York.

Shipe, D. 1971. Impulsivity and locus of control as predictors of achievement and adjustment in mentally retarded and borderline youth. Amer. J. Ment. Defic. 76:12—22.

Sidman, M., and L. T. Stoddard. 1966. Programming perception and learning for retarded children. *In* N. R. Ellis (ed.), International Review of Research in Mental Retardation, pp. 152—208. Academic Press, New York.

Skeels, H. M. 1941. A study of the effects of differential stimulation on mentally retarded children: A follow-up report. Amer. J. Ment. Defic. 46:340—350.

Skeels, H. M., and H. B. Dye. 1939. A study of the effects of differential stimulation on mentally retarded children. Proc. Amer. Assoc. Ment. Defic. 44:114—136.

Spivack, G., and M. Levine. 1957. The spiral after effect and reversible figures as measures of brain damage and memory. J. Personal. 25:211—227.

Sternlicht, M. 1966. Psychotherapeutic procedures with the retarded. *In* N. R. Ellis (ed.), International Review of Research in Mental Retardation. Vol. 2, pp. 279—354. Academic Press, New York.

Szasz, T. S. 1960. The myth of mental illness. Amer. Psych. 15:113—118.

Taylor, J. B. 1961. The Prediction of Rehabilitation Potential Among the Mentally Retarded. Office of Vocational Rehabilitation, Project No. RD-603. Goodwill Industries, Tacoma, Wash.

Throne, J. M. 1970. A radical behaviorist approach to diagnosis in mental retardation. Ment. Retard. 8:2—5.

Thurstone, L. L. 1938. Primary mental abilities. Psychomet. Mono. No. 1.

Tiffin, J. 1948. Examiner Manual for the Purdue Pegboard. Science Research Associates, Chicago.

Tizard, J. 1958. Longitudinal and follow-up studies. *In* A. Clarke and A. D. B. Clarke (eds.), Mental Deficiency: The Changing Outlook, pp. 422—449. Methuen, London.

Tredgold, R. F., and K. Soddy. 1956. A Textbook of Mental Deficiency. Williams & Wilkins, Baltimore.

Ullman, L. P., and L. Krasner. 1966. Case Studies in Behavior Modification. Holt, Rinehart, and Winston, New York.

Watson, L. S. 1967. Application of operant conditioning techniques to institutionalized severely and profoundly retarded children. Ment. Retard. Abstr. 4:1—18.

Wechsler, D. 1944. The Measurement of Adult Intelligence. Williams & Wilkins, Baltimore.

Wechsler, D. 1945. A standardized memory scale for clinical use. J. Psych. 19:87—95.

Wechsler, D. 1955. Manual for the Wechsler Adult Intelligence Scale. Psychological Corp., New York.

Wilson, J. D., and P. F. Spangler. 1974. The Peabody Individual Achievement Test as a clinical tool. J. Learn. Disab. 7(6):384—387.

Windle, C. 1962. Prognosis of mental subnormals. Amer. J. Ment. Defic. 66(Mono. Suppl. 5).

Work Samples Jewish Employment and Vocational Service, Philadelphia, Pa. 1968. Final Report. Experimental and demonstration project. Contract No. 82-40-67-40. Manpower Administration, U.S. Department of Labor, Washington, D.C.

Yates, A. J. 1954. The validity of some psychological tests of brain damage. Psych. Bull. 51:359–379.

Ziegler, W. A. 1949. Minnesota Rate of Manipulation Test: Manual. Educational Test Bureau, Minneapolis.

Zigler, E. 1966. Motivational determinants in the performance of retarded children. Amer. J. Orthopsych. 36:848–856.

Zigler, E. 1967. Familial mental retardation: A continuing dilemma. Science 155:292–298.

Zigler, E., and L. Phillips. 1961. Psychiatric diagnosis: A critique. J. Abnorm. Soc. Psych. 63:607–618.

Zisfein, L., and M. Rosen. 1974. Self-concept and mental retardation: Theory, measurement, and clinical utility. Ment. Retard. 12(4):15–19.

17 | Assessment of Counselor Performance

STANFORD E. RUBIN and KENNETH W. REAGLES

There is little reason to debate the value of appraising rehabilitation counselor performance because evaluation of performance is an inherent operation in all work settings where there are superiors and subordinates. As a consequence of this universal condition, it becomes highly significant to be concerned about the effectiveness of any appraisal system. The effectiveness of any system, of course, can only be determined by its ability to achieve its objectives. Three primary objectives for assessing counselor performance that would probably be readily agreed upon by most rehabilitation personnel are 1) to determine the most appropriate caseload assignment for each counselor, 2) to determine in-service training needs, and 3) to provide criteria for salary, promotions, and terminations. Achieving these goals would increase the likelihood of 1) an optimal work assignment for the counselor, 2) appropriate skill building opportunities for counselors, and 3) high counselor morale. An evaluation system's ability to meet the above goals will be greatly determined by two factors: the data that it yields and the appropriate utilization of that data.

DATA SOURCES

Three basic types of data have been utilized for the purposes of appraising employee performance. They are:

327

1. Ratings of employee traits (i.e., cheerfulness, initiative, etc)
2. Ratings of daily work behavior
3. Results of work efforts

Trait-based appraisal systems have been widely criticized in the personnel and industrual psychology literature (Lopez, 1968; McFarland, 1968; Strauss and Sayles, 1967). Four basic criticisms are:

1 They are too subjective (the "I like him" syndrome)
2. They have low statistical validity (they fail to measure what they purport to measure)
3. They strongly favor the conformist (they fail to recognize that "there is more than one way to skin a cat")
4. They provide little data on which change can be planned (it is difficult to change the personality of an employee)

Therefore, as can readily be concluded, although trait-based appraisal may be least costly to a rehabilitation agency in respect to expenditure of agency funds and supervisor time, it is also likely to be a waste of time if one is interested in achieving the goals listed in the introductory section.

The remaining two sources of data, daily work performance and results, hold more promise for meeting the objectives of an effective system for assessing counselor performance. They will be referred to as process criteria (measurement of counselor effectiveness on job tasks) and product criteria (measurement of client benefits) and will be discussed at length in the following two sections of this chapter.

MEASUREMENT OF
REHABILITATION COUNSELING PROCESS VARIABLES

Before one can seriously consider focusing on measuring counselor daily work behavior, at least three conditions must be present:

1. Significant job tasks can be specified
2. The extent of counselor deviation from accepted procedure on such job tasks can be accurately and objectively measured
3. Sufficient resources are available for measuring performance

Therefore, if assessment of performance is to be based upon rehabilitation counselor effectiveness on job tasks, one must have a comprehensive picture of what those tasks are. Also, accepting the ever present reality of limited resources, determination of the relative value of any particular counselor task must be possible. For example, one should be capable of rank ordering counselor tasks on a value dimension. The importance of a particular task would be greatly determined by its relationship to the achievement of agency goals: providing benefits to clients. Unfortunately, at this point little such relationship data exists. However, data does exist from Muthard and Salomone's (1969) rehabilitation counselor role and function study on the extent to which general agency, blind agency, and facility rehabilitation counselors consider eight factor analytically derived clusters of work activities to be a significant part of their job. The data suggest (p. 124) that, regardless of work setting, it would be most appropriate to measure counselor effectiveness in vocational counseling activities. However, if one had adequate staff time and resources for collecting additional data, the focus would be determined by the work setting of the counselor.

Unfortunately, the established technology for accurately and objectively measuring the extent of deviation from accepted procedures on such job tasks is at an infantile level. This conclusion is supported by the fact that at present the predominant system for measuring rehabilitation counselor performance is by the review of the client casefile folder (case review). Therefore, in order to clarify the low level of the state of the art a discussion of the case review system appears warranted.

The Case Review

The case review is usually conducted by the counselor's supervisor or a case review team established for such a purpose within the agency. When examining case records the focus of the case reviewer is usually guided by a list of items on a case review form. The following items are probably representative of the evaluation criteria of most state rehabilitation agencies with respect to case review:

1. Completion of appropriate forms
2. Promptness in contacting referral
3. Adequacy of diagnostic work-ups
4. Adequacy of vocational testing
5. Evidence of establishment of eligibility
6. Client advised of rights
7. Case movement
8. Adequacy of identification of needed services
9. Adequacy of how services will result in expendability
10. Adequacy of counselor contacts with clients
11. Evidence of counseling and client involvement in plan development
12. Client made aware of his responsibilities
13. Realistic vocational objective

14. Determination of economic need
15. Appropriateness of fund utilization
16. Effectiveness in provision of services, i.e., optimal speed, adequate supervision, appropriate use of other resources
17. Sufficiency of closure information
18. Agreement between VR objectives and placement
19. Adherence to the vocational rehabilitation agency procedural policies

If one considers the above as a nearly exhaustive list of the data required in all case folders by agency regulations, it can easily be concluded that review of the typical folder would be a greatly limited system for objectively assessing counselor performance in the vocational counseling area. This, of course, should come as no surprise, because the logical way to measure vocational counseling effectiveness would be through observation of counselor interview behavior.

The limitations of the case review are not restricted to assessing vocational counseling. Overall, there are three basic limitations in the present case review system that make its data questionable, regardless of the daily work behavior being assessed. The first limitation is a lack of a truly standardized system of case recording. This is supported by two research reports. Muthard and Salomone (1969) found that the "use of casefiles was not a feasible means of determining the activities performed by counselors." Miller (1963) found that casefiles provide an inadequate source of information for rating rehabilitation counselor performance. The second limitation is the absence of any evidence supporting a direct relationship between a counselor's actual performance and the data recorded in the casefile. Until such a relationship is empirically established, the validity of case review results will remain open to question. The third limitation pertains primarily to case reviews conducted by the counselor's immediate supervisor. Lopez (1968, p. 163) points out that supervisor ratings of employee performance are often loaded with so much subjectivity that they are relatively useless. He cites one study of supervisor ratings of the attendance and quantity of output of packagers in a food processing plant that found little relationship between the ratings and plant records of actual output and attendance. Rather, there appeared to be a greater relationship between the supervisors' ratings and how much they liked the employees. The negative effect of familiarity was also evidenced in Muthard and Miller's (1966) study of supervisor ratings of counselor case performance from observation of case files. The supervisors completed their ratings using a nine-item standard form. The intercorrelations among the nine scores on the Structured Case Review Blank for cases rated by supervisors with knowledge of the counselor's identity were much higher than the intercorrelations among the nine scores when supervisors did not know the identity of the counselor. This difference suggests that the "halo effect" influenced the ratings in a constant fashion.

Although it is possible that case review as a system for assessing counselor performance may always suffer from validity problems, these problems can be greatly reduced by the following:

1. Standardization of the content of all case records
2. Developing a case review form to be used by all reviewers in which all items are operationally defined
3. Restricting the items on the form to those in which a relationship between case record content and actual counselor behavior has been empirically established
4. Further limiting the items on the above form (point 3) to those daily work behaviors that have demonstrated a relationship with client outcome
5. Utilizing teams of trained raters who do not know the counselor personally

However, even if all of the above modifications are adopted, the case review data will still be less valid than data collected through direct observation of the counselor on daily work tasks, and the data can only be justified as superior to direct observation on the grounds of greater feasibility because of limited resources.

Objective Systems of Measuring Counselor Performance

Although the technology in the area of assessing rehabilitation counselor performance by means of direct observation is also limited at this time, ground has been broken that suggests that objective systems can be developed. On the basis of a comprehensive review of interview content analysis research (Campbell, 1962; Danskin, 1955; Hoffman, 1959; Wittmer, 1971) and the close examination of typescripts of a selected sample of interviews collected from practicing rehabilitation counselors, Richardson and Rubin (1973) developed the Rehabilitation Counseling Interview Subrole Behavior Scale (RCISBS). Studies have demonstrated that raters trained to use the RCISBS while listening to tape-recorded interviews can reliably allocate moment-to-moment counselor interview responses among the following 12 subrole categories:

1. Information giving—educational and occupational
2. Information giving—client based
3. Information seeking—specific

4. Information seeking—exploratory
5. Confrontation
6. Friendly discussion—rapport building
7. Supportive
8. Information giving—administrative
9. Information giving—structuring the relationship
10. Listening/client expression
11. Communication of values, opinions, and advice
12. Clarification, reflection, and restatement

Conclusions can be drawn from the resulting profiles regarding the predominant style of the counselor's interview performance (Bolton, 1974). Richardson, Rubin, and Bolton (1973) also demonstrated that rehabilitation counselor interpersonal skill levels could be reliably rated by trained raters listening to tape-recorded interviews. Such ratings could be utilized as a qualitative measure of rehabilitation counselor performance. This conclusion is supported by Muthard and Miller's (1966) finding that out of 28 evaluative criteria for counselors in state agencies, 18 either directly or indirectly reflected counselor ability to deal in interpersonal relationships.

Although costly to implement, it is not inconceivable that a state rehabilitation agency could collect tape-recorded work samples of counselor interview behavior that could then be rated for vocational and affective counseling effectiveness. Such a rating section could be operationalized through the creation of a permanent rating section within the central office program evaluation unit to which counselors would send tapes considered to be representative samples of their work. It is also conceivable that trained raters could arrange to accompany counselors periodically while the counselor conducted a specific job function, such as placement. Finally, it is not inconceivable that simulated experience based tests could be devised on which rehabilitation counselor performance could be rated. Of course, the more complex the task, the more difficult it would be to devise such role-played situations. Overall, any of the above systems of direct observation properly implemented could begin to provide a data base on which the state rehabilitation agency could make objective determinations of employee reward, in-service training needs, and appropriate assignment.

MEASUREMENT OF
REHABILITATION COUNSELING OUTCOME VARIABLES

Before one can seriously consider focusing on assessing counselor performance by means of measurement of client outcomes, at least three conditions must be present: 1) relevant outcomes must be specified, 2) these outcomes must be amenable to quantification so that counselors' performances can be compared, and 3) sufficient resources must be available for measuring the outcomes.

With the above criteria in mind a meaningful discussion of this issue can be developed through attention to the following dimensions of rehabilitation service outcome: 1) traditional outcome measures, 2) weighted closures, 3) sociopsychological measures, and 4) sustention of benefits.

Traditional Outcome Measures

Counselors have traditionally been evaluated on the basis of number of successful case closures: clients successfully returned to the work force each year (or habilitated). In recent years the success category has been expanded to include those clients closed as "unpaid family workers," "homemakers," or in "sheltered workshop employment" with the recognition that such outcomes of service were viable alternatives for people who would never be expected to enter the competitive labor market. In many agencies, however, the proportion of such noncompetitive labor market closures to the number closed in the competitive labor market has become an indirect measure of counselor performance. Other traditional measures of counselor performance have included change in client work status, earnings, and primary source of support from intake to closure. In recent years, total focus on traditional measures has received much criticism as criteria of counselor performance because of their failure to take caseload difficulty, sociopsychological client benefits, and sustention of benefits into account. Thus, while traditional indicators have served a useful purpose and will undoubtedly have a continuing role in future evaluation activities, they obviously leave much to be desired.

It can also be argued that a total focus on traditional measures, in addition to resulting in unfair judgments of the work of some counselors, produces several other unwanted effects. Several rehabilitation researchers (Miller and Barillas, 1967; Muthard and Miller, 1966; Silver, 1969) have argued that simply using the number of successful closures as the principal measure of rehabilitation counselor effort may lead counselors to prefer working with handicapped persons whose presenting conditions are uncomplicated. Dishart and Epstein's (1964) study of the screening practices of the state-federal rehabilitation agencies revealed that such a concern may indeed be legitimate. Although 68 out of the 98 agencies surveyed reported selecting cases on a first come, first served basis, a number of these agencies reported consideration of other factors in screening out cases. Among them were: motivational inadequacies, severity of disability, age, alcoholism, multiple disabilities, low intelligence, emotional inadequacies, length of work expectancy, type of disability, educational inadequacies, and the vocational objective of homemaker.

Weighted Closure Systems

The weighted closure movement is based on the rationale that counselors should receive differential credit for rehabilitated clients based on case difficulty. A number of researchers have focused on this area. Miller and Barillas (1967) developed a method of weighting successful closures with statistical estimates of case complexity, and Silver (1969) investigated the possibility of having counselors rate the effort that particular client problems require. Wallis and Bozarth (1971) developed two weighting schemes to distinguish among the complexity of cases accepted for rehabilitation services using a method that had been used earlier (Miller and Barillas, 1967). These two schemes used predictive variables of rehabilitation success such as age, education, disability type, and previous rehabilitation client status. Their findings revealed that nearly all clients accepted for services are eventually rehabilitated; thus, a plausible conclusion posited by the authors was that the most complex cases—the severely and multiply handicapped—are not accepted for services. Sermon (1972) developed an Index of Case Difficulty that was actually a ratio of the number of clients of any particular disability classification and the total number of clients rehabilitated nationally. When this ratio was multiplied by 10, ranges from 0.01 to 10 were possible. By summing the ratios over the number of cases in a caseload and dividing the sum by the number of cases in a caseload, an average (mean) weighted closure index may be derived. A disadvantage of this system is that the multiply-handicapped are classified, necessarily, as having a single disability. Thus, for the very complex cases the counselor still may not receive full credit. Another problem is that by tying the ratio solely to the disability classification, the contribution of other variables (e.g., age, race, skill levels, education, appearance, sex, previous employment history) is obviated. Presently no weighted closure system has yet received critical acclaim as the panacea for the counselor assessment problem. One reason is that they have all focused solely on client characteristics. Unfortunately, client characteristics do not reveal a full picture of necessary effort. Prevailing labor market conditions and the availability of rehabilitation resources are but two examples of other relevant variables. Interestingly, the Study Group of the Institute on Rehabilitation Issues charged with analyzing and critiquing existing systems for measuring rehabilitation outcome (Institute on Rehabilitation Issues, 1974) acknowledged the desirability of a weighted closure system but felt that the problems associated with weighted systems appear to be too complex to make its use realistic at this time. The Study Group felt that, as a minimum, client outcome should be assessed across the dimensions of vocational functioning and potential, economic independence, physical functioning, and psychosocial functioning (Institute on Rehabilitation Issues, 1974, p. 33). Such a recommendation was closely allied with the work of Lenhart and his colleagues in Oklahoma (Westerheide, Lenhart, and Miller, 1973), not surprisingly, because Lenhart was a member of the Study Group. The Oklahoma outcome measurement system is more of a comprehensive array of variables rather than of a weighted closure system, and it includes dimensions such as case difficulty, educational attainment, economic/vocational status, physical functioning, adjustment to disability, and social competency. It must be said that this system is, at present, the one that is most congruent with the state-federal VR program regulations. As such, it should be reviewed and considered for use by all who are planning evaluations of client change as a possible measure from which counselor competency may be inferred.

Sociopsychological Measures
All human service programs exist as a response to a segment of the nation's population who share a common base of unmet needs, needs that require the intervention of a wide variety of professional disciplines administered through a wide array of categorical human service programs. In the instance of vocational rehabilitation, the program exists to serve those people who, for a variety of reasons, have a physical or mental disability that constitutes a substantial handicap to employment and who may be expected· to benefit in terms of employability from the provision of vocational rehabilitaion services. As long as "employability" was defined simply in terms of the number of clients placed in competitive employment (as the regulations once required) the capacity to measure other potential client benefits was not necessary. However, over the years the definition of employability has been gradually broadened into "gainful employment," which, in addition to competitive employment, includes homemaking, family work (for which payment may be in kind rather than in cash), sheltered employment, homebound employment, or other gainful work. Furthermore, the Rehabilitation Act of 1973 (P.L. 93–112) specifies that those most severely handicapped—those whose needs for services are the most pronounced—are to be served first so that they may prepare for and engage in gainful employment. Therefore, the counselor is now being more greatly encouraged to work with the "whole person" during the rehabilitation process. The negative effects resulting from not doing so are evidenced in a recent study by Gay, Reagles, and Wright (1971). They revealed that the over-attention of rehabilitation counselors to the voca-

tional goals at the expense of consideration of other dimensions of potential client problems may be responsible for the failure of some clients to sustain themselves after the rehabilitation services have been terminated. If one accepts the value of this comprehensive emphasis, it appears that in addition to receiving credit for client economic benefits, the rehabilitation counselor should also be given credit for any improved client psychological functioning and physical functioning that can be associated with his case management activities.

Physical limitations associated with the onset of disability is a problem experienced by many people seeking rehabilitation services. Such limitations often result in reduced capacity for "gainful employment." When such is the case the rehabilitation counselor is expected to provide appropriate physical restoration services. The potential contribution of this service to the client's general well-being as well as his eventual vocational adjustment cannot be underplayed. From a discussion of studies concerned with the impact of physical dysfunction on client motivation, Barry and Malinovsky (1965, p. 7) concluded that clients who doubted whether their bodily needs would be met made only minimal progress toward achieving more general rehabilitation goals. When this additional criterion, physical restoration, is used to judge rehabilitation success, clients with physical limitations who somehow manage to find employment without having such limitations reduced to the greatest extent possible would be considered partial rather than complete rehabilitation successes.

Safilios-Rothschild (1970) points out that a disabled person can either accept the disability and its consequences, deny both of these phenomena, or exaggerate them. People who deny their disability are frequently frustrated because the unavoidable resulting limitations are not taken into consideration. Those who exaggerate their disabilities do not always take advantage of their residual abilities and capacities. Obviously then, the manner in which a person chooses to respond emotionally to his disability and incorporate it into his self-concept can influence both the immediate and long-range effects of rehabilitation services. Because the quality of one's self-concept is logically related to the likelihood of realistically accepting a disability, achieving positive change in a disabled person's self-concept is considered a viable concern of the rehabilitation counselor and therefore a valid evaluation criterion. There are a number of satisfactory measures of self-concept. Undoubtedly the most popular is the Tennessee Self-Concept Scale (Fitts, 1965). There are others that are more related to the population of persons with disabilities. The reader should consult a standard reference work such as Buros (1972) to determine which are most appropriate for specific purposes.

Overall, if one is to seriously consider multiple client benefits in respect to counselor assessment, sophisticated comprehensive measures of client change must be available. Fortunately, one such measure, the Human Service Scale (Reagles, Wright, and Butler, 1973), is presently available. The Human Service Scale was generated from the following rationale. If human service agencies—not just vocational rehabilitation— exist to meet the needs of particular dependent segments of the population, then an evaluation of how well agencies are fulfilling their purpose ought to include a measure of the extent to which client needs are met.

The Human Service Scale went through a comprehensive developmental process. Maslow's heirarchy of basic human needs provided the underlying theoretical rationale for its development. Over 300 multiple choice items were initially generated at the University of Wisconsin Regional Rehabilitation Research Institute (UW-RRRI) which seemed to reflect, to some extent, Maslow's need categories: physiological, safety and security, lovingness and belongingness, self-esteem, and self-actualization. These were then scrutinized for duplication. Eliminating some items and combining others resulted in a reduction to 150 items. The items were put into scale form and administered by over 200 rehabilitation counselors in 29 states to 1,018 clients who had been accepted for vocational rehabilitation services. The demographic characteristics of this group revealed that they were reasonably representative of clients served by the state-federal vocational rehabilitation program (Dishart, 1965), with the exception, naturally, of the near absence in the standardization group of the blind, retarded, and those with severe motor involvement.

The data yielded by the administration of these items were returned to the UW-RRRI where they were subjected to appropriate item and factor analyses. The outcome of these analyses yielded some very interesting results. First, the factor structure revealed that seven distinct need categories were apparent, instead of the five that Maslow had postulated. The need categories were labeled: physiological, emotional, economic security, family, social, economic self-esteem, and vocational self-actualization needs; the labels reflect the approximate relationship to Maslow's need categories. Second, the number of items was reduced from 150 to the present 80 items. Third, it was determined that the relationship among the need categories was not linear or heirarchal, as Maslow had postulated. Thus, the profile of need satisfaction yielded by the scale is presented as a spherical configuration.

In its present form the machine-scorable Human Service Scale lends itself nicely to program evaluation as a pre-post measure of client change. Furthermore, studies that are intended to determine the predictive validity of the scale are currently underway. When completed it is hoped that the scale may be used in a clinical sense; differential patterns of client need satisfaction at the time of intake may be translated into alternative patterns of intervention (rehabilitative services) to bring about desired outcomes. Such a model has a great deal of intuitive appeal because it maintains one of the basic attributes of the vocational rehabilitation program, viz., the one-to-one relationship of counselor and client in which the client's unique needs are translated into an equally unique plan of interventive rehabilitation services. By such a procedure, counselor performance may be more accurately measured; it is, so to speak, a marriage of the idiographic and nomothetic approaches; for nomothetic (normative) data are used to generate unique rehabilitation plans. Counselor performance can be inferred from the extent to which client change, i.e., need satisfaction, is optimized over the range of his caseload. Because normative data is available for a number of client characteristics (e.g., disability type) and contextual variables (e.g., rural versus urban settings), counselors who work with more difficult clients, the severely and multiply handicapped, for example, could be evaluated by comparison with counselors serving similar clients. As such, this approach to counselor evaluation includes the advantage of the weighted closure procedures.

Perhaps only one other evaluative technique offers advantages similar to the Human Service Scale. That is, the technique of Goal Attainment Scaling (Kiresuk and Sherman, 1968) in which individual behavior scales are constructed for each client. When the client changes as measured by the Goal Attainment Scales are transformed into standard scores for equivalency, they may be summed over clients for counselor or program evaluation purposes. This is certainly an appealing approach, but several disadvantages prevail. For example, who determines the goals to be achieved? The "degree of difficulty" is certainly a subjective process. Also, merely converting scale scores to standard scores does not negate the apparent summation of idiosyncratic client changes. Another difficulty concerns the reliability of scale construction; this refers to the observed inconsistency of different counselors arriving at substantially different scales from the same data about clients.

Sustention of Benefits and Client Satisfaction

Inherent in the philosophy of rehabilitation is the belief that as a result of receiving services a successfully rehabilitated person will maintain his adjustment and independent status into the future. However, follow-up studies of rehabilitated clients have revealed that the assumption of one-time services resulting in "permanent" rehabilitation is unrealistic for many disabled persons. This unfortunate reality could result from many conditions over which the counselor has little control, such as changing labor markets, the need for skill upgrading, and the dynamic nature of many disabling disease processes. Consequently, it may be argued that it is not fair to hold the rehabilitaiton counselor totally responsible for the client's sustention. Nonetheless, it may also be argued that the permanency of the impact of rehabilitation services constitutes a legitimate criterion for the evaluation of counselor performance. Legitimate because the truly effective counselor takes such factors into account at the time of rehabilitation planning so that the probability of sustention is enhanced. Legitimate, also because one of the nine federal evaluation standards is specifically concerned with sustention of client benefits.

The measurement of client sustention ideally encompasses three measurement points. The first point is at time of referral or intake. The second is at closure (termination of service), and the third is at follow-up, at least 6 months after closure. Such a longitudinal data collection scheme allows for the measurement of both client economic and psychosocial gains attributed to the impact of rehabilitation services. It also makes possible the measurement of sustention of gains following termination of services. Accomplishment of the latter is greatly dependent on advanced planning at time of client intake. At that point it will be necessary to obtain data from clients (addresses of family, friends, significant others, labor unions, social and religious clubs, etc.) that will increase the probability of locating them in the near and distant future.

Another aspect of follow-up studies, viz., the clients' expressed satisfaction with services, may also be thought of as a potential tool with which to make inferences about counselor competency. A variety of scales of client satisfaction have been generated of late (Grigg and Goodstein, 1957; Reagles, Wright, and Butler, 1970; Steffen, 1969). Many more attempts are currently under way as a result of the impetus provided by the creation of the evaluation standards by federal authorities, of which client satisfaction is a part. An issue within this measurement problem is when to measure client satisfaction. If measured too soon after services, one risks the measurement of some components of client dependency or what has been described as the "hello-goodby" phenomenon, while waiting too long risks diminished accuracy of client perceptions. A period of 6 months to 1 year has been recognized as acceptable.

MEASUREMENT OF COUNSELOR EFFICIENCY

Thus far, this chapter has restricted its focus to determination of counselor effectiveness. However, because most administrators are also concerned with counselor efficiency, it also deserves some attention.

Although not yet attempted, cost-benefit analysis is an investment appraisal technique that could be utilized as a measure of individual counselor efficiency. Basically, it compares all relevant costs and benefits in such a way that one is able to determine the return on a particular investment. The cost-benefit ratio is the primary tool of cost-benefit analysis. This ratio can be considered to be an index of investment effectiveness. Wright and Reagles (1971) developed the following cost-benefit ratio for vocational rehabilitation:

$$\frac{\text{Benefits accruing to VR clients that can be expressed in monetary terms}}{\text{Total dollar amount expended in behalf of VR clients}} =$$

$$\frac{\text{Benefits}}{\text{Costs}}$$

Serot (1972) has developed a benefit index and a cost index that are then utilized in a productivity index. The productivity index was designed as a tool for comparing the performance of different state agencies with disability mix controlled. However, the productivity index could be adapted as a comparative measure of the performance of counselors within a state rehabilitation agency. The adaptation process yields the following modified Serot indexes:

Counselor benefit index =

$$\frac{\begin{array}{l}\text{Average benefits accrued by Coun-}\\\text{selor A's disability group multiplied}\\\text{by the number of clients closed by}\\\text{Counselor A in that disability group}\\\text{(compute for each disability group}\\\text{and sum the results)}\end{array}}{\begin{array}{l}\text{Average benefits accrued by a dis-}\\\text{ability group agency-wide multi-}\\\text{plied by the number of clients}\\\text{closed by Counselor A in that}\\\text{disability group (compute for each}\\\text{disability group and sum the results)}\end{array}}$$

Counselor cost index =

Average dollar amount expended by
Counselor A on clients in a disability
group multiplied by the number of
clients closed by Counselor A in that

disability group (compute for each disability group and sum the results)

Average dollar amount expended agency-wide on clients in a disability group multiplied by the number of clients closed by Counselor A in that disability group (compute for each disability group and sum the results)

Counselor productivity index =

Counselor benefit index

Counselor cost index

Unfortunately, the above indexes contain limitations. For example, they fail to control for the effect of significant environmental influences, such as: 1) available community resources, 2) variations in local unemployment rates, 3) differential effectiveness of local placement personnel, and 4) variations in the local cost of purchased services. Of course, until a more comprehensive index is developed they could be applied conservatively with a counselor compared only with other counselors working under similar environmental conditions.

One of the real values of the Serot type system is its potential for more refined application as a measure of differential counselor efficiency. For example, the productivity index could be computed for each disability group separately for each counselor. Supervisors could then take into consideration counselor efficiency with specific disability groups when they are determining caseload assignments. Such individual disability efficiency ratios could be provided by computers in such a form that the data could be quickly disseminated.

Both the cost and difficulty level of implementing an on-going cost-benefit analysis program for purposes of assessing counselor performance would depend on the comprehensiveness of the design in respect to measuring costs and benefits. A very simple design that utilized only data normally collected for the R-300 form, such as total cost of services and change in earnings from intake to closure, would be rather easy to implement. On the other hand, a design that called for costs to be the sum of—1) rehabilitation agency service expenditures on a client, 2) counselor time spent with and for a client converted to dollars, 3) cost of services arranged by the counselor to be provided to the client by other state and federal agencies between intake and closure, and 4) loss of income to the client while in training—and called for benefits to include change in earnings from intake to follow-up one year after closure would obviously be more difficult and costly to implement. The personnel and equipment demands for this type of program should be minimal. Present program evaluation staff should be capable of setting up the program with the aid of a consulting economist.

SUMMARY

If a rehabilitation agency is to devise a comprehensive system for assessing counselor performance, multiple criteria should be used. These criteria should include: 1) an analysis of counselor case management style, 2) an analysis of client benefits, and 3) an analysis of counselor efficiency. A total focus on any one criterion would probably result in an inadequate system. Total reliance on efficiency measures precludes the possibility of determining either the quality of counselor daily performance or the extent of benefits experienced by his clients. Total reliance on process criteria precludes the possibility of demonstrating the effect of a counselor, as well as ever determining the significance of different process variables through their relationship with outcome criteria. Total dependence on the measurement of product for appraising employee performance has been criticized in the personnel psychology literature. These criticisms also have relevance for the problem of assessing rehabilitation counselor performance. For example, Lopez (1968, pp. 215 and 234) points out that even with respect to evaluating the performance of salesmen, output is rarely used as the sole criterion because of the influence of uncontrolled environmental variables.

Unfortunately, at present, most rehabilitation counselor evaluations are based on "traditional outcome measures" and/or case reviews. The limitations of these criteria were discussed earlier in this chapter. Fortunately, in the future, counselor evaluations will not be based solely on traditional outcome measures. While vocational rehabilitation program regulations may not be modified to directly bring about such a change, another development may: the evaluation standards developed to meet the demands of the Rehabilitation Act of 1973. For example, the published standards call for state rehabilitation agencies to collect data on the following:

1. "Percentage of homemakers for whom homemaking was the original goal"
2. "Percentage of clients who received training and who are placed in employment for which that training is relevant"

3. Client employment status and earnings at follow-up

4. "Number of clients who are satisfied with the adequacy and relevance of their rehabilitation training and services as reflected in the follow-up period"

At the heart of the dilemma of how to evaluate counselors lies one problem—measurement. As the goals of vocational rehabilitation programs become more clearly defined, researchers and evaluation experts will respond with more sophisticated measurement tools. One such tool, the Human Service Scale, has already been developed and was thoroughly described in the outcome section of this chapter.

The fact that the assessment of counselor performance is an organizational function cannot be ignored. Therefore, the efficacy of any assessment system is determined by the effectiveness with which the agency functions as a total organization. Agencies with a built-in capacity for utilizing counselor assessment data for management decisions are most likely to benefit from such evaluation systems. Assuming that such organizational capability is present, the potential impact of any program aimed at assessing counselor performance is greatly dependent upon a commitment on the part of the agency director and other agency professional staff to follow-up action based on the results. Such data utilization also will be facilitated if all relevant potential results have been anticipated and an implementation procedure for each is clearly delineated by the agency before the initiation of the system. The establishment of such clarity of purpose demands an ongoing dialogue between the designers of the evaluation system and agency management staff.

The smooth utilization of the results of such goal-oriented evaluation demands that administrators introduce counselors to the fact that assessment of their performance will be a continuous management function within the agency. Counselors should also be explicitly informed of the specific purposes of the appraisal system. Counselors must perceive the evaluation as a largely objective, nonthreatening experience that is intended for their personal growth. This should reduce counselor defensiveness, thereby facilitating both the implementation of the appraisal program and the utilization of its results. However, even with appropriate reassurances, counselors are only human, and many of them will be concerned with the effect such a program could have on promotions and salary increases as well as on the continution of their employment with the agency. Such a concern cannot help but create a degree of reluctance to accept a new evaluation program out of fear that the results might affect them negatively.

REFERENCES

Barry, J. R., and M. R. Malinovsky. 1965. Client motivation for rehabilitation: A review. Rehabilitation Research Monograph Series, No. 1. University of Florida, Gainesville.

Bolton, B. 1974. Three verbal interaction styles of rehabilitation counselors. Rehab. Counsel. Bull. 18:34–40.

Buros, O. K., ed. 1972. The Seventh Mental Measurement Yearbook. Gryphon Press, Highland Park, N. J.

Campbell, R. W. 1962. Counselor personality and background and his interview subrole behavior. J. Counsel. Psych. 9:329–334.

Danskin, D. G. 1955. Roles played by counselors in their interviews. J. Counsel. Psych. 2:22–27.

Dishart, M. 1965. Family adjustment in the rehabilitation plan. J. Rehab. 30 (1):42–43.

Dishart, M., and M. Epstein. 1964. Patterns of Rehabilitation Services Provided by the 90 State Vocational Rehabilitation Agencies of the U.S. National Rehabilitation Association Research Project, Washington, D.C.

Fitts, W. A. 1965. Manual for the Tennessee Self-Concept Scale. Counselor Recordings and Tests, Nashville.

Gay, D. A., K. W. Reagles, and G. N. Wright. 1971. Rehabilitation client sustention: A longitudinal study. Wisconsin Studies in Vocational Rehabilitation. Monograph XVI. University of Wisconsin Regional Rehabilitation Institute, Madison.

Grigg, A. E., and L. D. Goodstein. 1957. The use of clients as judges of the counselor's performance. J. Counsel. Psych. 4:31–36.

Hoffman, A. E. 1959. An analysis of counselor sub-roles. J. Counsel. Psych. 6:61–67.

Institute on Rehabilitation Issues. 1974. Assessment of Counselor Performance. Rehabilitation Services Administration, Washington, D.C.

Kiresuk, T. J., and R. E. Sherman. 1968. Goal attainment scaling: A general method for evaluating comprehensive community mental health programs. Comm. Ment. Health J. 4:443–453.

Lopez, F. M. 1968. Evaluating Employee Performance. Public Personnel Association, Chicago.

Maslow, A. H. 1952. The S-I Test: A Measure of Psychological Security–Insecurity. Consulting Psychologists Press, Palo Alto.

McFarland, D. E. 1968. Personnel Management: Theory and Practice. Macmillan, New York.

Miller, L. A. 1963. A study of case review criteria for evaluating rehabilitation counselor performance. Unpublished doctoral dissertation, University of Iowa, Iowa City.

Miller, L., and M. Bàrillas. 1967. Using weighted closures as a more adequate measure of counselor and agency effort in rehabilitation. Rehab. Counsel. Bull. 11 (2):117–121.

Muthard, J. E., and L. A. Miller. 1966. The Criteria Problem in Rehabilitation Counseling. College of Education, University of Iowa, Iowa City.

Muthard, J. E., and P. R. Salomone. 1969. The roles and functions of rehabilitation counselors. Rehab. Counsel. Bull. 13, Special Issue, Oct. pp. 81–168.

Reagles, K. W., G. N. Wright, and J. Butler. 1970. Correlates of client satisfaction in an expanded vocational rehabilitation program. Wisconsin Studies in Vocational Rehabilitation. Monograph XII. University of Wisconsin Regional Rehabilitation Research Institute, Madison.

Reagles, K. W., G. N. Wright, and A. J. Butler. 1973. Human Service Scale. Human Service Systems, Madison, Wis.

Richardson, B. K., and S. E. Rubin. 1973. Rehabilitation Counseling Interview Subrole Behavior Scale. University of Arkansas Rehabilitation Research and Training Center, Fayetteville.

Richardson, B. K., S. E. Rubin, and B. Bolton. 1973. Counseling interview behavior of empirically derived subgroups of rehabilitation counselors. Arkansas Studies in Vocational Rehabilitation. Series I, Monograph VII. Arkansas Rehabilitation Research and Training Center, University of Arkansas, Fayetteville.

Safilios-Rothschild, C. 1970. The Sociology and Social Psychology of Disability and Rehabilitation. Random House, New York.

Sermon, D. T. 1972. The Difficulty Index: An Expanded Measure of Counselor Performance. Minnesota DVR, St. Paul.

Serot, D. E. 1972. Indices of cost, output and productivity for use in evaluating rehabilitation services programs. Project for cost-benefit analysis and evaluation of rehabilitation services. Working Paper No. 187/RS013. Institute of Urban and Regional Development, Berkeley, Calif.

Silver, D. L. 1969. A look at evaluation of VR counselor performance. J. Rehab. 35 (6):13–14.

Steffen, R. D. 1969. Development of a client satisfaction scale. Unpublished master's thesis, University of Wisconsin, Madison.

Strauss, G., and L. R. Sayles. 1967. Personnel: The Human Problems of Management. Prentice-Hall, Englewood Cliffs, N. J.

Wallis, J. H., and J. D. Bozarth. 1971. Development and evaluation of weighted DVR case closures. Rehab. Res. Pract. Rev. 2(3), Summer, pp. 55–60.

Westerheide, W. J., L. Lenhart, and M. C. Miller. 1973. Field Test of a Services Outcome Measurement Form: Case Difficulty. Monograph II. Department of Institutions, Social and Rehabilitation Services, Oklahoma City.

Wittmer, J. 1971. An objective scale for content analysis of the counselor's interview behavior. Counsel. Ed. Superv. 10:283–290.

Wright, G. N., and K. W. Reagles. 1971. The economic impact of an expanded program of vocational rehabilitation. Wisconsin Studies in Vocational Rehabilitation. Series 2, Monograph XV. Regional Rehabilitation Research Institute, University of Wisconsin, Madison.

Author Index

Subject Index